CANCER ETIOLOGY, DIAGNOSIS AND TREATMENTS

PHOTODYNAMIC THERAPY

FUNDAMENTALS, APPLICATIONS AND HEALTH OUTCOMES

CANCER ETIOLOGY, DIAGNOSIS AND TREATMENTS

Additional books in this series can be found on Nova's website under the Series tab.

Additional e-books in this series can be found on Nova's website under the e-book tab.

CANCER ETIOLOGY, DIAGNOSIS AND TREATMENTS

PHOTODYNAMIC THERAPY

FUNDAMENTALS, APPLICATIONS AND HEALTH OUTCOMES

ADRIAN G. HUGO
EDITOR

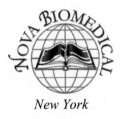

New York

NOTICE TO THE READER

The Publisher has taken reasonable care in the preparation of this book, but makes no expressed or implied warranty of any kind and assumes no responsibility for any errors or omissions. No liability is assumed for incidental or consequential damages in connection with or arising out of information contained in this book. The Publisher shall not be liable for any special, consequential, or exemplary damages resulting, in whole or in part, from the readers' use of, or reliance upon, this material. Any parts of this book based on government reports are so indicated and copyright is claimed for those parts to the extent applicable to compilations of such works.

Independent verification should be sought for any data, advice or recommendations contained in this book. In addition, no responsibility is assumed by the publisher for any injury and/or damage to persons or property arising from any methods, products, instructions, ideas or otherwise contained in this publication.

This publication is designed to provide accurate and authoritative information with regard to the subject matter covered herein. It is sold with the clear understanding that the Publisher is not engaged in rendering legal or any other professional services. If legal or any other expert assistance is required, the services of a competent person should be sought. FROM A DECLARATION OF PARTICIPANTS JOINTLY ADOPTED BY A COMMITTEE OF THE AMERICAN BAR ASSOCIATION AND A COMMITTEE OF PUBLISHERS.

Additional color graphics may be available in the e-book version of this book.

Library of Congress Cataloging-in-Publication Data

ISBN: 978-1-63463-857-9

Library of Congress Control Number: 2014959221

Published by Nova Science Publishers, Inc. † New York

CONTENTS

PREFACE

Photodynamic therapy (PDT) is a well-established clinical modality for cancer, cardiovascular, ophthalmic, dermatological, and dental diseases. PDT is based on the activation of photosensitizer agents with specific wavelength of light, which results in energy transfer cascades that ultimately yield cytotoxic reactive oxygen species that can render cell death. This book discusses the fundamentals, applications and health outcomes of photodynamic therapy.

Chapter 1 - Photodynamic therapy (PDT) has evolved over last century and is now becoming a more widely used medical tool having gained regulatory approval for the treatment of various diseases such as cancer and macular degeneration. PDT is based on the activation of photosensitizer agents with specific wavelength of light, which results in energy transfer cascades that ultimately yield cytotoxic reactive oxygen species that can render cell death. Although this modality has significantly improved the quality of life and survival time of many patients, it still offers significant potential for further improvement. For example, due to the tendency of most photosensitizer molecules to be poorly soluble and to form nonphotoactive aggregates, delivery vehicles have become of great importance. The use of different types of nanoparticles as photosensitizer carriers is a promising approach because these nanomaterials can satisfy all the requirements for an ideal PDT agent. This review describes some of the main types of nanoparticles that are currently in use for PDT applications. Recent advances in the use of multifunctional nanoparticles as carriers of photosensitizer molecules are highlighted. Novel strategies for designing photosensitizer delivery systems with improved PDT efficacy are described. Finally, the authors summarize exciting new results concerning the improvement of light tissue penetration for PDT through two-photon excitation and upconversion nanoparticles.

Chapter 2 - Photodynamic therapy (PDT) with minimal invasion has emerged as one of the important therapeutic modalities for cancer, which combines the use of low energy light with a photosensitizer. Despite its multifaceted advantages, PDT has not yet become the mainstream of cancer intervention mainly due to its insufficient therapeutic efficacy, low selectivity of currently available photosensitizers, and limited light penetration for deep tumor tissues. Recognition of these challenges has greatly motivated the efforts in adopting nanotechnology for improving the design and delivery of photosensitizer, increasing the intensity of photodynamic reaction, and enhancing light penetration and absorption. A variety of nanomaterials have been employed in PDT, serving as either passive carriers or active participants. This review will discuss about the state-of-art approaches and future perspectives of the applications of nanomaterials in PDT.

Chapter 3 - Evidence indicates that good clinical outcomes and excellent cosmesis can be achieved with topical dermatological photodynamic therapy (PDT) when treating licensed superficial malignant and premalignant lesions with protoporphyrin IX (PpIX) precursors. Topical dermatological PDT protocols have been standardised for clinical practice to good effect but the mechanism of action underlying the photodynamic process is complex and opportunities still exist to further improve outcomes and widen the application of this modality.

By providing copious amounts of PpIX precursors exogenously it is possible to manipulate the innate capacity of neoplastic cells to synthesise and accumulate PpIX more rapidly than their surrounding normal cells. This naturally occurring photosensitiser (PpIX) can then be activated by red light of 635 nm to produce (in the presence of molecular oxygen) necrosis and apoptosis via Type I and II photochemical reactions. Non-invasive monitoring of PpIX fluorescence and oxygen saturation during clinical PDT of licensed dermatological lesions has provided increased understanding of this process *in situ*, thus identifying opportunities for further improvement.

Chapter 4 - The increasing incidence of cancer and the search for the development of more effective therapies with minimal side effects have prompted studies to find alternative new treatments. Among new therapies, PhotoDynamic Therapy (PDT) appears a promising modality in cancer treatment with the lowest rates of side effects over traditional modalities as surgery, ionizing radiation and chemotherapy. PDT is currently used in the clinic for the treatment of several types of tumors, i.e. lung, gastrointestinal tract, head and neck, bladder, prostate, non melanoma skin cancers, and actinic keratosis but also for non oncology applications in ophthalmology, dermatology, cardiology, virus inactivation and blood purification.

PDT exploits the interaction between light, tissue molecular oxygen and PhotoSensitizer (PS). These three components are mandatory for the photodynamic reaction that produces Reactive Oxygen Species (ROS) which by interacting with neighboring lipids and proteins, cause acute injury to tumor microvascular, blood vessel blockage, cell death and immune responses.

This has brought about an active pursuit of new PDT agents that can be optimized for the unique set of photophysical characteristics that are required for a successful clinical agent. Many of the PS under investigation are already commercially available, but most of them show prolonged skin phototoxicity, extended retention in the host organism, low extinction coefficient and absorption peak at short wavelengths, low photostability, limited range of solvent conditions and loss of photodynamic activity in aqueous media. In particular, the majority of PS in the clinical use or under preclinical study are hydrophobic and strongly aggregate in aqueous media, thus resulting in a reduction of the photosensitizing efficacy.

The recent application of NanoMaterials (NMs) in biomedicine offers excellent prospects for circumventing these PSs drawbacks. For examples, the aggregation tendency may be minimized by using a nanostructured photosensitive molecular structure. The selective release and accumulation of PSs at the targeted tissue can be enhanced by using nanocarriers. Among the many NMs already exploited in oncomedicine, like polymeric NanoParticles (NPs), dendrimers, liposomes, polymersomes, polymeric micelles, nanospheres, fullerenes, Quantum Dots (QDs), SuperParamagnetic Iron Oxide NanoParticles (SPIONs) and metallic and non-metallic NPs, researchers are searching for the most suitable NM for PDT use. Liposomes, polymeric NPs, gold NPs, QDs and UpConvertingNanoParticles (UCNPs) are particularly promising to circumvent photobleaching and low tissue penetration of PSs.

In this chapter the authors will overview the most important and recent developments of NMs for cancer PDT.

Chapter 5 - Photodynamic therapy (PDT) is a treatment option indicated for various therapeutic protocols, such as local infections, bacteria, fungi and cancer. In veterinary medicine, studies are also being carried out to make the PDT a safe and effective treatment option for animals. In the literature, there are reports of studies about this therapeutic modality demonstrating encouraging clinical results using different classes of photosensitizers and types of light sources. PDT is based on chemical activation of a substance through visible light, generating oxygen radicals and causing destruction of the target tissue or cell without developing resistance. Although studies in the literature reporting the use of PDT with their advantages and disadvantages, it is still considered as a new and promising treatment for neoplastic and non-neoplastic diseases, and its potential, either as single treatment or in combination with conventional therapy, has much yet to be explored. This chapter attempts to provide the reader, succinctly, the advance of photodynamic therapy in veterinary medicine until today, seeking a cure for potentially fatal diseases or even better quality of life for the veterinary patient. Many of these discoveries become a chance to be applied in humans due to similarities in the etiopathogeny of some diseases.

Chapter 6 - Number of studies and advances in health has been made in the discovery of new photosensitizers (PS) proposed as potentially useful in photodynamic therapy (PDT) for the treatment of various diseases. Photodynamic therapy has been known and applied for over a hundred years, and it is used in the treatment of malignant and nonmalignant diseases, through the interaction of three factors: photosensitizer, light source and oxygen. These factors act intrinsically, so photodynamic effect not occurring separately. The photosensitizer administered to the patient, topically or systemically, plays a key role in the development of PDT. The photosensitizer agent is responsible for capturing light and its transformation into energy, resulting in factors capable of destroying the target, it's cannot exert toxicity beyond the affected area. Thus, researches are presented in constant development to find the photosensitizer as close to optimal. In this chapter, the reader will have access to information concerning the photosensitizer in PDT.

Chapter 7 - The effects of combined administration of doxorubicin (DOX) and vincristine (VCR), with 5-aminolevulinic acid photodynamic treatment (ALA-PDT), were analyzed in sensitive murine leukemic cell lines (LBR-) and DOX and VCR chemoresistant LBR-D160 and LBR-V160 cell lines. Low doses of DOX and VCR increased anti-cancer effect of ALA-PDT in LBR-cells. Decrease in cell survival was higher when the combination VCR + ALA-PDT was used compared to DOX + ALA-PDT. Resistant cell lines LBR-D160 and LBR-V160 were sensitive to ALA-PDT; however, no changes occured when combining therapies. Thus, ALA-PDT can overcome drug resistance and is a good candidate for using treating multidrug resistant (MDR) cells.

This combined treatment were evaluated in a murine model. For this purpose, BALB/c mice were inoculated with LBR-cells previously treated with DOX or VCR plus ALA-PDT. 30 days after treatment animals were sacrificed and tumoral infiltration analyzed in many tissues: liver, kidney, spleen, lung, brain, timus, lymph nodes. Histologic studies revealed that in control animals inoculated with LBR-cells without any treatment, infiltration reached 87%

in all the tissues analyzed. Animals inoculated with LBR-cells treated with only ALA-PDT, showed 50% of organs infiltrated. When animals were inoculated with cells treated with DOX or VCR, tumor infiltration was found in 87.5% and 75% of organs, respectively. In the case of inoculation with LBR- cells treated with DOX or VCR plus ALA-PDT, no evidence of tumor infiltration was observed in any of the tissues. These results show the beneficial effect of combining therapies, suggesting the potential therapeutic alternative in leukemic patients, additionaly bringing the possibility of diminishing chemotherapy dose, thus minimizing undesirable drug side effects.

Chapter 8 - Classical photodynamic therapy, as it has evolved in the span of nearly a century, is based on the interaction between red light and a macrocycle resulting in the subsequent activation of molecular oxygen to a highly reactive and cytotoxic singlet species. This approach has the fundamental clinical drawbacks of nonspecific bystander tissue effects and local inflammation due to necrosis. Over the last two decades an alternative approach has emerged with the potential to overcome both these limitations and it involves the use of thiated nucleoside mimics of thymidine which promise tumour selective localization and exclusive apoptotic cell killing. In this chapter the authors survey the development of this technology from synthesis to clinical applications.

The Open University is incorporated by Royal Charter (RC 000391), an exempt charity in England & Wales and a charity registered in Scotland(SC 038302). The Open University is authorised and regulated by the Financial Conduct Authority.

Chapter 9 - The use of a photodynamic therapy (PDT) is hampered in some cases by the inability to create a sufficient concentration of photosensitizer (PS) in a tumor or the inability to deliver effectively laser radiation in some localization of malignant neoplasms. A number of nosological forms of the primary tumor and its metastases (in brain, peripheral parts of the lung, pancreas, liver, kidney, and bone tissue) are not available for exposure to light, which not only limits the possibilities for PDT application but also reduces in general the effectiveness of cancer care.

One promising way to improve this situation with PDT is the creation of hybrid polymer nanosystems (HPNS) containing nanostructures from the nanoparticles (NPs) and PS, which activation is carried out without the constraints and can easily penetrate to any depth in the human body using an ionizing radiation (X-ray or gamma radiation). Under the action of ionizing radiation, NPs generate light in the spectral range required for PS activation. The nanostructures can go into the tumor itself or the blood stream with a special media such as NPs-containing colloids.

The motivation for this work was synthesizing the novel HPNSs based on zinc selenide (ZnSe) nanoparticles, stabilized by biocompatible water-soluble polymers, and a new generation PS - the Photodithazine (PD) under different conditions of their preparation. The results of PD clinical trials have demonstrated a high clinical potential of the drug, exhibiting good solubility in water and physiological media and high absorption selectivity for tumor. The author's research focuses on designing water-soluble, stable in the biological environment and non-toxic HPNS. Perspective applications of prepared HPNS include, for example, their use as fluorescent cellular labels, deep-tissue and tumor imaging agents, and sensitizers for PDT in cancer treatment.

The paper briefly covers the morphology, crystalline and electronic structure of novel ZnSe-and PD-containing HPNS, their spectral characteristics and bioactivity. The combination of atomic-force microscopy (AFM), high-resolution electron microscopy

(HREM), X-ray diffraction (XRD), X-ray photoelectron spectroscopy (XPS), differential scanning calorimetry (DSC), infra-red spectroscopy (IR), photoluminescence (PL), and UV-vis spectroscopy methods are used.

The authors' research is oriented towards the development of new generation of drugs for selective PDT in oncology.

Chapter 10 - Verteporfin is a light-activated photosensitizing drug administered in a liposomal properties formulation. It is preferentially taken up by neovascular endothelium cells that have increased expression of low-density lipoprotein receptors. It is activated by non-thermal laser light to obtain endothelial damage and closure of neovascular structures.

Ocular photodynamic therapy (PDT) was approved and introduced as a novel treatment for choroidal neovascularization related to age-related macular degeneration, pathologic myopia and ocular histoplasmosis syndrome.

Other ocular pathologies had also used PDT with some remarkable results. These extended applications include choroidal neovascularization (CNV) secondary to choroiditis and retinochoroiditis, angioid streaks, central serous chorioretinopathy, retinal angiomatous proliferation, parafoveal telangiectasia or CNV associated with macular dystrophy and idiopathic CNV, as well as diseases unrelated to CNV, such as choroidal hemangioma, retinal hamartoma, choroidal melanoma and angiomatous lesions secondary to systemic diseases.

To date, with the introduction of various anti-Vascular endothelial growth factor (VEGF) and VEGF trap therapy, the role of PDT has certainly changed. It still has an important role in some diseases, such as chronic central serous chorioretinopathy and polypoidal choroidal vasculopathy. It might also maintain a role in combination therapy due to its unique properties of selective vascular targeting.

In: Photodynamic Therapy
Editor: Adrian G. Hugo

ISBN: 978-1-63463-857-9
© 2015 Nova Science Publishers, Inc.

Chapter 1

MULTIFUNCTIONAL NANOPARTICLES IN PHOTODYNAMIC THERAPY: RECENT DEVELOPMENTS

Juan L. Vivero-Escoto

Department of Chemistry, University of North Carolina at Charlotte,
Charlotte, North Carolina, US
The Center for Biomedical Engineering and Science,
University of North Carolina at Charlotte, Charlotte, North Carolina, US

ABSTRACT

Photodynamic therapy (PDT) has evolved over last century and is now becoming a more widely used medical tool having gained regulatory approval for the treatment of various diseases such as cancer and macular degeneration. PDT is based on the activation of photosensitizer agents with specific wavelength of light, which results in energy transfer cascades that ultimately yield cytotoxic reactive oxygen species that can render cell death. Although this modality has significantly improved the quality of life and survival time of many patients, it still offers significant potential for further improvement. For example, due to the tendency of most photosensitizer molecules to be poorly soluble and to form nonphotoactive aggregates, delivery vehicles have become of great importance. The use of different types of nanoparticles as photosensitizer carriers is a promising approach because these nanomaterials can satisfy all the requirements for an ideal PDT agent. This review describes some of the main types of nanoparticles that are currently in use for PDT applications. Recent advances in the use of multifunctional nanoparticles as carriers of photosensitizer molecules are highlighted. Novel strategies for designing photosensitizer delivery systems with improved PDT efficacy are described. Finally, we summarize exciting new results concerning the improvement of light tissue penetration for PDT through two-photon excitation and upconversion nanoparticles.

1. INTRODUCTION

Photodynamic therapy (PDT) is a well-established clinical modality for cancer, cardiovascular, ophthalmic, dermatological, and dental diseases. In the particular case of cancer, a variety of cancer treatments including cancer of the oesophagous, papillary bladder, lung and melanoma have been clinically approved using PDT. [1-4] The underlying principle of PDT is the selective uptake of a photosensitizer (PS) agent that localizes to a specific tissue/tumor cell type, followed by irradiation with light of the appropriate wavelength to activate the PS (Figure 1). [1, 5, 6] Upon activation, the PS interacts with molecular oxygen and generates singlet oxygen ($^1O_2$) and reactive oxygen species (ROS), leading to the destruction of cancer cells by necrotic and/or apoptotic mechanisms. [7] PDT is a less invasive method than traditional therapies for treating cancer because of its relative specificity and selectivity, together with the absence of harmful side effects typically encountered with chemotherapy or radiotherapy. Nevertheless, PDT is currently being used primarily to treat skin diseases and easily accessible cancerous and pre-cancerous lesions. [2, 3, 8] One reason for this limited clinical repertoire is the complication associated with the delivery of PSs. Traditionally, PSs such as porphyrins and phthalocyanines have dominated the field. [6, 9] However, these PS agents have several drawbacks such as low water solubility, poor light absorption, cutaneous photosensitivity, and reduced selectivity for targeted tissues. Ideally, PSs should meet several requirements: (1) chemical stability, (2) water-solubility, (3) high quantum yield of $^1O_2$ generation, (4) biocompatibility in the absence of light, (5) tumor selectivity, (6) rapid accumulation in target tumor tissues, (7) rapid clearance from the body and (8) a high molar absorption coefficient in the long wavelength (700-900 nm) that can penetrate deeper tissues. [10, 11] Although some of those features, such as molar and wavelength absorption can be easily modified, other aspects, such as manipulation of the pharmacokinetics, tumor selectivity, accumulation and clearance, are not so easily controlled. [12] Therefore the search for novel nanoparticle-based delivery methods with the ability to fulfill the necessary chemical, physical and biological requirements of an ideal photosensitizer is a burgeoning area of research. [13-15]

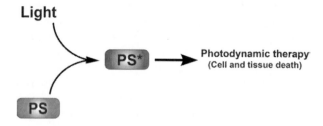

Figure 1. Schematic representation of the principle behind PDT.

2. TYPES OF NANOMATERIALS USED FOR PDT

The nanoparticulate platforms that have been extensively explored for PDT are predominantly based on organic or inorganic materials. Organic nanoparticles such as liposomes, natural polymers, polymeric micelles and dendrimers have been extensively used in drug delivery applications. [16] These delivery vehicles have also been used for delivering PSs for photodynamic cancer treatment. In addition to organic nanoparticles, various inorganic nanomaterials with interesting structures as well as unique photophysical, physical and chemical properties have also been explored to deliver PS agents. Inorganic nanoparticles based on silica, semiconductor materials, iron oxide, gold and carbon have been broadly used in PDT. Interestingly, some of these platforms are not only used to carry PS molecules; but due to their photophysical properties, they can be used as the PS agent themselves. Both types of PS delivery platforms have been systematically summarized in a number of previous review articles; [3, 11-15, 17-22] in this chapter, I only briefly introduce several major classes of organic and inorganic nanocarriers for PDT applications.

2.1. Liposomes

Liposomes have been the most successful nanoparticle platform for biomedical applications, with several formulations clinically available. [17] These nanoparticles are composed of an aqueous core surrounded by a phospholipid bilayer and have been used to deliver a variety of therapeutic, imaging and photosensitizer agents. [23-25] Liposomes have also been extensively used in PDT due to their high loading capacity and flexibility for modification. [18, 19] For instance, the photofrin encapsulated liposomes exhibited significantly higher photodynamic efficacy against a human glioma implanted in rat brain as compared to photofrin only. [26] As a commercial product of liposomal PDT agent, Visudyne containing verteporfin, abenzoporphyrin derivative, has been approved for the treatment of age-related macular degeneration (AMD), which is caused by abnormal choroidal neovascularization. [27] Recently, Park and co-workers reported the use of membrane fusogenic liposomes (MFLs) as organelle-specific delivery system to localize the hydrophobic PSs selectively into the plasma membrane. [28] Zinc phthalocyanine (ZnPc) was used as a PS because its lipophilicity to allow the membrane localization and strong phototoxicity upon NIR irradiation. The ZnPc molecules were delivered selectively into the plasma membrane by the MFLs. The authors demonstrated that the selective delivery of ZnPc into the plasma membrane can significantly enhance the therapeutic efficacy of PDT. According to the report, the ZnPc molecules delivered in the plasma membrane induced substantial membrane disruption upon irradiation, thereby leading to acute necrosis-like cell death.

2.2. Natural Polymeric Particles

There have been many reports on the use of natural degradable polymeric particles as delivery vehicles for PDT. [29, 30] Commonly used natural degradable polymers include alginate, chitosan, dextran, albumin, ferritin, gelatin, collagen agars, and others. Yoon et al. used hyaluronic acid nanoparticles (HANPs) containing Ce6 for simultaneous imaging and PDT. [31] Self-assembled HANPs were synthesized by chemical conjugation of aminated 5β-cholanic acid, PEG, and black hole quencher3 (BHQ3) to the HA polymers. Ce6 was readily loaded into HANPs by a simple dialysis method, resulting in Ce6-loaded hyaluronic acid nanoparticles (Ce6-HANPs). After intravenous (iv) injection into the tumor bearing mice,

Ce6-HANPs could efficiently reach the tumor tissue via the passive targeting mechanism and specifically enter tumor cells through the receptor-mediated endocytosis based on the interactions between HA on nanoparticles and CD44, the HA receptor on the surface of tumor cells. Upon laser irradiation, Ce6 that was released from the nanoparticles generated fluorescence and $^1O_2$ inside tumor cells, resulting in effective suppression of tumor growth (Figure 2).

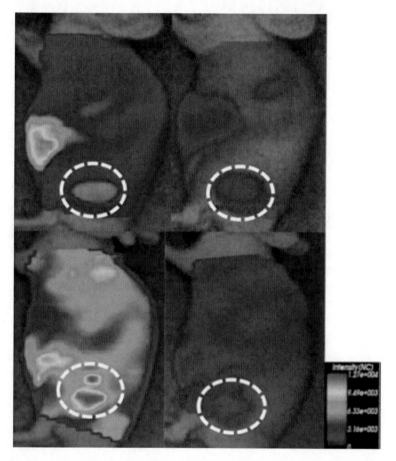

Figure 2. *In vivo* photodynamic imaging with Ce6-HANPs. Whole body fluorescence images of HT29 tumor-bearing mice treated with free Ce6 (top) and Ce6-HANPs (bottom). White circles indicate tumor sites. Reprinted with permission of Ref. 31.

2.3. Polymeric Micelles

The development of nano-formulated polymeric micelles to carry PSs has emerged as a promising technique because of the biocompatibility and the accessibility for multi-functionalization of NPs. [11, 13, 32] These platforms usually follow two strategies to carry the PSs either by physical entrapment and/or covalent bond to the hydrophobic cores. Polymers such as poly(ethylene glycol)-poly(caprolactone) (PEG-PCL), pluronics, PEGylated lipids and many others have been used to encapsulate PSs. Wilson and co-workers investigated the formulation of hydrophobic protoporphyrin IX (PpIX) with MePEG5000-b-

PCL4100 [methoxy poly (ethylene glycol)-b-poly (caprolactone)] diblock copolymers and compared their PDT response to that of free PpIX. [33] The authors studied the photophysical and photochemical properties of the polymeric PpIX micelles by measuring absorbance and fluorescence spectra, PpIX-loading efficiency and stability, the micelle particle size and morphology, as well as $^1O_2$ luminescence and lifetime. *In vitro* PDT results showed that the PpIX micelles have markedly increased photocytotoxicity over that with free PpIX by nearly an order of magnitude at the highest light dose used. These findings suggest that diblock copolymer micelles have great potential as a drug delivery system for hydrophobic photodynamic sensitizers.

2.4. Dendrimers

Dendrimers and other hyper-branched organic polymers have also been extensively evaluated for their potential in imaging and drug delivery applications. [34-37] Photosensitizers can be attached at the periphery of the dendrimers branches or have been encapsulated in the core of a dendrimers in a similar way than drugs and imaging agents. Lai et al. evaluated the effects of phthalocyanine-encapsulated dendrimers doxorubicin-loaded polymeric micelle nanoparticles to overcome drug resistance. [38] The platform was studied in drug resistance MCF-7 cells and a xenograft model. The experiments demonstrated that the nanoparticle-mediated PDT elicited remarkably effective endosomal-lysosomal release and nuclear accumulation of doxorubicin, which killed doxorubicin-resistant cells *in vitro*. In animal experiments, the PS-loaded nanoparticle combined with doxorubicin showed higher antitumor activity than the nanoparticle alone. Thus, this platform is an innovative photosensitizer formulation that not only improves the effectiveness and safety of PDT but also overcomes drug resistance to chemotherapy.

2.5. LBL Microcapsules/Vesicles

Layer by layer (LBL) microcapsules or vesicles can also be used to encapsulate a wide variety of therapeutic agents including PS molecules for PDT. [39-42] In general, those capsules are prepared by the sequential deposition of oppositely charged polyelectrolytes onto charged templates using the so-called LBL method. Son et al. reported the preparation of hollow nanocapsules by the LBL technique. [43] Adendrimerporphyrin (DP) was introduced not only as the PS molecule but also to offer negative charges, the latter of which could be utilized in the deposition of counter-charged polymers by LBL. After removal of the template core, stable hollow nanocapsules were successfully obtained and used for combined PDT and chemotherapy. Overall, LBL-based hollow nanoparticles could serve as an interesting platform to develop PDT nanoagents usually with multiple functions.

2.6. Semiconducting Quantum Dots (QDs)

The archetypical inorganic nanoparticles, QDs are nanomaterials generally composed of elements from either groups II and VI or III and V. [44-48] They display unique optical properties, including sharp and symmetrical emission spectra, high quantum yields, broad absorption spectra, good chemical and photostability, and tunable size-dependent emission wavelengths. [47] As a result, they have been evaluated extensively for use as optical imaging probes both *in vitro* and *in vivo*. Compared with molecular PSs, some properties of QDs are very attractive for PDT applications: they can be targeted to specific pathological areas; their emission can be broadly tuned (UV to IR) simply by size and composition, and they are stable *in vivo* for very long periods of time without degradation. [49-51] Moreover, it has been found that QDs can produce $^1O_2$ under direct photoactivation (Figure 3). In 2003, Burda et al. employed hydrophobic-capped CdSe QDs dissolved in oxygen saturated toluene and observed noticeable $^1O_2$ production under light irradiation with an efficiency at 5%. [52] They found that this low quantum efficiency for $^1O_2$ production by QDs was due to ultrafast carrier trapping, nonradiative carrier relaxation, and the large hydrodynamic size of QDs. However, conventional PS molecules based on porphyrins with small hydrodynamic size and long-living triplet state can produce $^1O_2$ at much higher efficiencies (>75%). To utilize the photostability of QDs and improve the production of $^1O_2$, several QD-PS hybrids have been developed as a new generation of PS agents for PDT. [53] In such hybrid QD-PS systems, the excited singlet and triplet states of PS drugs are indirectly generated by nonradioactive energy transfer, also known as fluorescence resonance energy transfer (FRET). Because of the indirect photoactivation, photobleaching of PS drugs could be minimized. Burda et al. reported on the applicability of semiconductor CdSe QDs for PDT. [52] The authors synthesized and functionalized CdSe QDs (average diameter of 5 nm) with silicon phthalocyanine (Pc4) PS agents through an alkyl amino group on the photosensitizer's axial substituent. The CdSe QD emission at 568 nm was used to activate the Pc4 photosensitizer. The combination of semiconductor QDs and PSs enabled the use of an excitation wavelength where the PS molecule alone does not absorb. Their results demonstrated that CdSe QDs could be used to sensitize a PDT agent via the FRET mechanism.

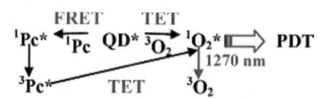

Figure 3. Schematics of the $^1O_2$ generation in QD-based PDT systems. Printed with permission of Ref. 52.

Following the first investigation of QD-PS system by Burda, many researchers were attracted to the energy transfer properties of covalent and non-covalent QD-PS systems composed of CdSe, CdSe/CdS/ZnS, CdSe/ZnS, and CdTe QDs as energy donors and various chromophores such as porphyrins, phthalocyanines, inorganic complexes and other organic dyes as energy acceptors. [53-55] Depending on the energy acceptor, the QD-PS systems can be classified into QD-phthalocyanines, QD-porphines, QD-organic dyes, and QD-inorganic dyes. Careful design of QD-PS complexes will allow effective delivery into tumors, efficient generation of ROS, and image-guided PDT. However, the potential toxicity of QDs containing heavy metal elements could be a major obstacle toward clinical use of QDs-PS complexes. [49, 51] Recently, to overcome this issue, Nann and co-workers have coupled a less toxic InP/ZnS QDs to the photosensitizer chlorin e6 (Figure 4). [56] The authors studied in detail the spectroscopic properties of these hybrids. Moreover, the PDT efficacy of the QD/chlorin e6 hybrids has been assessed against a breast cancer (MDA-MB-231) cell line using a colorimetric MTT assay (Figure 4). The spectroscopic investigations of the hybrid system showed that the energy transfer between the QDs and photosensitizer is the rate-determining step for the production of $^1O_2$. When comparing the $^1O_2$ production activities of the chlorin e6 photosensitizer, it was found that the rate of production of $^1O_2$ of the hybrid was slightly inferior to that of the free PS agent. This result was strengthened by the *in vitro* measurements, where similar cell viability was found for both the free chlorin e6 and QD/chlorin e6 hybrids.

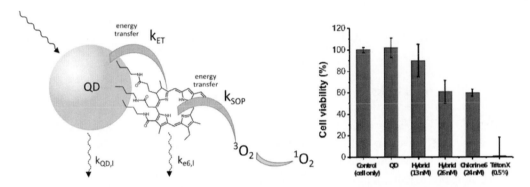

Figure 4. Energy transfer pathways in QD/chlorin e6 hybrids (left). Cell viability represented as percentage of viable cells after 3 h treatment with QDs, chlorin e6, and the QD/chlorin e6 hybrid following UV irradiation (0.033 J·cm^{-2}) assessed with a MTT assay (right). Printed with permission of Ref. 56.

2.7. Iron Oxide Nanoparticles

Another class of inorganic nanoparticles that have been evaluated for PDT applications are metal oxides, such as superparamagnetic iron oxide nanoparticles (SPIONPs). [57-61] Iron oxide nanoparticles have been used as contrast agents for magnetic resonance imaging (MRI), magnetic hyperthermia, and targeted drug delivery via magnetic attraction. One of the very few types of FDA approved inorganic-based nanomaterials for *in vivo* use is polymer-coated SPIONPs agents for MRI. In past years many different groups have explore the use of SPIONPs in the delivery of PS molecules and MR imaging guided PDT. [62-68] Recently, Albericio and co-workers developed a method for the preparation of SPIO nanoparticle–porphyrin (SPION-TPP) conjugates through click chemistry, which can be used as novel theranostic nanoagents for PDT. [69] Upon light irradiation, SPION-TPP nanoconstructs promote a photodynamic effect *in vitro* in murine amelanotic melanoma B78-H1 cells, with IC_{50} values in the region of 800 nM, similarly to unbound TPP, whereas they remained non-cytotoxic in the dark. To improve the cellular uptake, the authors conjugated a well-known cell-penetrating peptide (TAT peptide) to the SPIONP-TPP nanoparticles. The new nanoconstructs showed lower IC_{50} values (in the region of 500 nM) and a clear dose–response effect. These results showed that TAT-conjugated SPIONP-TPP nanoparticles are efficient nanodevices both for tracking drugs by means of magnetic resonance imaging (MRI)-based techniques and for treating cancer cells through PDT, thus functioning as promising theranostic nanoagents. Liu et al. loaded chlorin e6 (Ce6), a widely used PS molecule in PDT, on polyethylene glycol (PEG) functionalized iron oxide nanoclusters (IONCs), obtaining IONC-PEG-Ce6 as a theranostic agent for dual-mode imaging guided and magnetic targeting enhanced *in vivo* PDT. [70] Without noticeable dark toxicity, IONC-PEG-Ce6 exhibits significantly accelerated cellular uptake compared with free Ce6, and thus offers greatly improved *in vitro* photodynamic cancer cell killing efficiency under a low-power light exposure. Interestingly, the authors in this report demonstrated an enhancement of PDT effect due to the presence of the magnetic field (MF). The *in vivo* PDT experiment achieved high therapeutic efficacy with dramatically delayed tumor growth after just a single injection and the MF-enhanced photodynamic treatment. Considering the biodegradability and non-toxicity of iron oxide, the IONC-PEG-Ce6 nanoparticles developed in this work may be a useful multifunctional agent promising in photodynamic cancer treatment under magnetic targeting.

2.8. Gold Nanoparticles

Metallic nanoparticles such as Au, Ag, and Pt, possess many fascinating properties, and have been widely explored for applications in biomedicine. [71-74] In particular, Au nanoparticles (AuNPs) with controllable morphologies have been extensively used for drug delivery and biological imaging applications as they can be engineered to exhibit strong absorption in the NIR region. [75-79] AuNPs have also been explored for photothermal therapy, where absorbed light by small gold nanoparticles (10–30 nm) is rapidly converted into thermal energy to lead to hyperthermia and cell death. AuNPs can also be used as PS delivery systems for PDT. [80-85] Kim and co-workers developed a multifunctional PDT platform by using AuNPs as water soluble and biocompatible nanocarriers to allow the delivery of a PS agent to a tumor site for PDT action. [86] The authors modified 17.6 nm citrate-stabilized AuNPs with folic acid (FA)-conjugated biocompatible block copolymers through a bidentate dihydrolipoic acid (DHLA) linker. Then, the PS molecule, pheophorbide a (Pheo), was conjugated to the stable vectors through a pH-sensitive linkage. Confocal microscopy, flow cytometry assay, and bio-TEM measurements were used for determining the cellular uptake of Pheo and AuNPs in HeLa cells. The FA–PEG–AuNPs–Pheo showed 99.16% cellular uptake and exhibited an excellent phototoxicity compared to free Pheo and FA-unconjugated nanoparticles at pH 6.4. Recently, the effect of 5-aminolevulinic acid (ALA) and ALA combined with gold nanoparticles (ALA–AuNPs) for PDT on human cervical HeLa cancer cell line was compared. [87] The authors found that ALA–AuNPs combination can enhance ROS production and then induce higher phototoxicity. The results showed that ALA–AuNPs combinations induced cell death via ROS mediated apoptosis after PDT.

Interestingly, $^1O_2$ can also be generated from AuNPs without the presence of PS molecules. In 2011, Hwang et al. reported that $^1O_2$ could be formed through plasmonical excitation of metal nanoparticles, including Au, Ag and Pt. [88] Direct evidence include the observation of phosphorescence emission of $^1O_2$ at approximately 1268 nm, hydroperoxidation of olefins, fluorescence of a selective $^1O_2$ sensor, and the quenching of $^1O_2$ phosphorescence with sodium azide. However, those nanoparticles were not tested *in vitro*. In a recent work, Gao and co-workers reported the use of gold nanocages (AuNCs) as intrinsic inorganic PSs mediating generation of ROS by plasmon-enabled photochemistry under near-infrared (NIR) one/two-photon irradiation. [82] The authors demonstrated the production of three main radical species, namely, $^1O_2$, superoxide radical anion ($O_2\bullet$), and hydroxyl radical ($\bullet$OH) by applying electron spin resonance spectroscopy. The existence of hot electrons from irradiated AuNCs was confirmed by a well-designed photoelectrochemical experiment based on a three-electrode system. The authors also compared AuNCs' ROS generation efficiency in different surface chemical environments under one/two-photon irradiation and verified that, compared with one photon irradiation; two-photon irradiation could bring about much more ROS. Furthermore, *in vitro*, under two-photon irradiation, ROS can trigger mitochondrial depolarization and caspase protein up-regulation to initiate tumor cell apoptosis (Figure 5). This report showed that the combination of plasmon-mediated ROS generation and hyperthermia can be tuned to optimize anticancer PDT.

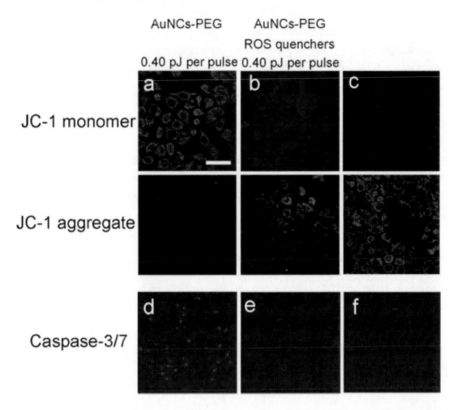

Figure 5. CLSM images of mitochondrial membrane potential (JC-1 staining) of cells pretreated with AuNCs-PEG in the absence (a) or presence (b) of 250 µMROS quenchers under NIR two-photon irradiation at 0.40 pJ per pulse; (c) control cells. CLSM images of caspase-3/7 activity of cells pretreated with AuNCs-PEG in the absence (d) or presence (e) of 250 µM ROS quenchers under NIR two-photon irradiation at 0.40 pJ per pulse; (f) control cells. Scale bar is 50 µm. Printed with permission from Ref. 82.

Carbon-based Nanoparticles

There are several carbon-based nanoparticles currently tested in biomedical applications including fullerenes, carbon nanotubes (CNTs), graphene and carbon dots. [89-91] Fullerenes were discovered in 1985, they are typically composed of 60 carbon atoms arranged in a soccer-ball structure. [92] The condensed aromatic rings presented in fullerenes lead to an extended π–conjugated system of molecular orbitals and therefore to significant absorption of visible light. Fullerenes are found to be able to generate ROS upon illumination, suggesting a promising role in PDT. [93-96] As non-functionalized fullerenes are highly hydrophobic, surfaces modified with some functional groups attached to fullerenes are thus needed to make them more soluble in water and biological solutions. Phototoxicity of fullerenes has been demonstrated since 1993, Tokuyama et al. used carboxylic acid-functionalized fullerenes in HeLa cells and demonstrated the phototoxic effect of fullerenes. [97] To improve the solubility of fullerenes (C60) in water, Diao and co-workers explore a non-covalent approach using cyclodextrins (CDs) as a suitable solubilizing agent. CDs can provide hydrophobic cavities in aqueous solutions for C60 to form inclusion complexes because of their suited cavity size. [98] In this report, γ-CDs was chosen as the host polymer because of its high water-solubility and right cavity size for C60 (Figure 6). The supramolecular interactions between host and guest molecules significantly preserved the integrity of C60, which is critical for many biomedical applications. The authors also evaluated the ability of a C60 inclusion complex with γ-CDs (C60–γ-CDs) to generate $^1O_2$ under ultraviolet A (UVA) irradiation. C60–γ-CDs could efficiently generate $^1O_2$ species, and be regarded as a safe inclusion complex due to the low cell toxicity without UVA irradiation. γ-CDs not only imparted solubility to the hydrophobic C60 in aqueous solution with less aggregation, but also increased biocompatibility efficiently. Finally, the authors tested the phototoxicity of the C60 supramolecular complex. C60–γ-CDs with high water solubility and $^1O_2$ generation ability showed great phototoxicity for B17-F10 melanoma cells (Figure 6). These results confirmed that a CD-functionalized methodology of fullerenes without any chemical modification can be advantageous to develop fullerene-based supramolecular complexes for PDT applications.

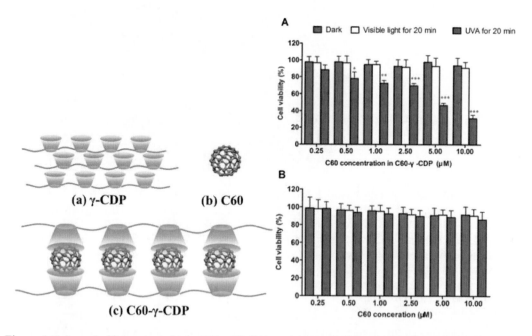

Figure 6. Schematic illustration of (a) γ-CDs, (b) C60, and (c) C60-γ-CDs (left). Effect of different concentrations of (A) C60-γ-CDs and (B) C60 exposure on the viability of B16-F10 cells irradiated with UVA and cool white light as measured by the MTT assay (right). Printed with permission of Ref. 98.

In vivo PDT for tumor treatment has also been demonstrated using fullerenes as the PS agents. Tabata et al. demonstrated fullerene-based PDT of tumors in animal experiments. In this work, fullerene was functionalized with PEG, not only to acquire colloidal stability, but also to enable preferential accumulation and prolonged retention of fullerene in the tumor tissue. [99] As compared to the commercial agent Photofrin; C60-PEG platform, administered by intravenous injection, offered a stronger tumor suppressive effect under exposure to the visible light. Fullerene derivatives have been demonstrated to be effective PS agents in PDT cancer treatment. However, the major disadvantage of fullerene is that they have to be excited with light with short wavelengths in the UV or blue regions, which has very limited tissue penetration. Other carbon nanomaterials, including CNTs, graphenes and carbon dots have also been applied in PDT. In a recent report, Zhang and co-workers investigated the application of modified CNTs as PS agents. The authors synthesized and characterized two types of nanomaterials; CNTs functionalized covalently with polyethylenimine (PEI) (CNT-PEI) and non-covalently functionalized with polyvinylpyrrolidone (PVP-K30) (CNT-PVP-K30). [100] The photophysical and phototoxic properties of both materials were successfully tested. The authors demonstrated that these materials induce ROS-dependent DNA cleavage after irradiation with visible light. *In vitro*, no cytotoxic damage was detected in B16-F10 cells; however after illumination, both CNT materials shown a dramatic increase in the cytotoxicity of cells as an indication of the PDT effect. To investigate the *in vivo* PDT efficacy of CNT-PEI and CNT-PVP-K30, comparative efficacy studies were conducted in B16-F10 tumor-bearing mice. The authors found that the CNT-PEI with illumination treatment group had tumor growth inhibition (TGI) of 45%, which is significantly more effective than CNT-PVP-K30 and the control groups ($p < 0.05$). These results suggested that CNT-PEI nanomaterial can be used as a photosensitizer in PDT to achieve *in vivo* tumor treatment efficacy.

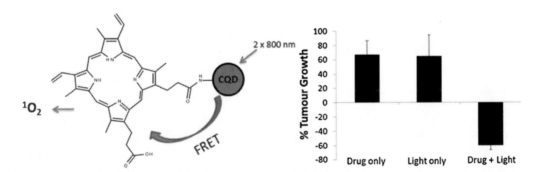

Figure 7. Schematic representation of the PpIX-CQD conjugate illustrating indirect excitation of the PpIX upon two-photon excitation of the CQD (left). Plot of % tumor growth after 4 days in tumor bearing mice who received the following treatments: PpIX-CQD only (Drug only); two-photon irradiation at 800 nm (Light only); and PpIX-CQD and two-photon irradiation at 800 nm (Drug + Light) (right). Printed with permission of Ref. 102.

Carbon quantum dots (CQDs) have recently emerged as novel carbon materials showing great potential in nanomedicine and bioapplications. [101] One of the attractive features of CQDs is their high two-photon absorption cross section, which is three orders of magnitude greater than conventional dye based photosensitizers. In this context, several groups have employed CQDs to improve PDT by indirect two-photon excitation through FRET from

CQDs to the PS molecules. [102-104] Recently, Callan and co-workers used this strategy in the design of a protoporphyrin IX (PpIX)-CQDs conjugate. [102] PpIX, which contains carboxylic acid functionality, was attached to CQDs (4.65 nm, diameter) at three different loading ratios using standard carbodiimide chemistry. The authors showed the successful generation of $^1O_2$ through a FRET mediated process in the PpIX-CQD nanoparticles. HeLa cells were used to determine the phototoxicity of this system. The results showed a significant reduction in viability for those cells treated with PpIX-CQDs and two-photon light compared with those treated with the nanoparticles alone. The authors also evaluated this platform *in vivo* using a syngenic radiation-induced fibrosarcoma (RIF-1) mouse tumor model. Four days after treatment with PpIX-CQDs and two-photon light, tumor on animals treated with the nanoconstruct and light regressed and were found to be 60% smaller than the original pre-treatment size. Moreover, the authors noticed that even 13 days post treatment the tumors had still not reached their pre-treatment size. Based on their results, it is suggested that PS-CQDs conjugates, in combination with two-photon excitation, can have significant value as a potential treatment of deep-seated tumors using PDT. Chen at al. also followed a similar approach to design PS-CQD nanoconstructs, in their case they used 5,10,15,20-tetrakis(1-methyl-pyridinio) porphyrin tetra(p-toulenesulfonate) (TMPyP) as PS agent and 8 nm in diameter CQDs. [105] The authors demonstrated the efficient production of $^1O_2$ under irradiation of NIR fs lasers. *In vitro* experiments also showed the efficient TMPyP-CQDs FRET mediated PDT treatment of HeLa cells under two-photon excitation of 700 nm fs laser beam with a low power density of 160 mW/mm^2.

3. NANOPARTICLES AS DELIVERY SYSTEMS FOR CHEMO AND PHOTODYNAMIC THERAPY

The novel properties of nanomaterials make them a promising avenue to overcome most of the shortcomings for the delivery of common PSs. Numerous advantages can be introduced by using nanoparticles as PS delivery systems: (i) they can carry large payloads of PS molecules; (ii) their surface and composition can be tailored to develop multifunctional (e.g. target-specific, theranostic) and biodegradable systems; and (iii) their small size allows deep penetration into tissues and ready internalization by cells. [11, 12, 22] Several platforms have been used as PS nanocarriers such as liposomes, micelles, polymers, silica-, and gold-nanoparticles. [3, 19, 106] Clinical interest in the use of nanomaterials as PS delivery platforms was confirmed in 2000 with FDA approval of the liposomal formulation Visudyne® for the treatment of classic subfoveal choroidal neovascularization due to age-related macular degeneration. [107] Various other formulations (e.g. Fospeg®, Foslip®) are being evaluated in pre-clinical and clinical trials. [21, 108] Several critical design parameters from the synthesis of nanoparticles as anticancer drug delivery systems can be applied to the development of PS nanocarriers. [16] For example: (1) controlling the size of the nanovehicles (50 – 200 nm) to facilitate vascular margination and extravasation into tumors; (2) increasing the blood circulation time of nanoparticles to allow for increased contact of PS nanocarriers with the tumor site, thereby enhancing the possibility of passive-mediated accumulation within the tumor stroma; (3) maximizing the amount of drug encapsulated into the nanocarrier to enhance the therapeutic effect; (4) endowing controlled release capabilities to maintain desirable therapeutic action solely and specifically at the target site; and (5) activating cell-targeting abilities to facilitate receptor-mediated intracellular uptake. Different platforms both organic and inorganic nanoparticles have been used as PS delivery systems. Certainly, this is a relatively mature field, which has been systematically summarized in a number or previous review articles. [3, 11, 13, 15, 20, 21, 32] In this section, I will only briefly introduce recent reports in this area of PDT. Light-harvesting conjugated polyelectrolytes (CPEs) with –delocalized backbones have been widely used in biological sensing and imaging applications. [109-112] Recently, it has also been reported that CPEs with specific structures can generate ROS efficiently under light irradiation. Liu and co-workers used this platform to develop a drug delivery system based on a PEGylated CPE, which can be used not only as a matrix for drug delivery but also as a photosensitizing unit for PDT. [113, 114] In addition to therapeutic function, the inherent fluorescence of CPE also provides the opportunity for image-guided chemo- and photodynamic therapy. Liu and co-workers developed a PEGylated CPE that can easily self-assemble into NPs in aqueous media, which can easily encapsulated commonly used hydrophobic chemotherapeutic drugs, such as paclitaxel (PTX). [114] To improve the target-ability of this system cyclic arginine-glycine-aspartic acid (cRGD) tripeptide, which can target integrin $\alpha_v\beta_3$ overexpressed cancer cells, was incorporated onto the self-assembled NPs for targeted cancer therapy. The PTX-PEG-CPE nanoparticles have an average diameter of about 100 nm, with the absorption and emission maxima at 502 and 598 nm, respectively. The lethal doses concentration (LD_{50}) value for the combination therapy to U87-MG cells is 12.7 μg/mL, which is much lower than that for solely PDT (25.5 μg/mL) or chemotherapy (132.8 μg/mL). The drug delivery system based on PEG-CPE platform is simple to design and synthesize, which offers new opportunities for image-guided combination therapy. The same group also developed ROS-responsive doxorubicin (DOX)-loaded PEG-CPE platform for targeted and image-guided on-demand PDT and chemotherapy. [113] In this system, DOX was conjugated to a PEG-CPES using thioketal groups (ROS-cleavable linker) (Figure 8). Recent reports show that thioketal groups can be readily cleaved by ROS. The obtained ROS-responsive DOX-PEG-CPE nanoparticles were further functionalized with cRGD to enhance their targetability toward cancer cells. Under irradiation with light, these materials can generate ROS efficiently for PDT. Meanwhile, the generated ROS can quickly cleave the linker that covalently attaches DOX to the NPs for specific on-demand drug release. The authors investigated the successful ROS production upon irradiation with light using dichlorofluorescein diacetate as ROS-sensitive probe. The release of ROS-responsive release of DOX was monitored by HPLC after light irradiation of 0.1 W/cm^2 for 15 min. The authors tested the therapeutic properties of this platform *in vitro* using breast cancer cell line (MDA-MB-231 and MCF-7). The investigators demonstrated that the combination of cRGD and light-triggered chemotherapy and PDT clearly makes it a very efficient light controlled cancer therapy system.

Zhang et al. also developed a stimuli-responsive delivery system for DOX. The authors synthesized a DOX-loaded poly(ethyleneimine) (PEI) functionalized fullerene (C60-PEI-DOX) to facilitate combined chemo and photodynamic therapy in one system. [115] Moreover, DOX was covalently conjugated onto C60-PEI by the pH-sensitive hydrazine linkage. The authors showed that the release of DOX from C60-PEI-DOX followed a strong dependence on the pH conditions. The researchers also tested this platform *in vivo* using a tumor (B16-F10 cells)-bearing mice. To evaluate the biodistribution of C60-PEI-DOX particles CdSe/ZnS QDs were injected as contrast imaging agents. Compared with free DOX in an *in vivo* murine tumor model, C60-PEI-DOX afforded higher antitumor efficacy without obvious toxic effects to normal organs. The authors observed better tumor targeting efficacy and 2.4-fold greater amount of DOX released in the tumor than in normal tissues using C60-PEI-DOX nanoparticles. This system also showed high antitumor efficacy during PDT. The ability of C60-PEI-DOX platform to combine local specific chemotherapy with external PDT significantly improved the therapeutic efficacy of the cancer treatment.

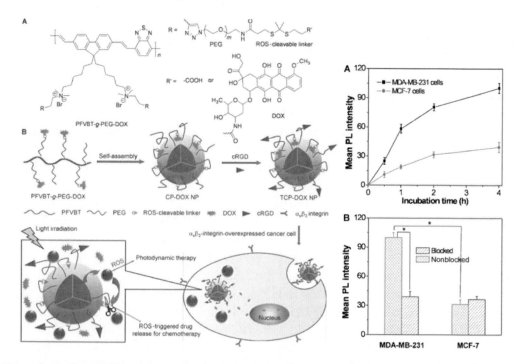

Figure 8. A) Chemical structure of DOX-PEG-CPE and B) schematic illustration of the light-regulated ROS-activated on-demand drug release and the combined chemo–photodynamic therapy (left). Evaluation of the targeting of DOX-PEG-CPE to different cancer cells. A) Integrated photoluminescence (PL) intensity of DOX-PEG-CPE in MDA-MB-231 and MCF-7 cells at different incubation time. B) PL intensity of DOX-PEG-CPE in MDA-MB-231 and MCF-7 cells with and without pretreatment with cRGD (50 μm) (right). Printed with permission of Ref. 113.

4. DESIGNING DELIVERY SYSTEMS FOR ENHANCED PHOTODYNAMIC THERAPY

The design of PS delivery systems has taken advantage from the strategies developed for drug delivery platforms, which were mentioned in the previous section. Nevertheless, it is important to note that designing PS nanovehicles is associated with its own particular challenges. [12, 20] For instance, for PDT it is desire that the nanoparticles are produced in an optically transparent form to avoid light absorption from the nanocarrier itself. Moreover, the platform should help to stop the PSs from dimerizing and aggregating as occurs in the free state. These forms are ineffective to produce $^1O_2$ due to the self-quenching of the excited states. [116-119] Consequently, it is critical to develop novel synthetic strategies to afford PS-loaded nanoparticulate platforms that not only carry a large quantity of PSs, but also demonstrate an effective PDT response. In addition; another problem associated with PS loaded into nanoparticles is the consequent trapping of the produced $^1O_2$ inside the nanoparticle matrix. Also, the presence of solid nanocarriers can slow down the out-diffusion of the generated ROS. [81] The lifetime and diffusion distance of $^1O_2$ under physiological conditions are 1-3 µs and 2-4 x 10^{-6} cm^{2}s^{-1}, respectively.[2] Therefore, under these conditions, the diffusion distance of $^1O_2$ is predicted to be limited to approximately 40 nm. The inhibited $^1O_2$ escaping from the nanomaterials to the cytoplasm would largely reduce their cell killing capability. [120] Consequently, it is critical to develop novel synthetic strategies to afford PS-loaded nanoparticulate platforms that not only carry a large quantity of PSs, but also demonstrate an effective PDT response.

Different strategies have been developed to improve the PS loading and PDT effect in nanoparticulate PS delivery platforms. We have developed polysilsesquioxane (PSilQ) nanoparticles as a novel alternative for the efficient delivery of PSs. [121, 122] We envision several advantages of PSilQ nanomaterials as PS carriers such as carrying a large payload of PS molecules; their surface and composition can be tailored to develop multifunctional devices (e.g. biodegradable and target-specific); and due to their small size, nanoparticles can penetrate deep into tissues and be readily internalized by cells. We recently reported on the design of PSilQ NPs that are degraded under specific conditions found inside the cells such as reducing environment, pH and enzymatic cleavage. Before being degraded, PSs are inactive inside the nanoparticles due to aggregation; however, once the platform is internalized by cells and under the right conditions, it releases the PSs as individual units maximizing the generation of $^1O_2$ production (Figure 9). We synthesized and tested *in vitro* a PSilQ system that contains PpIX agents chemically attached through a redox-responsive linker (RR-PpIX-PSilQ-NPs). [121, 122] The linker has a disulfide bond that can be broken under reducing conditions such as those found in cancer cells. We hypothesized that after internalization by cancer cells, the disulfide bond will be broken releasing the PpIX agents in monomeric form. We synthesized RR-PpIX-PSilQ NPs by a reverse microemulsion method using a quaternary emulsion system; in a similar way, a non-degradable PpIX-PSilQ material was synthesized as control sample. The structural characterization of these particles showed a high aggregation under physiological conditions according to DLS data due to the hydrophobic nature of the nanoparticles, the surface charge is slightly negative based on ζ-potential measurement (-7.7 to -14.3 mV) and a high loading of PpIX molecules (43-46 % wt.) was determined according to thermogravimetric analysis. The redox-responsive properties in solution showed that the degradation and subsequent release of PpIX agents is triggered by the addition of reducing agents such as dithiothreitol (DTT). We tested the dark toxicity and phototoxicity of this system *in vitro* by MTS assay using HeLa cells. Both materials, RR-PpIX-PSilQ and PpIX-PSilQ NPs, showed minimal toxicity in the absence of light. However, under light irradiation RR-PpIX-PSilQ-NPs showed a much higher phototoxicity than the control sample as an indication of the intracellular release of PpIX photoactive molecules (Figure 9). Overall, our data proved that by developing redox-responsive PSilQ materials with a high content of photosensitizers, which selectively release PS agents inside the cells, the PDT efficacy can be improved. We were interested in demonstrating that the PpIX agents are indeed been released inside the HeLa cells upon reducing environment. For that, we developed a two-labeled approach using solid silica nanoparticles (SiNPs) embedded with fluorescein dye and functionalized on the exterior surface with RR-PpIX linker. [121] The RR-PpIX-Si-NPs and the corresponding control material did not show cytotoxicity under dark conditions. But, upon light irradiation the RR-PpIX-Si-NPs showed at least twice higher phototoxicity than control sample, this performance is similar to the one observed with RR-PSilQ-NPs. Confocal microscopy allowed us to investigate the localization of the RR-PpIX-SiNPs inside HeLa cells. By developing the two-labelled platform with FITC-marking the SiNPs and PpIX on the exterior surface, we were able to keep track of the intracellular release of PpIX molecules. The confocal micrographs for the RR-PpIX-SiNPs showed the fluorescence in the green channel and the red channel in separated spot as an indication that the SiNPs are not co-localized with PpIX molecules as an indication that the redox-responsive linker has been broken releasing the PpIX agents. The confocal micrographs only showed spots in the green channel, which demonstrated that, the PpIX molecules are still attached to the SiNPs. These results further confirm that indeed the intracellular degradation of RR-PpIX nanoparticles is responsible for the improvement on the PDT efficacy.

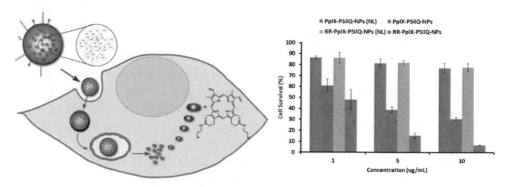

Figure 9. Schematic representation of the cellular internalization, redox-responsive release and phototoxic effect of RR-PpIX-PSilQ NPs (left). Phototoxicity of PpIX-PSilQ NPs (blue) and RR-PpIX-PSilQ NPs (green) in the absence of light, and PpIX-PSilQ NPs (red) and RR-PpIX-PSilQ NPs (purple) after light exposure (right). Printed with permission from Ref. 122.

Other groups have reported similar results using other types of PS delivery platforms. Huh and co-workers reported on the synthesis and application *in vitro* and *in vivo* of a second generation PDT agent (pheophorbide A, PheoA) conjugated with glycol chitosan (GC) polymer via bioreducible disulfide linkages. [119] The developed polymer self-assembled to form spherical NPs (PheoA-ss-CNPs) about 200 nm in size. The photoactivity and therapeutic efficacy of the bioreducible NPs were compared with non-reducible NPs (PheoA-CNPs) *in vitro*. The photoactivity of both NPs was prohibited by the self-quenching effect. However, it was restored by the instantaneous dissociation of NPs because of the cleavage of disulfide bonds when exposed to an intracellular reductive environment. The bioreductible NPs showed rapid cellular uptake and significantly higher phototoxicity than the non-reducible NPs did. The *in vivo* imaging results showed that the bioreducible NPs selectively accumulated to the tumor site through the EPR effect and prolonged circulation. The results of *in vivo* therapeutic efficacy in the tumor-bearing mice showed that a significantly decreased tumor volume was observed for PDT with PheoA-ss-CNPs. Roder and co-workers developed nanoparticulate formulations of human serum albumin (HSA) as carriers for PSs. [123, 124] This HSA carrier system has the advantage that once it is endocytosed by cells and taken up to the lysosomes, the nanoparticle is decomposed by enzymatic cleavage and low pH and as a result releases the

PS as individual units. The authors used pheophorbide as PS agent for this work. The photophysical properties such as quantum yield and fluorescence life time of the Pheo-HSA nanoparticles revealed interaction among PS and HSA nanoparticles. For the same reason, the $^1O_2$ quantum yield for the materials is significantly lower compared to Pheo molecule. Pheo-HSA nanoparticles cause a much lower phototoxicity than free Pheo molecules in Jurkat cells after 1 h incubation due to their lower $^1O_2$ quantum yield. Interestingly, after 24 h incubation Pheo-HSA materials reached higher levels of phototoxicity that free Pheo molecules although the cellular uptake is equivalent for HSA-bonded Pheo and free Pheo. More than 90% of the dead cells were apoptotic rather that necrotic similar to free Pheo. As mentioned above, the reason for this increase in the PDT effect is because the biodegradable HSA carrier platform is decomposed inside lysosomes and as a result releases the Pheo molecules.

Another approach to enhance the PDT effect is by designing nanomaterials with frameworks that keep PSs well-isolated to avoid aggregation and self-quenching of the excited states and porous structures that provide a pathway for facile diffusion of $^1O_2$ out of the nanoparticle interior to exert their cytotoxic effects on cancer cells. Kopelman and co-workers have developed methylene blue (MB)-loaded polyacrylamide nanoparticles (MB-PAA NPs) by two different methods, encapsulation and chemical conjugation. The MB-PAA-NPs were found to be biocompatible and biodegradable nanocarriers; moreover the NP matrix was easily modified with targeting moieties and successfully protected the MB from reduction/conversion by bioenzymes. [125] For making the MB-PAA-NPs, the conjugation approach was found to be the most efficient method, demonstrated by higher loading, negligible leaching of MB from the nanocarriers, and by better PDT efficacy. Probably this effect is due to a more homogeneous distribution of the conjugated MB molecules inside PAA-NP matrix. However, upon increasing the PS loading, the MB-PAA-NPs showed an upper limit for the generation of $^1O_2$. The production of $^1O_2$ initially increased with MB loading, but then peaked and decreased. This limitation on the PDT efficacy of the MB-PAA-NPs is probably due to aggregation of MB dyes and self-quenching of produced excited states and/or ROS inside the nanocarriers. These drawbacks can be overcome by modifying the NP matrix structure through the use of longer cross-linkers. This is expected to allow 1) longer distances between the conjugated MB moieties, 2) higher oxygen permeability, and 3) a lower collision probability between the produced ROS. Following these ideas, the authors synthesized a new version of MB-PAA-NPs that contain longer cross linkers than the previous version of the nanomaterials. [120] The authors investigated the amount of $^1O_2$ generated by using two ROS sensing dyes, ADPA and singlet oxygen sensor green (SOSG). It was determined after these experiments that the new version of MB-PAA-NPs produced 1.44 times more $^1O_2$ than the previous one. The authors also tested the PDT efficacy of this platform in vitro using C6 cancer cells. Interestingly, the material with the highest amount of $^1O_2$ generated, correlates with the most rapid killing of the C6 cancer cells and a linear relationship was found between the generation of $^1O_2$ in solution and the half maximal inhibitory time (IT_{50}) for PDT killing. By using silica nanoparticles; Li and co-workers developed "dense" and "loose" silica nanomaterials to carry MB (MB-SiNPs) (Figure 10). [81] The dense silica NPs were synthesize using the traditional Stöber method, this type of material is characterized as tight trapping of MB into the nanocarriers with little drug leakage. The "loose" MB-SiNPs were synthesized by introducing MB molecules into SiO$_2$ during the NP growth at controlled experimental conditions. The authors showed that by creating a radial concentration gradient of MB in the NP, MB release occurs simultaneously with the

SiO$_2$ carrier decomposition, as driven by drug molecule diffusion. Compared to conventional dense MB-SiNPs, the loose MB-SiNPs had higher ^{1}O$_2$ or MB diffusion capability as the NPs themselves would undergo self-decomposition accompanied by facile MB release in a physiological environment (Figure 10). The experimental results suggested that trapping MB into the dense SiNP matrix suppressed all types of generated ROS. This was mainly due to the difficulty in ^{1}O$_2$ out-diffusion from the MB-SiNPs in the dense SiO$_2$ matrix. Contrary, loose MB-SiNPs showed enhanced generation of ROS. These findings provide a general guideline for the design of SiNPs for PDT applications.

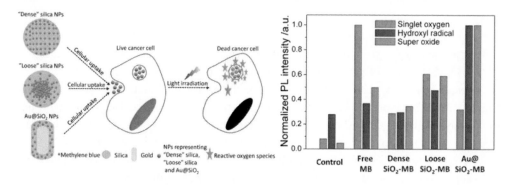

Figure 10. Schematic illustration of design of dense MB-SiNPs, loose MB-SiNPs and MB-Au-SiNPs for performing PDT *in vitro* (left). Quantitative comparison of various ROS generated including singlet oxygen, hydroxyl radical and superoxide in various MB loaded SiNPs in aqueous solution (right). Printed with permission from Ref. 81.

5. NANOPARTICLES AS ENERGY TRANSDUCERS

As mentioned in this chapter, PDT has many advantages such as minimally invasive, can be locally applied onto a specific area by selective irradiation, and can be repeated as often as required. A major drawback of PDT is that it needs to use poor tissue-penetrating light like visible or UV light, for the activation of the PS agent. [14, 20, 126] Therefore, the use of PDT is mostly limited to surface tumors such as skin and the treatment of large or deep-seated tumors is severely hampered. The delivery of light for PDT through body tissue implicates processes of refraction, reflection, absorption and scattering. Scattering of light in tissue has the most pronounced effect on light intensity and directionality. Besides scattering, absorption of light quanta is most relevant for the loss of light intensity with penetration depth. The most important chromophores in tissue are water, oxyhemoglobin and deoxyhemoglobin, melanin and cytochromes. The absorption spectra of these molecules define the optical window for PDT in tissue. [127] Consequently, a significant effort is currently devoted to develop new PDT strategies that can utilize NIR (700-1000 nm) light. This wavelength threshold offers deep tissue penetration in the "transparency window" and exhibits low toxicity to normal cells and tissue. For example, clinical treatment with Photofrin, a hematoporphyrin derivative for excitation at 630 nm, the light penetration depth is approximately 3-5 mm, depending on the tissue. The use of PSs with absorption peaks at wavelengths > 700 nm (or even higher) should, at least, double the penetration depth and thus enable treatment of thicker tumors. [128]

We have already described in this chapter the excellent features of nanomaterials for delivering PS agents effectively to diseased sites. However, some nanomaterials have intrinsic physicochemical properties, which can be harnessed to trigger light-induced reactions. In this way, the nanoparticles can convert inert chemical compounds to active cytotoxic species in a spatially and temporally controlled manner to damage or destroy malignant tissues. [128, 129] In recent years, a promising strategy being pursued involves the use of upconverting nanoparticles (UCNPs) and two-photon absorption (TPA) nanomaterials that can harvest and convert low-energy light into electrons or visible/UV light, thereby facilitating the transformation of PDT into a viable therapy for the treatment of depth and ticker tumors. [130-133] In addition, these nanoscale antennas can also be exploited as nanoplatforms for delivery of the PS to specific tissues and cellular compartments and for imaging the effect of the treatment using multimodal approaches.

5.1. Two-photon Exciting Nanoparticles

TPA is the simultaneous absorption of two photons of identical or different frequencies to excite a molecule from one state (usually the ground state) to a higher energy electronic state. Different to UCNPs, two-photon excitation (TPE) requires extremely high power densities that can only be readily achieved with femtosecond (fs) lasers. [15] Using TPA materials, the window for excitation can be extended into the NIR region, thereby making the process more viable to be used to treat deep lesions. Lo and co-workers constructed a mesoporous silica encapsulated gold nanorods (GNRs) system for two-photon activated PDT. [134] Two-photon enhanced plasmonic resonance energy transfer (PRET) from GNRs has considerable potential for PDT because of its high resolution, low photo-damage, good biocompatibility and low attenuation by water and biomaterials, enhancing photon penetration depth in tissue. Moreover, the mesoporous silica shell deposited around the GNRs not only provided a large surface area for conjugating therapeutic moieties, but also served as platform for intra-particle/plasmonic energy transfer between the GNRs and the PS molecules. The authors incorporated Pd-meso-tetra(4-carboxyphenyl) porphyrin (PdTPP) into the mesopores of the GNR-MSS nanoparticles. The authors observed substantial phototoxic effect in both *in vitro* cells and *in vivo* murine models of breast cancer. This novel platform is a promising nanosystem for the efficient *in vivo* tracking and PDT of malignancies in deep tissues. Following a similar approach Xu and co-workers developed a silica-based GNR nanoparticle for one- and two-photon imaging and PDT (Figure 11). [135] The authors systematically investigated the GNR enhancement of one- and two-photon excitation fluorescence of a porphyrin, T790. The separation distance between the GNR and T790 PS was varied by adjusting the silica shell thickness from 13 to 42 nm. The optimum one- and two-photon excitation fluorescence enhancement was found to occur at shell thickness of 34 and 20 nm, with enhancement factors of 2.1 and 11.8, respectively. The GNR-Si NPs that displayed enhanced two-photon excitation fluorescence were also found to exhibit significantly improved $^1O_2$ generation capability under two-photon excitation. The authors demonstrated the improved two-photon cell imaging and PDT effect in HepG2 cancer cells (**Figure 11**). QDs are excellent materials for FRET processes, in the majority of cases, acting as the donor molecules. Chen et al. synthesized a conjugated of QDs and sulfonated aluminum phthalocyanine (AlPcS) for two-photon excitation PDT. [15] QDs have a very high two-photon absorption cross section that allows them to be excited by an unfocused 800 nm fs laser beam with a low power density. FRET allows the transfer of energy to the conjugated AlPcS to afford $^1O_2$ generation. The authors observed that the QD-AlPcS can effectively destroy KB and HeLa cancer cells under the irradiation of the 800 nm unfocused fs laser beam with a power density of 92 mW/mm^2.

TPE mediated PDT is able to increase the penetration depth of the PDT illumination light in tissue and allow for treatment of thicker malignancies. However, this technique requires the use of a pulsed laser as the light source to excite focused small areas to obtain sufficient instant energy needed for two-photon excitation, and thus may have limited value for real clinical applications. [15]

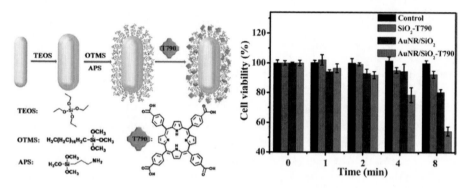

Figure 11. Schematic procedure for preparation of T790-GNRs-SiNPs (left). Time-dependent cell viability of HepG2 cancer cells after incubation with T790-GNRs-SiNPs and T790-SiNPs under femtosecond laser illumination at 800 nm (two-photon excitation) (right). Printed with permission of Ref. 135.

5.2. Upconversion Nanoparticles

UCNPs are usually lanthanide-doped nanocrystals, which have the ability to emit photons in the UV and visible region upon NIR irradiation. Typically, UCNPs are composed of a host matrix with a low concentration of dopant lanthanide elements. [129, 131] Although one lanthanide element is sufficient to achieve UC, in terms of the absorption of light, a single type of lanthanide is not enough to have useful system. For this reason, the UCNPs are often doped with different lanthanides to increase the efficacy of UC. As compared to traditional down-conversion fluorescence, the NIR light excited upconversion luminescence (UCL) of UCNPs exhibits improved tissue penetration depth, higher photochemical stability, and is free of autofluorescence background, making them widely explored nanoprobes in biomedical imaging in recent years. Many groups have demonstrated *in vitro* PDT and recent reports have shown *in vivo* PDT using UCNPs. [13, 15, 128, 129, 131] In an early study by Zhang and co-workers, UCNPs were coated with a porous, thin layer of silica doped with merocyanine-540 PS, and conjugated with a tumor-targeting antibody for the targeted PDT to kill MCF-7/AZ breast cancer cells. [136] Shi and co-workers developed a multifunctional nanotheranostic system containing Gd-UCNPs core, mesoporous silica shell, and a hollow cavity in between (UCMSNPs). The platform has been simultaneously used for MR/UCL biomodal imaging and in situ tri-modal therapy. [137] The authors loaded hematoporphyrin

(HP) a PS agent and docetaxel (Dtxl) an anticancer drug to achieve synergetic chemo-/radio-/photodynamic therapy upon NIR excitation and X-ray irradiation. Both *in vitro* and *in vivo* tests showed the excellent colloidal stability and biocompatibility of the as-synthesized UCMSNPs. In addition, upon NIR excitation and X-ray irradiation, synergetic chemo-/radio-/photodynamic therapy was achieved by the co-delivery of radio-/photo-sensitizer HP and radiosensitizer/chemodrug Dtxl via UCMSNPs, which produces remarkably enhanced therapeutic effects relative to any individual treatment, and consequently leads to the satisfactory therapeutic efficacy for tumor elimination. Zhang et al. fabricated a highly efficient nanophotosensitizer, which consists of UCNP and Zn(II)-phthalocyanine (ZnPc). [138] The authors observed a high $^1O_2$ production that can form the enhancement of the 660 nm upconversion emission of $NaYF4:Yb^{3+},Er^{3+}$ UCNP with 25% Yb^{3+} doping. Moreover, UCNPs were covalent attached to ZnPc which significantly shortened the distance and enhanced the FRET between both components. The high $^1O_2$ generation lead to a secure and efficient PDT treatment, as evidenced by the in vivo test where UCNPs-ZnPc of 50 mg per kg body weight was locally injected into the tumor in mice, a low 980 nm radiation dose of 351 J/cm^2 (0.39 W/cm^2) and short irradiation duration of 15 min were sufficient to perform image-guided PDT and caused the tumor inhibitory ratio of approximately 80.1%. Gu and co-workers developed a similar UCNPs-ZnPc platform, but coated with folic acid modified chitosan polymer to enhance the target ability and biocompatibility of the final nanoconstruct (Figure 12). [139] Confocal microscopy and NIR small animal imaging demonstrated the enhanced tumor-selectivity of the nanoplatform to cancer cells that overexpressed folate receptor. ROS generation in cancer cells under a 1cm tissue was higher upon excitation of UCNPs-ZnPc with the 980 nm light than that with 660 nm irradiation. *In vivo* PDT treatments for deep-seated tumors demonstrated that NIR light-triggered PDT based on the nanoparticles possessed remarkable therapeutic efficacy with tumor inhibition ratio up to 50% compared with conventional visible light-activated PDT with a noticeable reduced tumor inhibition ratio of 18%. These results indicate that the multifunctional FA-chitosan UCNPs-ZnPc system is a promising PDT agent for deep-seated tumor treatment. Liu et al. developed a charge-reversible Mn^{2+} doped UCNPs for pH sensitive *in vivo* PDT. A layer-by-layer (LbL) self-assembly strategy was employed to load multiple layers of Ce6 conjugated polymers onto UCNOs via electrostatic interactions. [140] By further coating with an outer layer of charge-reversible polymer, the obtained nanoparticles were negatively charged and PEG coated under pH 7.4, and could be converted to have a positively charged naked surface at pH 6.8. As the result, significantly enhanced *in vitro* cell internalization and *in vivo* tumor retention of those nanoparticles were observed, leading to the remarkably improved NIR-induced PDT efficacy both *in vitro* and *in vivo*. The authors' results suggested the great potential of tumor acidity-targeted *in vivo* dual modal imaging and therapy using environmentally responsive nanomaterials.

UCNPs with the unique upconversion optical properties have significant potential in PDT. However, still remain a number of challenges in this field. The low quantum yield of UCL emission of UCNPs is an important issue that needs to be addressed. Moreover, the potential long-term toxicity of various types of UCNPs still needs to be studied and understood. [15]

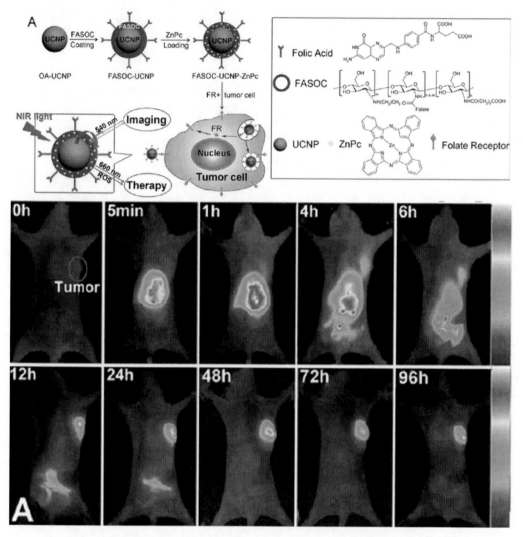

Figure 12. Schematic representation of the synthesis of FA-UCNPs-ZnPc nanoconstruct and folate-mediated binding of tumor cells with folate receptor expression (left and middle). Fluorescence images of nude mice bearing Bel-7402 tumors with intravenously injection of ICG-labeled FA-UCNPs-ZnPc (right). Printed with permission of Ref. 139.

CONCLUSION

Photodynamic therapy (PDT) has emerged as one of the important therapeutic options in management of cancer and other diseases. PDT offers a unique set of advantages over traditional radio- and chemotherapy such as the absence of harmful side effects, minimally invasive and cost-effective. It can be administered more than once for continued disease management with low risk of resistance. However, it is currently limited by insolubility and aggregation of current PS agents in physiological conditions, poor selectivity, the limited light penetration into tissues, a degree of oxygen dependence, and difficulty in prescribing the correct light dosimetry for each situation. Nanomaterials offer solutions for some of these difficulties. Nanoparticles can carry PS molecules to overcome issues of hydrophobicity;

moreover, these nanoplatforms have the appropriate size for passive targeting to tumor tissues by the enhanced permeability and retention (EPR) effect. [16] The selective accumulation of nanoparticle-based PS delivery systems can be enhanced by surface modification with targeting agents such as antibodies or small molecules. The use of nanoparticles as energy transducers such as two-photon exciting and upconversion nanomaterials allows activation with low energy light which can deeply penetrate tissues. The rational design of nanoparticle-based PS delivery systems is critical to enhance the PDT effect. Nanoparticles that transport a high amount of PS agents inside cancer cells and release them as individual PS units upon internal (reducing environment, pH or enzymatic cleavage) or external (light, ultrasound or alternating magnetic field) conditions are ideal to improve the therapeutic outcome of PDT.

Combination therapy is without doubt the future approach for cancer therapies. Combined treatments such as chemo- and photodynamic therapy will target different cellular/molecular pathways, increasing the efficiency of destroying cancer cells. Moreover, there has recently been an explosion of interest in developing platforms that combine diagnostic and therapeutic abilities ("theranostic") in the same material. Therefore, the development of multifunctional nanocarriers that enable different therapeutic mechanisms for cancer combination therapy and theranostic capabilities is a burgeoning area of research.

However, despite the tremendous amount of promising results reported in the past few years in this field, much work still need to be done before these multifunctional nanoparticle-based PS platforms can be translated toward clinical applications. One of the major issues is the long-term toxicology of the nanomaterials, especially those inorganic systems that are not biodegradable. Although progress has been made in the development of nanoparticles as energy transducers, great efforts are still required to develop new generations of PDT agents that can be more efficiently excited by the NIR light. Certainly issues such as the oxygen dependence of PDT and the difficulty in prescribing the correct light dosimetry for each situation have not been fully addressed by nanotechnology. I envision that the rapid growth in nanotechnology we have seen in the last decade is only going further continue in the coming years, and I expect that the application of nanotechnology to potentiate PDT will also continue to grow.

REFERENCES

[1]   Celli, J. P.; Spring, B. Q.; Rizvi, I.; Evans, C. L.; Samkoe, K. S.; Verma, S.; Pogue, B. W.; Hasan, T.: Imaging and Photodynamic Therapy: Mechanisms, Monitoring, and Optimization. *Chemical Reviews (Washington, DC, United States)* 2010, *110*, 2795-2838.

[2]   O'Connor, A. E.; Gallagher, W. M.; Byrne, A. T.: Porphyrin and nonporphyrin photosensitizers in oncology: preclinical and clinical advances in photodynamic therapy. *Photochemistry and Photobiology* 2009, *85*, 1053-1074.

[3]   Chatterjee Dev, K.; Fong Li, S.; Zhang, Y.: Nanoparticles in photodynamic therapy: an emerging paradigm. *Advanced drug delivery reviews* 2008, *60*, 1627-37.

[4]   Sharman, W. M.; Allen, C. M.; van Lier, J. E.: Photodynamic therapeutics: basic principles and clinical applications. *Drug Discovery Today* 1999, *4*, 507-517.

[5] Juarranz, A.; Jaen, P.; Sanz-Rodriguez, F.; Cuevas, J.; Gonzalez, S.: Photodynamic therapy of cancer. Basic principles and applications. *Clinical & Translational Oncology* 2008, *10*, 148-154.

[6] Josefsen, L. B.; Boyle, R. W.: Unique diagnostic and therapeutic roles of porphyrins and phthalocyanines in photodynamic therapy, imaging and theranostics. *Theranostics* 2012, *2*, 916-966.

[7] Robertson, C. A.; Evans, D. H.; Abrahamse, H.: Photodynamic therapy (PDT): A short review on cellular mechanisms and cancer research applications for PDT. *Journal of Photochemistry and Photobiology, B: Biology* 2009, *96*, 1-8.

[8] Detty, M. R.; Gibson, S. L.; Wagner, S. J.: Current Clinical and Preclinical Photosensitizers for Use in Photodynamic Therapy. *Journal of Medicinal Chemistry* 2004, *47*, 3897-3915.

[9] Ethirajan, M.; Chen, Y.; Joshi, P.; Pandey, R. K.: The role of porphyrin chemistry in tumor imaging and photodynamic therapy. *Chemical Society Reviews* 2011, *40*, 340-362.

[10] Yano, S.; Hirohara, S.; Obata, M.; Hagiya, Y.; Ogura, S.-i.; Ikeda, A.; Kataoka, H.; Tanaka, M.; Joh, T.: Current states and future views in photodynamic therapy. *Journal of Photochemistry and Photobiology, C: Photochemistry Reviews* 2011, *12*, 46-67.

[11] Bechet, D.; Couleaud, P.; Frochot, C.; Viriot, M.-L.; Guillemin, F.; Barberi-Heyob, M.: Nanoparticles as vehicles for delivery of photodynamic therapy agents. *Trends in Biotechnology* 2008, *26*, 612-621.

[12] Master, A.; Livingston, M.; Sen Gupta, A.: Photodynamic nanomedicine in the treatment of solid tumors: Perspectives and challenges. *Journal of Controlled Release* 2013, *168*, 88-102.

[13] Gupta, A.; Avci, P.; Sadasivam, M.; Chandran, R.; Parizotto, N.; Vecchio, D.; de Melo Wanessa, C. M. A.; Dai, T.; Chiang Long, Y.; Hamblin Michael, R.: Shining light on nanotechnology to help repair and regeneration. *Biotechnology advances* 2013, *31*, 607-31.

[14] Voon, S. H.; Kiew, L. V.; Lee, H. B.; Lim, S. H.; Noordin, M. I.; Kamkaew, A.; Burgess, K.; Chung, L. Y.: In Vivo Studies of Nanostructure-Based Photosensitizers for Photodynamic Cancer Therapy. *Small* 2014, Ahead of Print.

[15] Cheng, L.; Wang, C.; Feng, L.; Yang, K.; Liu, Z.: Functional nanomaterials for phototherapies of cancer. *Chemical reviews* 2014, *114*, 10869-939.

[16] Petros, R. A.; De Simone, J. M.: Strategies in the design of nanoparticles for therapeutic applications. *Nature Reviews Drug Discovery* 2010, *9*, 615-627.

[17] Torchilin, V. P.: Recent advances with liposomes as pharmaceutical carriers. *Nature Reviews Drug Discovery* 2005, *4*, 145-160.

[18] Derycke, A. S. L.; de Witte, P. A. M.: Liposomes for photodynamic therapy. *Advanced Drug Delivery Reviews* 2004, *56*, 17-30.

[19] Chen, B.; Pogue Brian, W.; Hasan, T.: Liposomal delivery of photosensitising agents. *Expert opinion on drug delivery* 2005, *2*, 477-87.

[20] Huang, Y.-Y.; Sharma, S. K.; Dai, T.; Chung, H.; Yaroslavsky, A.; Garcia-Diaz, M.; Chang, J.; Chiang, L. Y.; Hamblin, M. R.: Can nanotechnology potentiate photodynamic therapy? *Nanotechnology Reviews* 2012, *1*, 111-146.

[21] Paszko, E.; Ehrhardt, C.; Senge, M. O.; Kelleher, D. P.; Reynolds, J. V.: Nanodrug applications in photodynamic therapy. *Photodiagnosis and Photodynamic Therapy* 2011, *8*, 14-29.

[22] Chouikrat, R.; Seve, A.; Vanderesse, R.; Benachour, H.; Barberi-Heyob, M.; Richeter, S.; Raehm, L.; Durand, J. O.; Verelst, M.; Frochot, C.: Non polymeric nanoparticles for photodynamic therapy applications: recent developments. *Current Medicinal Chemistry* 2012, *19*, 781-792.

[23] Torchilin, V. P.: Surface-modified liposomes in γ-[ray scintigraphic] and MR-imaging. *Advanced Drug Delivery Reviews* 1997, *24*, 301-313.

[24] Tseng, Y.-C.; Mozumdar, S.; Huang, L.: Lipid-based systemic delivery of siRNA. *Advanced Drug Delivery Reviews* 2009, *61*, 721-731.

[25] Sadasivam, M.; Avci, P.; Gupta, G. K.; Lakshmanan, S.; Chandran, R.; Huang, Y.-Y.; Kumar, R.; Hamblin, M. R.: Self-assembled liposomal nanoparticles in photodynamic therapy. *European Journal of Nanomedicine* 2013, *5*, 115-129.

[26] Jiang, F.; Lilge, L.; Grenier, J.; Li, Y.; Wilson, M. D.; Chopp, M.: Photodynamic therapy of U87 human glioma in nude rat using liposome-delivered photofrin. *Lasers in surgery and medicine* 1998, *22*, 74-80.

[27] Zacks David, N.; Ezra, E.; Terada, Y.; Michaud, N.; Connolly, E.; Gragoudas Evangelos, S.; Miller Joan, W.: Verteporfin photodynamic therapy in the rat model of choroidal neovascularization: angiographic and histologic characterization. *Investigative ophthalmology & visual science* 2002, *43*, 2384-91.

[28] Kim, J.; Santos, O. A.; Park, J.-H.: Selective photosensitizer delivery into plasma membrane for effective photodynamic therapy. *Journal of Controlled Release* 2014, *191*, 98-104.

[29] Duncan, R.: Polymer conjugates as anticancer nanomedicines. *Nature Reviews Cancer* 2006, *6*, 688-701.

[30] Maham, A.; Tang, Z.; Wu, H.; Wang, J.; Lin, Y.: Protein-Based Nanomedicine Platforms for Drug Delivery. *Small* 2009, *5*, 1706-1721.

[31] Yoon, H. Y.; Koo, H.; Choi, K. Y.; Lee, S. J.; Kim, K.; Kwon, I. C.; Leary, J. F.; Park, K.; Yuk, S. H.; Park, J. H.; Choi, K.: Tumor-targeting hyaluronic acid nanoparticles for photodynamic imaging and therapy. *Biomaterials* 2012, *33*, 3980-3989.

[32] Sibani, S. A.; McCarron, P. A.; Woolfson, A. D.; Donnelly, R. F.: Photosensitiser delivery for photodynamic therapy. Part 2: systemic carrier platforms. *Expert Opinion on Drug Delivery* 2008, *5*, 1241-1254.

[33] Li, B.; Moriyama, E. H.; Li, F.; Jarvi, M. T.; Allen, C.; Wilson, B. C.: Diblock copolymer micelles deliver hydrophobic protoporphyrin IX for photodynamic therapy. *Photochemistry and Photobiology* 2007, *83*, 1505-1512.

[34] Lee, C. C.; MacKay, J. A.; Frechet, J. M. J.; Szoka, F. C.: Designing dendrimers for biological applications. *Nature Biotechnology* 2005, *23*, 1517-1526.

[35] Jang, W.-D.; Koh, W.-G.: Biomedical applications of dendrimer porphyrin or phthalocyanine. *Nanobiomaterials* 2014, 81-108.

[36] Mintzer, M. A.; Grinstaff, M. W.: Biomedical applications of dendrimers: a tutorial. *Chemical Society Reviews* 2011, *40*, 173-190.

[37] Svenson, S.; Tomalia, D. A.: Dendrimers in biomedical applications-reflections on the field. *Advanced Drug Delivery Reviews* 2005, *57*, 2106-2129.

[38] Lu, H.-L.; Syu, W.-J.; Nishiyama, N.; Kataoka, K.; Lai, P.-S.: Dendrimer phthalocyanine-encapsulated polymeric micelle-mediated photochemical internalization extends the efficacy of photodynamic therapy and overcomes drug-resistance in vivo. *Journal of Controlled Release* 2011, *155*, 458-464.

[39] Ai, H.; Jones, S. A.; Lvov, Y. M.: Biomedical applications of electrostatic layer-by-layer nano-assembly of polymers, enzymes, and nanoparticles. *Cell Biochemistry and Biophysics* 2003, *39*, 23-43.

[40] Reum, N.; Fink-Straube, C.; Klein, T.; Hartmann, R. W.; Lehr, C.-M.; Schneider, M.: Multilayer Coating of Gold Nanoparticles with Drug-Polymer Coadsorbates. *Langmuir* 2010, *26*, 16901-16908.

[41] Ungun, B.; Prud'homme, R. K.; Budijono, S. J.; Shan, J.; Lim, S. F.; Ju, Y.; Austin, R.: Nanofabricated upconversion nanoparticles for photodynamic therapy. *Optics Express* 2009, *17*, 80-86.

[42] Yoon, H.-J.; Lim Tae, G.; Kim, J.-H.; Cho Young, M.; Kim Yong, S.; Chung Ui, S.; Kim Jung, H.; Choi Byoung, W.; Koh, W.-G.; Jang, W.-D.: Fabrication of multifunctional layer-by-layer nanocapsules toward the design of theragnostic nanoplatform. *Biomacromolecules* 2014, *15*, 1382-9.

[43] Son, K. J.; Yoon, H.-J.; Kim, J.-H.; Jang, W.-D.; Lee, Y.; Koh, W.-G.: Photosensitizing Hollow Nanocapsules for Combination Cancer Therapy. *Angewandte Chemie, International Edition* 2011, *50*, 11968-11971, S11968/1-S11968/6.

[44] Smith, A. M.; Duan, H.; Mohs, A. M.; Nie, S.: Bioconjugated quantum dots for in vivo molecular and cellular imaging. *Advanced Drug Delivery Reviews* 2008, *60*, 1226-1240.

[45] Samir, T. M.; Mansour, M. M. H.; Kazmierczak, S. C.; Azzazy, H. M. E.: Quantum dots: heralding a brighter future for clinical diagnostics. *Nanomedicine (London, United Kingdom)* 2012, *7*, 1755-1769.

[46] Chen, C.; Peng, J.; Sun, S.-R.; Peng, C.-W.; Li, Y.; Pang, D.-W.: Tapping the potential of quantum dots for personalized oncology: current status and future perspectives. *Nanomedicine (London, United Kingdom)* 2012, *7*, 411-428.

[47] Li, Z.-H.; Peng, J.; Chen, H.-L.: Bioconjugated quantum dots as fluorescent probes for biomedical imaging. *Journal of Nanoscience and Nanotechnology* 2011, *11*, 7521-7536.

[48] Torchynska, T.; Vorobiev, Y.: Semiconductor II-VI quantum dots with interface states and their biomedical applications. *Advanced Biomedical Engineering* 2011, 143-182.

[49] Tsoi, K. M.; Dai, Q.; Alman, B. A.; Chan, W. C. W.: Are Quantum Dots Toxic? Exploring the Discrepancy Between Cell Culture and Animal Studies. *Accounts of Chemical Research* 2013, *46*, 662-671.

[50] Ragusa, A.; Zacheo, A.; Pellegrino, T.; Manna, L.: Quantum dot nanoparticles: properties, surface functionalization, and their applications in biosensing and imaging. *Nanostructured Materials for Biomedical Applications* 2009, 151-221.

[51] Yaghini, E.; Seifalian, A. M.; MacRobert, A. J.: Quantum dots and their potential biomedical applications in photosensitization for photodynamic therapy. *Nanomedicine (London, United Kingdom)* 2009, *4*, 353-363.

[52] Samia, A. C. S.; Chen, X.; Burda, C.: Semiconductor quantum dots for photodynamic therapy. *J. Am. Chem. Soc.* 2003, *125*, 15736-15737.

[53] Biju, V.; Mundayoor, S.; Omkumar, R. V.; Anas, A.; Ishikawa, M.: Bioconjugated quantum dots for cancer research: Present status, prospects and remaining issues. *Biotechnol. Adv.* 2010, *28*, 199-213.

[54] Valanciunaite, J.; Klymchenko, A. S.; Skripka, A.; Richert, L.; Steponkiene, S.; Streckyte, G.; Mely, Y.; Rotomskis, R.: A non-covalent complex of quantum dots and chlorin e6: efficient energy transfer and remarkable stability in living cells revealed by FLIM. *RSC Advances* 2014, *4*, 52270-52278.

[55] Chou, K.-L.; Meng, H.; Cen, Y.; Li, L.; Chen, J.-Y.: Dopamine-quantum dot conjugate: a new kind of photosensitizers for photodynamic therapy of cancers. *Journal of Nanoparticle Research* 2013, *15*, 1348/1-1348/9, 9 pp.

[56] Charron, G.; Stuchinskaya, T.; Edwards, D. R.; Russell, D. A.; Nann, T.: Insights into the Mechanism of Quantum Dot-Sensitized Singlet Oxygen Production for Photodynamic Therapy. *Journal of Physical Chemistry C* 2012, *116*, 9334-9342.

[57] Laurent, S.; Forge, D.; Port, M.; Roch, A.; Robic, C.; Vander Elst, L.; Muller Robert, N.: Magnetic iron oxide nanoparticles: synthesis, stabilization, vectorization, physicochemical characterizations, and biological applications. *Chemical reviews* 2008, *108*, 2064-110.

[58] Amstad, E.; Textor, M.; Reimhult, E.: Stabilization and functionalization of iron oxide nanoparticles for biomedical applications. *Nanoscale* 2011, *3*, 2819-2843.

[59] Chen, B.; Wu, W.; Wang, X.: Magnetic iron oxide nanoparticles for tumor-targeted therapy. *Current Cancer Drug Targets* 2011, *11*, 184-189.

[60] Tran, P. H.-L.; Tran, T. T.-D.; Vo, T. V.; Lee, B.-J.: Promising iron oxide-based magnetic nanoparticles in biomedical engineering. *Archives of Pharmacal Research* 2012, *35*, 2045-2061.

[61] Xu, C.; Sun, S.: New forms of superparamagnetic nanoparticles for biomedical applications. *Advanced Drug Delivery Reviews* 2013, *65*, 732-743.

[62] Ding, J.; Zhao, J.; Cheng, K.; Liu, G.; Xiu, D.: In vivo photodynamic therapy and magnetic resonance imaging of cancer by TSPP-coated Fe3O4 nanoconjugates. *Journal of Biomedical Nanotechnology* 2010, *6*, 683-686.

[63] Lee, D. J.; Park, G. Y.; Oh, K. T.; Oh, N. M.; Kwag, D. S.; Youn, Y. S.; Oh, Y. T.; Park, J. w.; Lee, E. S.: Multifunctional poly (lactide-co-glycolide) nanoparticles for luminescence/magnetic resonance imaging and photodynamic therapy. *International Journal of Pharmaceutics (Amsterdam, Netherlands)* 2012, *434*, 257-263.

[64] Ling, D.; Park, W.; Park, S.-j.; Lu, Y.; Kim, K. S.; Hackett, M. J.; Kim, B. H.; Yim, H.; Jeon, Y. S.; Na, K.; Hyeon, T.: Multifunctional Tumor pH-Sensitive Self-Assembled Nanoparticles for Bimodal Imaging and Treatment of Resistant Heterogeneous Tumors. *J. Am. Chem. Soc.* 2014, *136*, 5647-5655.

[65] Mbakidi, J. P.; Drogat, N.; Granet, R.; Ouk, T.-S.; Ratinaud, M.-H.; Riviere, E.; Verdier, M.; Sol, V.: Hydrophilic chlorin-conjugated magnetic nanoparticles-Potential anticancer agent for the treatment of melanoma by PDT. *Bioorganic & Medicinal Chemistry Letters* 2013, *23*, 2486-2490.

[66] Wang, D.; Fei, B.; Halig, L. V.; Qin, X.; Hu, Z.; Xu, H.; Wang, Y. A.; Chen, Z.; Kim, S.; Shin, D. M.; Chen, Z.: Targeted Iron-Oxide Nanoparticle for Photodynamic Therapy and Imaging of Head and Neck Cancer. *ACS Nano* 2014, *8*, 6620-6632.

[67] Wang, F.; Chen, X.-L.; Zhao, Z.-X.; Tang, S.-H.; Huang, X.-Q.; Lin, C.-H.; Cai, C.-b.; Zheng, N.-F.: Synthesis of magnetic, fluorescent and mesoporous core-shell-structured

nanoparticles for imaging, targeting and photodynamic therapy. *Journal of Materials Chemistry* 2011, *21*, 11244-11252.

[68]   Yoon, H.-J.; Lim, T. G.; Kim, J.-H.; Cho, Y. M.; Kim, Y. S.; Chung, U. S.; Kim, J. H.; Choi, B. W.; Koh, W.-G.; Jang, W.-D.: Fabrication of Multifunctional Layer-by-Layer Nanocapsules toward the Design of Theranostic Nanoplatform. *Biomacromolecules* 2014, *15*, 1382-1389.

[69]   Thandu, M.; Rapozzi, V.; Xodo, L.; Albericio, F.; Comuzzi, C.; Cavalli, S.: "Clicking" porphyrins to magnetic nanoparticles for photodynamic therapy. *ChemPlusChem* 2014, *79*, 90-98.

[70]   Li, Z.; Wang, C.; Cheng, L.; Gong, H.; Yin, S.; Gong, Q.; Li, Y.; Liu, Z.: PEG-functionalized iron oxide nanoclusters loaded with chlorin e6 for targeted, NIR light induced, photodynamic therapy. *Biomaterials* 2013, *34*, 9160-9170.

[71]   Arvizo, R. R.; Bhattacharyya, S.; Kudgus, R. A.; Giri, K.; Bhattacharya, R.; Mukherjee, P.: Intrinsic therapeutic applications of noble metal nanoparticles: past, present and future. *Chemical Society Reviews* 2012, *41*, 2943-2970.

[72]   Soh, J. H.; Gao, Z.: Metal nanoparticles in biomedical applications. *Complex-Shaped Metal Nanoparticles* 2012, 477-519.

[73]   Stanley Rosarin, F.; Mirunalini, S.: Nobel metallic nanoparticles with novel biomedical properties. *Journal of Bioanalysis & Biomedicine* 2011, *3*, 085-091.

[74]   Tiwari, P. M.; Vig, K.; Dennis, V. A.; Singh, S. R.: Functionalized gold nanoparticles and their biomedical applications. *Nanomaterials* 2011, *1*, 31-63.

[75]   Fratoddi, I.; Venditti, I.; Cametti, C.; Russo, M. V.: Gold nanoparticles and gold nanoparticle-conjugates for delivery of therapeutic molecules. Progress and challenges. *Journal of Materials Chemistry B: Materials for Biology and Medicine* 2014, *2*, 4204-4220.

[76]   Gupta, V.; Gupta, A. R.; Kant, V.: Synthesis, characterization and biomedical applications of nanoparticles. *Science International* 2013, *1*, 167-174, 8 pp.

[77]   Liu, A.; Ye, B.: Application of gold nanoparticles in biomedical researches and diagnosis. *Clinical Laboratory (Mainz, Germany)* 2013, *59*, 23-36.

[78]   Raghavendra, R.; Arunachalam, K.; Annamalai, S. K.; Arunachalam, A. M.: Diagnostics and therapeutic application of gold nanoparticles. *International Journal of Pharmacy and Pharmaceutical Sciences* 2014, *6*, 74-87, 14 pp.

[79]   Sumbayev, V. V.; Yasinska, I. M.; Gibbs, B. F.: Biomedical applications of gold nanoparticles. *Recent Advances in Electrical Engineering Series* 2013, *9*, 342-348.

[80]   Cheng, Y.; Doane, T. L.; Chuang, C.-H.; Ziady, A.; Burda, C.: Near infrared light-triggered drug generation and release from gold nanoparticle carriers for photodynamic therapy. *Small* 2014, *10*, 1799-1804.

[81]   Chu, Z.; Zhang, S.; Yin, C.; Lin, G.; Li, Q.: Designing nanoparticle carriers for enhanced drug efficacy in photodynamic therapy. *Biomaterials Science* 2014, *2*, 827-832.

[82]   Gao, L.; Liu, R.; Gao, F.; Wang, Y.; Jiang, X.; Gao, X.: Plasmon-Mediated Generation of Reactive Oxygen Species from Near-Infrared Light Excited Gold Nanocages for Photodynamic Therapy in Vitro. *ACS Nano* 2014, *8*, 7260-7271.

[83]   Seo, S.-H.; Kim, B.-M.; Joe, A.; Han, H.-W.; Chen, X.; Cheng, Z.; Jang, E.-S.: NIR-light-induced   surface-enhanced   Raman   scattering   for   detection   and

photothermal/photodynamic therapy of cancer cells using methylene blue-embedded gold nanorod@SiO2 nanocomposites. *Biomaterials* 2014, *35*, 3309-3318.

[84] Shiao, Y.-S.; Chiu, H.-H.; Wu, P.-H.; Huang, Y.-F.: Aptamer-Functionalized Gold Nanoparticles As Photoresponsive Nanoplatform for Co-Drug Delivery. *ACS Applied Materials & Interfaces* 2014, Ahead of Print.

[85] Yang, Y.; Hu, Y.; Du, H.; Wang, H.: Intracellular gold nanoparticle aggregation and their potential applications in photodynamic therapy. *Chem. Commun. (Cambridge, U. K.)* 2014, *50*, 7287-7290.

[86] Zhao, L.; Kim, T.-H.; Ahn, J.-C.; Kim, H.-W.; Kim, S. Y.: Highly efficient "theranostics" system based on surface-modified gold nanocarriers for imaging and photodynamic therapy of cancer. *Journal of Materials Chemistry B: Materials for Biology and Medicine* 2013, *1*, 5806-5817.

[87] Oo, M. K. K.; Yang, X.; Du, H.; Wang, H.: 5-aminolevulinic acid-conjugated gold nanoparticles for photodynamic therapy of cancer. *Nanomedicine (London, United Kingdom)* 2008, *3*, 777-786.

[88] Vankayala, R.; Sagadevan, A.; Vijayaraghavan, P.; Kuo, C.-L.; Hwang, K. C.: Metal Nanoparticles Sensitize the Formation of Singlet Oxygen. *Angewandte Chemie, International Edition* 2011, *50*, 10640-10644, S10640/1-S10640/6.

[89] Kolosnjaj, J.; Szwarc, H.; Moussa, F.: Toxicity studies of fullerenes and derivatives. *Advances in experimental medicine and biology* 2007, *620*, 168-80.

[90] Li, H.; Song, S. I.; Song, G. Y.; Kim, I.: Non-covalently functionalized carbon nanostructures for synthesizing carbon-based hybrid nanomaterials. *Journal of Nanoscience and Nanotechnology* 2014, *14*, 1425-1440.

[91] Zhang, Y.; Petibone, D.; Xu, Y.; Mahmood, M.; Karmakar, A.; Casciano, D.; Ali, S.; Biris, A. S.: Toxicity and efficacy of carbon nanotubes and graphene: the utility of carbon-based nanoparticles in nanomedicine. *Drug Metabolism Reviews* 2014, *46*, 232-246.

[92] Singh, S. B.; Singh, A.: The third allotrope of carbon: fullerene an update. *International Journal of ChemTech Research* 2013, *5*, 167-171.

[93] Constantin, C.; Neagu, M.; Ion, R.-M.; Gherghiceanu, M.; Stavaru, C.: Fullerene-porphyrin nanostructures in photodynamic therapy. *Nanomedicine (London, United Kingdom)* 2010, *5*, 307-317.

[94] Ikeda, A.: Photodynamic therapy using fullerenes as photosensitizer. *Bio Industry* 2012, *29*, 13-19.

[95] Sharma, S. K.; Chiang, L. Y.; Hamblin, M. R.: Photodynamic therapy with fullerenes in vivo: reality or a dream? *Nanomedicine (London, United Kingdom)* 2011, *6*, 1813-1825.

[96] Sharma, S. K.; Huang, Y.-Y.; Mroz, P.; Wharton, T.; Chiang, L. Y.; Hamblin, M. R.: Fullerenes in photodynamic therapy. *Nanomaterials for the Life Sciences* 2011, *9*, 419-448.

[97] Tokuyama, H.; Yamago, S.; Nakamura, E.; Shiraki, T.; Sugiura, Y.: Photoinduced biochemical activity of fullerene carboxylic acid. *J. Am. Chem. Soc.* 1993, *115*, 7918-19.

[98] Zhang, W.; Gong, X.; Liu, C.; Piao, Y.; Sun, Y.; Diao, G.: Water-soluble inclusion complex of fullerene with γ-cyclodextrin polymer for photodynamic therapy. *Journal of Materials Chemistry B: Materials for Biology and Medicine* 2014, *2*, 5107-5115.

[99] Liu, J.; Ohta, S.-I.; Sonoda, A.; Yamada, M.; Yamamoto, M.; Nitta, N.; Murata, K.; Tabata, Y.: Preparation of PEG-conjugated fullerene containing Gd3+ ions for photodynamic therapy. *Journal of Controlled Release* 2007, *117*, 104-110.

[100] Wang, L.; Shi, J.; Liu, R.; Liu, Y.; Zhang, J.; Yu, X.; Gao, J.; Zhang, C.; Zhang, Z.: Photodynamic effect of functionalized single-walled carbon nanotubes: a potential sensitizer for photodynamic therapy. *Nanoscale* 2014, *6*, 4642-4651.

[101] Wang, Y.; Hu, A.: Carbon quantum dots: synthesis, properties and applications. *Journal of Materials Chemistry C: Materials for Optical and Electronic Devices* 2014, *2*, 6921-6939.

[102] Fowley, C.; Nomikou, N.; McHale, A. P.; McCaughan, B.; Callan, J. F.: Extending the tissue penetration capability of conventional photosensitisers: a carbon quantum dot-protoporphyrin IX conjugate for use in two-photon excited photodynamic therapy. *Chem. Commun. (Cambridge, U. K.)* 2013, *49*, 8934-8936.

[103] Generalov, R.; Christensen, I. L.; Chen, W.; Sun, Y.-P.; Kristensen, S.; Juzenas, P.: Generation of singlet oxygen and other radical species by quantum dot and carbon dot nanosensitizers. *Proceedings of SPIE* 2009, *7380*, 738072/1-738072/9.

[104] Huang, P.; Lin, J.; Wang, X.; Wang, Z.; Zhang, C.; He, M.; Wang, K.; Chen, F.; Li, Z.; Shen, G.; Cui, D.; Chen, X.: Light-Triggered Theranostics Based on Photosensitizer-Conjugated Carbon Dots for Simultaneous Enhanced-Fluorescence Imaging and Photodynamic Therapy. *Advanced Materials (Weinheim, Germany)* 2012, *24*, 5104-5110, S5104/1-S5104/18.

[105] Wang, J.; Zhang, Z.; Zha, S.; Zhu, Y.; Wu, P.; Ehrenberg, B.; Chen, J.-Y.: Carbon nanodots featuring efficient FRET for two-photon photodynamic cancer therapy with a low fs laser power density. *Biomaterials* 2014, *35*, 9372-9381.

[106] Couleaud, P.; Morosini, V.; Frochot, C.; Richeter, S.; Raehm, L.; Durand, J.-O.: Silica-based nanoparticles for photodynamic therapy applications. *Nanoscale* 2010, *2*, 1083-1095.

[107] Allison, R. R.; Sibata, C. H.: Oncologic photodynamic therapy photosensitizers: a clinical review. *Photodiagnosis and Photodynamic Therapy* 2010, *7*, 61-75.

[108] Senge, M. O.; Brandt, J. C.: Temoporfin (foscan, 5,10,15,20-tetra(m-hydroxyphenyl)chlorin)-A second-generation photosensitizer. *Photochemistry and Photobiology* 2011, *87*, 1240-1296.

[109] An, L.; Liu, L.; Wang, S.; Bazan, G. C.: An Optical Approach for Drug Screening Based on Light-Harvesting Conjugated Polyelectrolytes. *Angewandte Chemie, International Edition* 2009, *48*, 4372-4375.

[110] Chi, C.; Chworos, A.; Zhang, J.; Mikhailovsky, A.; Bazan, G. C.: Anatomy and growth characteristics of conjugated polyelectrolyte/DNA aggregates. *Advanced Functional Materials* 2008, *18*, 3606-3612.

[111] Jeong, J.-E.; Woo, S.-J.; Le, V. S.; Choi, H.; Woo, H. Y.: Combination of conjugated polyelectrolytes and biomolecules: A new optical platform for highly sensitive and selective chemo- and biosensors. *Macromolecular Research* 2014, *22*, 461-473.

[112] Ngo, A. T.; Cosa, G.: Assembly of Zwitterionic Phospholipid/Conjugated Polyelectrolyte Complexes: Structure and Photophysical Properties. *Langmuir* 2010, *26*, 6746-6754.

[113] Yuan, Y.; Liu, J.; Liu, B.: Conjugated-polyelectrolyte-based polyprodrug: targeted and image-guided photodynamic and chemotherapy with on-demand drug release upon

irradiationwith a single light source. *Angewandte Chemie, International Edition* 2014, *53*, 7163-7168.

[114] Yuan, Y.; Liu, B.: Self-Assembled Nanoparticles Based on PEGylated Conjugated Polyelectrolyte and Drug Molecules for Image-Guided Drug Delivery and Photodynamic Therapy. *ACS Applied Materials & Interfaces* 2014, *6*, 14903-14910.

[115] Shi, J.; Liu, Y.; Wang, L.; Gao, J.; Zhang, J.; Yu, X.; Ma, R.; Liu, R.; Zhang, Z.: A tumoral acidic pH-responsive drug delivery system based on a novel photosensitizer (fullerene) for in vitro and in vivo chemo-photodynamic therapy. *Acta Biomaterialia* 2014, *10*, 1280-1291.

[116] Bae, B.-c.; Na, K.: Self-quenching polysaccharide-based nanogels of pullulan/folate-photosensitizer conjugates for photodynamic therapy. *Biomaterials* 2010, *31*, 6325-6335.

[117] Lovell, J. F.; Chen, J.; Jarvi, M. T.; Cao, W.-G.; Allen, A. D.; Liu, Y.; Tidwell, T. T.; Wilson, B. C.; Zheng, G.: FRET Quenching of Photosensitizer Singlet Oxygen Generation. *Journal of Physical Chemistry B* 2009, *113*, 3203-3211.

[118] Lee, S. J.; Koo, H.; Lee, D.-E.; Min, S.; Lee, S.; Chen, X.; Choi, Y.; Leary, J. F.; Park, K.; Jeong, S. Y.; Kwon, I. C.; Kim, K.; Choi, K.: Tumor-homing photosensitizer-conjugated glycol chitosan nanoparticles for synchronous photodynamic imaging and therapy based on cellular on/off system. *Biomaterials* 2011, *32*, 4021-4029.

[119] Oh, I.-h.; Min, H. S.; Li, L.; Tran, T. H.; Lee, Y.-k.; Kwon, I. C.; Choi, K.; Kim, K.; Huh, K. M.: Cancer cell-specific photoactivity of pheophorbide a-glycol chitosan nanoparticles for photodynamic therapy in tumor-bearing mice. *Biomaterials* 2013, *34*, 6454-6463.

[120] Yoon, H. K.; Lou, X.; Chen, Y.-C.; Koo Lee, Y.-E.; Yoon, E.; Kopelman, R.: Nanophotosensitizers Engineered to Generate a Tunable Mix of Reactive Oxygen Species, for Optimizing Photodynamic Therapy, Using a Microfluidic Device. *Chemistry of Materials* 2014, *26*, 1592-1600.

[121] Vivero-Escoto, J. L.; Vega, D. L.: Stimuli-responsive protoporphyrin IX silica-based nanoparticles for photodynamic therapy in vitro. *RSC Advances* 2014, *4*, 14400-14407.

[122] Vivero-Escoto, J. L.; DeCillis, D.; Fritts, L.; Vega, D. L.: Porphyrin-based polysilsesquioxane nanoparticles to improve photodynamic therapy for cancer treatment. *Proceedings of SPIE* 2014, *8931*, 89310Z/1-89310Z/10.

[123] Preuss, A.; Chen, K.; Hackbarth, S.; Wacker, M.; Langer, K.; Roeder, B.: Photosensitizer loaded HSA nanoparticles II: In vitro investigations. *International Journal of Pharmaceutics* 2011, *404*, 308-316.

[124] Chen, K.; Preuss, A.; Hackbarth, S.; Wacker, M.; Langer, K.; Roeder, B.: Novel photosensitizer-protein nanoparticles for Photodynamic therapy: Photophysical characterization and in vitro investigations. *Journal of Photochemistry and Photobiology, B: Biology* 2009, *96*, 66-74.

[125] Hah, H. J.; Kim, G.; Lee, Y.-E. K.; Orringer, D. A.; Sagher, O.; Philbert, M. A.; Kopelman, R.: Methylene blue-conjugated hydrogel nanoparticles and tumor-cell targeted photodynamic therapy. *Macromolecular Bioscience* 2011, *11*, 90-99.

[126] Allison, R. R.; Bagnato, V. S.; Cuenca, R.; Downie, G. H.; Sibata, C. H.: The future of photodynamic therapy in oncology. *Future Oncology* 2006, *2*, 53-71.

[127] Plaetzer, K.; Krammer, B.; Berlanda, J.; Berr, F.; Kiesslich, T.: Photophysics and photochemistry of photodynamic therapy: fundamental aspects. *Lasers in medical science* 2009, *24*, 259-68.

[128] Arguinzoniz, A. G.; Ruggiero, E.; Habtemariam, A.; Hernandez-Gil, J.; Salassa, L.; Mareque-Rivas, J. C.: Light Harvesting and Photoemission by Nanoparticles for Photodynamic Therapy. *Particle & Particle Systems Characterization* 2014, *31*, 46-75.

[129] Shanmugam, V.; Selvakumar, S.; Yeh, C.-S.: Near-infrared light-responsive nanomaterials in cancer therapeutics. *Chemical Society Reviews* 2014, *43*, 6254-6287.

[130] Park, Y. I.; Lee, K. T.; Suh, Y. D.; Hyeon, T.: Upconverting nanoparticles: a versatile platform for wide-field two-photon microscopy and multi-modal in vivo imaging. *Chemical Society Reviews* 2014, Ahead of Print.

[131] Shen, J.; Zhao, L.; Han, G.: Lanthanide-doped upconverting luminescent nanoparticle platforms for optical imaging-guided drug delivery and therapy. *Advanced Drug Delivery Reviews* 2013, *65*, 744-755.

[132] Belfield, K. D.; Yao, S.; Bondar, M. V.: Two-photon absorbing photonic materials: from fundamentals to applications. *Advances in Polymer Science* 2008, *213*, 97-156.

[133] Ogawa, K.; Kobuke, Y.: Design of two-photon absorbing materials for molecular optical memory and photodynamic therapy. *Organic & Biomolecular Chemistry* 2009, *7*, 2241-2246.

[134] Chen, N.-T.; Tang, K.-C.; Chung, M.-F.; Cheng, S.-H.; Huang, C.-M.; Chu, C.-H.; Chou, P.-T.; Souris, J. S.; Chen, C.-T.; Mou, C.-Y.; Lo, L.-W.: Enhanced plasmonic resonance energy transfer in mesoporous silica-encased gold nanorod for two-photon-activated photodynamic therapy. *Theranostics* 2014, *4*, 798-807, 10 pp.

[135] Zhao, T.; Yu, K.; Li, L.; Zhang, T.; Guan, Z.; Gao, N.; Yuan, P.; Li, S.; Yao, S. Q.; Xu, Q.-H.; Xu, G. Q.: Gold Nanorod Enhanced Two-Photon Excitation Fluorescence of Photosensitizers for Two-Photon Imaging and Photodynamic Therapy. *ACS Applied Materials & Interfaces* 2014, *6*, 2700-2708.

[136] Zhang, P.; Steelant, W.; Kumar, M.; Scholfield, M.: Versatile Photosensitizers for Photodynamic Therapy at Infrared Excitation. *J. Am. Chem. Soc.* 2007, *129*, 4526-4527.

[137] Fan, W.; Shen, B.; Bu, W.; Chen, F.; He, Q.; Zhao, K.; Zhang, S.; Zhou, L.; Peng, W.; Xiao, Q.; Ni, D.; Liu, J.; Shi, J.: A smart upconversion-based mesoporous silica nanotheranostic system for synergetic chemo-/radio-/photodynamic therapy and simultaneous MR/UCL imaging. *Biomaterials* 2014, *35*, 8992-9002.

[138] Xia, L.; Kong, X.; Liu, X.; Tu, L.; Zhang, Y.; Chang, Y.; Liu, K.; Shen, D.; Zhao, H.; Zhang, H.: An upconversion nanoparticle - Zinc phthalocyanine based nanophotosensitizer for photodynamic therapy. *Biomaterials* 2014, *35*, 4146-4156.

[139] Cui, S.; Yin, D.; Chen, Y.; Di, Y.; Chen, H.; Ma, Y.; Achilefu, S.; Gu, Y.: In Vivo Targeted Deep-Tissue Photodynamic Therapy Based on Near-Infrared Light Triggered Upconversion Nanoconstruct. *ACS Nano* 2013, *7*, 676-688.

[140] Yuan, Y.; Min, Y.; Hu, Q.; Xing, B.; Liu, B.: NIR photoregulated chemo- and photodynamic cancer therapy based on conjugated polyelectrolyte-drug conjugate encapsulated upconversion nanoparticles. *Nanoscale* 2014, *6*, 11259-11272.

In: Photodynamic Therapy
Editor: Adrian G. Hugo

ISBN: 978-1-63463-857-9
© 2015 Nova Science Publishers, Inc.

Chapter 2

RECENT ADVANCES IN NANOMEDICINE FOR PHOTODYNAMIC THERAPY OF CANCER

*Yamin Yang and Hongjun Wang**

Department of Chemistry, Chemical Biology and Biomedical Engineering
Stevens Institute of Technology, Hoboken, NJ, US

ABSTRACT

Photodynamic therapy (PDT) with minimal invasion has emerged as one of the important therapeutic modalities for cancer, which combines the use of low energy light with a photosensitizer. Despite its multifaceted advantages, PDT has not yet become the mainstream of cancer intervention mainly due to its insufficient therapeutic efficacy, low selectivity of currently available photosensitizers, and limited light penetration for deep tumor tissues. Recognition of these challenges has greatly motivated the efforts in adopting nanotechnology for improving the design and delivery of photosensitizer, increasing the intensity of photodynamic reaction, and enhancing light penetration and absorption. A variety of nanomaterials have been employed in PDT, serving as either passive carriers or active participants. This review will discuss about the state-of-art approaches and future perspectives of the applications of nanomaterials in PDT.

1. OVERVIEW OF PHOTODYNAMIC THERAPY (PDT)

The term of "photodynamic" was first introduced by Von Tappeiner in 1904 to describe the oxygen-dependent chemical reactions induced by photosensitization, [1] which formulates the basis for photodynamic therapy (PDT), a special form of photochemotherapy with the combination of light, oxygen and a photosensitizing drug. During PDT, two individually non-toxic components, *i.e.*, photosensitizer and administrated light, are involved. Photosensitizers are the photosensitive molecules that can be excited by the light of a particular wavelength and then transfer the energy to neighboring molecular oxygen for singlet oxygen formation.

* Tel.: +1 201 216 5556; Fax: +1 201 216 8240; E-mail: Hongjun.Wang@stevens.edu.

Consequently, the highly reactive and unstable singlet oxygen species destroy target cells *via* apoptotic or necrotic process or the combination. [2–4] In recognition of the minimally invasive nature, PDT has been extensively explored for possible use in treating various diseases since 1980's. [5]

1.1. Major Components of PDT

1.1.1. Photosensitizer

Photosensitizers are chemical compounds that can absorb the photonic energy of light with a specific wavelength. Several commercially available photosensitizers are listed in Table 1 with their molecule structures and the typical maximum absorption wavelength. Among them, porphyrins, as the first-generation photosensitizers, were identified in the mid-nineteenth century and are the most extensively studied, officially approved, and commonly used in clinics. [6, 7] Photofrin, a complex mixture of more active porphyrin oligomers, mainly comprises of hematoporphyrin derivative (HpD). Photofrin is now approved for the treatment of lung and esophageal cancer in the United States, for the prophylactic treatment of bladder cancer in Canada, and for the treatment of several other cancers worldwide. [8] However, several major drawbacks of Photofrin are also recognized, including: the difficulty of reproduction, limited selectivity for tumor tissue, long-lasting cutaneous photosensitivity and complexity, poor absorption of tissue-penetrating red light, and low molar absorption coefficient (1170 $M^{-1}cm^{-1}$). To achieve the therapeutic efficacy, therefore, high concentrations of photosensitizer and high doses of light must be delivered to the tumors, which cause unwanted side effects. [7]

Table 1. Types of commercially available photosensitizers

Class	Molecular structure	Typical *max.* absorption (nm)
Porphyrins		630 nm
Chloro aluminium sulphonated phthalocyanine (AlPcS)		675 nm

Class	Molecular structure	Typical *max.* absorption (nm)
Zinc phthalocyanine (ZnPc)		675 nm
5-Aminola-evulinic acid (ALA)		630 nm
Indocyanine green (ICG)		800 nm
Chlorine e6		654 nm
Hypericin		590 nm

The limitations of Photofrin have motivated the development of versatile second-generation photosensitizers such as porphyrin-like macrocycles, phthalocyanines, benzoporphyrins, verteporfin, and so on. [9, 10] Water-soluble derivatives of phthalocyanines can be readily synthesized through substitution of the ring with moieties such as sulphonic acid, carboxylic acid and amino groups. The incorporation of Zn or Al into the phthalocyanine macrocycle (e.g., zinc phthalocyanines, ZnPc4; chloro aluminium sulphonated phthalocyanine, AlPcS) can provide a long-life triplet state with high photodynamic efficacy. Compared to first-generation photosensitizers, derivatives of phthalocyanines own particular advantages, such as 1) negligible dark-toxicity, 2) selective retention and high selectivity in some tumors, and 3) increased wavelength for excitation with enhanced cytotoxic efficiency. [11] However, low purification capability (a mixture of mono- , di-, tri- and tetrasulphonated derivatives) and easy aggregation in the aqueous media are the recognized challenge with this category of photosensitizers. [12]

Besides administration of exogenous photosensitizer, there is also an alternative way to stimulate the cellular synthesis of endogenous photosensitizers by intracellular metabolism. For instance, 5-Aminolaevulinic acid (5-ALA) is a precursor of a natural photosensitizer of protoporphyrin IX (PpIX). Administration of exogenous 5-ALA can lead to the build-up of phototoxic levels of PpIX. As a matter of fact, 5-ALA is the only clinically approved photosensitizer precursor. 5-ALA, a polar molecule exists as a charged zwitterion at the physiologic pH, accounting for its low lipid solubility and reduced bioavailability. Clinical evidence has shown an increased accumulation of 5-ALA-induced PpIX in tumor tissues with low demonstrated side effects. Further modifications of 5-ALA are also made to extend its clinical use by improving its cellular permeability and increasing the stability and selectivity. [13]

Additionally, many other types of photosensitizers (indocyanine green, chlorine e6, hypericin, and so on) have been approved by FDA for the use as the fluorescence contrast agents in diagnostic imaging and as effective reagents in photodynamic therapy. [14, 15] Ideally, the photosensitizing molecules should be amphiphilic, allowing for prolonged circulation in the blood and entry to the cells through the phospholipid membrane. In addition, it should have a high molar absorption coefficient in the red region of visible lights to increase tissue penetration for clinical applications. [16]

1.1.2. Light

During the PDT, delivery of sufficient light to activate photosensitizers is an essential step toward successful formation of singlet oxygen species. In this regard, great efforts have been made to investigate various light delivery systems for PDT and a significant improvement has been made in last 20 years. In general, the typical light sources used include: 1) broadband light beam produced by incoherent lamps, 2) focused light beam with a specific wavelength produced by lasers, 3) light emitting diodes (LEDs), and 4) fluorescent light sources. [17] Due to the inexpensiveness and easy handling, broadband light is often used for PDT of large lesions especially with regard to a limited difference in treatment efficacy between broadband and laser light sources. [18, 19] As traditional lasers are expensive and relatively immobile, the use of semiconductor diode lasers and LED array lasers is a convenient option for clinical utility. The treatment of deep internal organs is normally realized with the use of endoscopes and optical fibers for guided light delivery. [17]

Along with the advances in light delivery systems, the increase of light penetration depth can further extend the utility of PDT for treating deep diseased tissues, where optical scattering and light absorption dominate and significantly interfere with light delivery efficiency. In the human body, the tissue chromophores (e.g., hemoglobin) and water are the major absorbers of visible and infrared light, respectively. Interestingly, they have the lowest optical absorption coefficients in the NIR region around 650-900 nm. [20] In this case, the light of NIR region is more transparent with better tissue penetration, reaching as deep as 500 μm or even centimeters. NIR light is also less harmful to cells and tissues and can thus reduce the risk of inadvertent tissue destruction. [21] Therefore, future efforts should be made to develop NIR-based PDT for tumors in the deep anatomical location. In conjunction with the fact that NIR light with the wavelength above 800 nm does not have sufficient energy to activate photosensitizers for forming singlet oxygen, where the triplet state of activated photosensitizer is below the energy level of singlet oxygen, [22] thus, NIR in the range of 650-800 nm may be better light sources.

1.1.3. Tissue Oxygen

In addition to photosensitizer and light, PDT efficacy is also closely related to the intracellular oxygen level, which is always required to form the active species (*i.e.*, singlet oxygen) upon interaction with the excited photosensitizer. However, it should be noted that the PDT efficacy is not always in a linear proportion to the tissue oxygen concentration, that is, simply increasing respiratory oxygen may not correspondingly enhance the PDT tumor destruction. [23]

1.2. Clinical Treatment Procedure of PDT

Depending on the type of cancer or lesions and their anatomical location, photosensitizers can be administrated *via* intravenous injection, local injection or topically applied to the skin. A waiting time of 4-72 hours is often required for photosensitizers to be cleared from normal tissues but preferentially retained in the rapidly growing tissues with neoplastic cells (*i.e.* tumor cells). [22] Afterwards, light irradiation with abovementioned light sources is performed onto the diseased tissues for photosensitizer activation and singlet oxygen formation. The overall treatment procedures are minimally invasive with limited traumatic effect and no need for hospitalization.

1.3. Photodynamic Reaction Mechanism

As depicted in Figure 1, excitation of the photosensitizer can trigger a series of photophysical reaction. Briefly, following the absorption of light (photonic energy), the photosensitizer (^{1}PS) is excited from an electronically stable ground singlet state ($^1S_0$) to an excited singlet state ($^1S_1$), becoming ^{1}PS* with the lifetime of 10^{-8}-10^{-9} s. It then decays back to the ground state with the release of energy in the form of fluorescence (photon emission) or undergoes intersystem crossing to a longer-lived excited triplet state (^{3}PS*) (with a lifetime of 10^{-3} s). The excited triplet state photosensitizer can follow two kinds of reactions (either Type I or Type II reaction mechanism) to transfer the energy to other biomolecules. [24]

In Type I reaction, the excited photosensitizer can react directly with a substrate, such as the cell membrane or a molecule, and produce ions, or electron/hydrogen extraction from a substrate molecule to form radicals. These radicals then react rapidly, usually with oxygen molecule, to produce highly reactive oxygen species (ROS) such as superoxide and peroxide anions. [25]

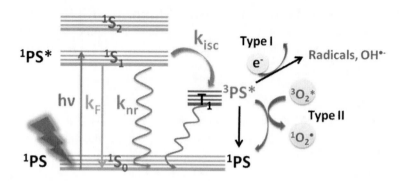

Figure 1. A simplified diagram of various energy levels of a photosensitizing molecule during the photoexcitation. $^1S_0$, $^1S_1$, and $^1S_2$ represent the singlet electronic states of the molecule. Absorption of a photon (depicted by $h\nu$) results in the excitation of the absorbing molecule from the ground singlet state, $^1S_0$, to the first excited singlet state, $^1S_1$. Photochemistry may occur from $^1S_1$ directly or from the first triplet excited state, T_1, which is generated after intersystem crossing. The molecule can relax back to the ground state $^1S_0$ from either $^1S_1$ or T_1, radiatively or nonradiatively. k_{nr}, k_{isc}, and k_F represent the rate constant for nonradiative decay, intersystem crossing, and fluorescence, respectively. In general, with conventional light sources, only S_1 and T_1 are populated. With high-intensity, pulsed irradiation, or with two-wavelength excitation, the upper excited states, such as S_2, may also be populated, giving rise to different photochemistry.

In Type II reaction, the triplet state photosensitizer interacts directly with oxygen molecules in proximity and transfers its energy to create an excited singlet state oxygen molecule ($^1O_2$). Singlet oxygen is a very aggressive species and will immediately react with any nearby biomolecules. [26] The quantum yield of free radicals heavily depends on the type of photosensitizer chosen. [22]

Energy transfer allows the transition of excited photosensitizer to its ground singlet state. The relaxed photosensitizer is able to repeat the process of energy transfer to oxygen many times. Both Type I or Type II reactions occur simultaneously, and the ratio between these two processes depends on the type of photosensitizer used, the concentrations of substrate and oxygen, as well as the binding affinity of the photosensitizer to the substrate. Most photosensitizers for PDT are efficient producers of $^1O_2$ in simple chemical systems, and it is assumed, although impossible to measure directly, that Type II photochemistry is the dominant mechanism for PDT in most circumstances with cells and tissues. [25]

1.4. Effects of PDT on Tumors

It is now accepted that PDT-mediated tumor destruction *in vivo* mainly involves three routes. Firstly, the PDT-generated ROS, $^1O_2$ in particular, can kill tumor cells directly. Secondly, PDT also damages the tumor-associated vasculature, leading to tumor infarction. Finally, PDT can activate an immune response against tumor cells. [27]

In the first circumstances, cell killing occurs through apoptosis and/or necrosis. [28] Apoptosis, a normal physiologic process, is essential for tissue development and involution, as well as tissue homeostasis. In contrast, cell necrosis leads to cell lysis due to the loss of the integrity of plasma membrane, which consequently triggers tissue inflammation. PDT-generated ROS can induce apoptosis, necrosis, or a combination; however, apoptosis has been recognized as the more prominent form of cell death in response to PDT as evidenced in many cell cultures, where DNA fragmentation and chromatin condensation are measured. [29]

PDT-triggered apoptosis is closely associated with the intracellular localization and binding sites of photosensitizer. [29] Photoactivation of a mitochondrion-localized photosensitizer causes the release of cytochrome c. The released cytochrome c becomes part of the "apoptosome" complex to generate active caspase-9, which then cleaves and activates caspase-3. Caspase-3 is the major effector caspase and is responsible for cleavage and activation of other caspases, especially caspases-6, -7, and -8. The effector caspases cleave numerous proteins, including nuclear lamins, leading to nuclear breakdown; poly ADP ribose polymerase (PARP) and DNA-dependent protein kinase (DNA-PK), resulting in inhibition of DNA repair; inhibitor of caspase-activated DNase (ICAD), releasing active CAD to degrade DNA; and other proteins that affect cell structure and adhesion. In the cases with the participation of Fas and tumor necrosis factor receptor (TNFR), the cell surface death receptors, binding to their respective ligands, lead to activation of caspase-8, which can in turn result in the activation of caspase-3, independent of mitochondrial involvement. Caspase-8 cleaves the Bcl-2 homolog Bid to produce the pro-apoptotic fragment tBid, which can act on mitochondria to cause cytochrome c release.

Besides the critical function of mitochondria, other intracellular organelles are also involved in photodynamic reaction. Photoactivation of lysosome-bound photosensitizers can cause the release of cathepsins, which can cleave Bid to promote apoptosis. Damage to the endoplasmic reticulum (ER) by PDT causes the release of Ca^{2+}, which can promote apoptosis. Apoptosis is also controlled by members of the Bcl-2 family that either promote or inhibit the process. In addition to Bid, shown here are the anti-apoptotic proteins Bcl-2 and Bcl-xL, blocking PDT-induced apoptosis by inhibiting caspase activation, and the pro-apoptotic Bax that has been proposed to promote mitochondrial reactions, including cytochrome c release.

Now a number of evidences have also demonstrated the absence of apoptosis during PDT-induced cell death. At a high PDT dose, excessive damage occurs to the cells, resulting in cell lysis or the destruction of components of the apoptotic pathways. [29]

1.5. Key Functions of Mitochondria in PDT Efficacy

During PDT, the intracellular location of photoactivated ROS formation plays a critical role in determining the efficacy of PDT. Since the mid-1990s, efforts have been made to develop photosensitizers localized to subcellular organelles, such as mitochondria, plasma membrane, lysosomes and nuclei. [9] Among them, mitochondria have been proposed to be the most effective subcellular targets for photodamage. Numerous reports have implicated the importance of mitochondria as PDT targets. [9] Photosensitizers that localize to mitochondria are more efficient in killing cells than those localizing to other intracellular sites. [30, 31] Localization of therapeutics into mitochondria can be realized by utilizing the electrochemical potential gradient across the mitochondrial membrane. Normally, cationic lipophilic photosensitizers such as the krytocyanine dye N,N'-bis(2-ethyl-1,3-dioxolane)-kryptocyanine (EDKC) and rhodamine-123 as well as methylene blue derivatives (MBD) have a high opportunity to accumulate in the mitochondria. Photosensitizers with negative charge such as

Photofrin, or neutral charge such as Pc4 can also accumulate in mitochondria, but may bind to various mitochondrial constituents. [29, 32]

1.6. Advantages and Challenges with Current PDT

1.6.1. Advantages of PDT

The major advantages of PDT over other therapies such as surgery, radiotherapy and chemotherapy include 1) minimal invasiveness, 2) low morbidity, 3) relative simplicity, and 4) good patient tolerability for repeated application to the same site. [33] PDT appears to be able to overcome or bypass many of the barriers that limit the effectiveness of ionizing radiation and chemotherapy toward cell killing. [29] PDT also exhibits its intrinsic specificity for cancer therapy. Initially, photosensitizers are taken up by both normal healthy cells and hyperproliferating cancer cells, but retained longer in the cancer cells. The tumor selectivity increases to some extend with the lipophilic characteristics of photosensitizers. Due to the particular presence of a large number of low-density lipoprotein membrane receptors in neoplastic cells, hydrophobic photosensitizers that strongly bind to lipoproteins can accumulate in the malignant tissue with a distinct selectivity. Lower pH over the tumor region may also favor the uptake of photosensitizers by tumor cells. In addition, PDT can be confined to specific location by locally administering the photosensitizers with restricted mobility and by delivering the light irradiation to the diseased region only. [22, 34]

1.6.2. Challenges with Current PDT

Clinically, PDT is mainly applied to those tissues located in the superficial regions of the body, such as skin cancer, superficial epidermal lesions, superficial mucosal lesions, and this is particularly true when considering the limited light penetration. With the development of endoscopes and fiber optic catheters, light can be delivered to various locations of internal organs, which significantly extend the application of PDT to treat cancers ranging from the head, neck, pancreas, to prostate, and so on. [35, 36] Increasing efforts are also under the way to further explore the utility of PDT for more organs. Despite the intriguing advantages, several unmet challenges are identified while applying PDT to cancerous tissues far beneath the surface.

First of all, traditional photosensitizers suffer from several limitations such as poor selectivity, the need for a large quantity to achieve high efficiency, and a high cutaneous photosensitivity. [37] Most photosensitizers used are lipophilic and they intend to aggregate in an aqueous environment, which can significantly reduce the quantum yield of singlet oxygen. [38] In this regard, it would be highly beneficial to develop a delivery system that can protect the hydrophobic photosensitizer and meanwhile provide an optimal environment for photosensitizer administration in a monomeric form. In addition, the maximum absorbance wavelength of currently approved PDT photosensitizers are in the visible spectral regions below 700 nm, which has very limited tissue penetration depth, only a few millimeters, implying the suitability of current PDT treatment for topical lesions. Clearly, further improvement is necessary for efficient delivery of photosensitizers at therapeutic concentrations to target cells but with minimal uptake by non-target cells and for the administration of light with sufficient penetration depth and doses to targeted areas, which can increase the specificity and efficiency of PDT.

2. NANOMATERIALS AND THEIR APPLICATIONS IN PDT

The emergence of nanotechnology has shed promising light to improve the potency of PDT efficacy for cancer destruction while minimizing the collateral toxicity to nonmalignant cells. [39–41] Nanomaterials, normally referring to the materials with at least one dimension less than 100 nm, exhibit several recognized superior characteristics, including: 1) small size and large surface to volume ratio, 2) unique physiochemical properties at nanoscale, and 3) multifunctionality encompassing both detective and therapeutic capabilities. [42]

Broadly, the use of nanomaterials in PDT can be divided into two major categories based on the functions, *i.e.*, as carriers of photosensitizers and/or as active participants in photodynamic reaction. Based on the material composition, they can be further divided into (a) biodegradable nanoparticles, such as liposomes, micelles, polymeric nanoparticles, and (b) non-polymeric nanoparticles such as gold nanoparticles. Active participating nanoparticles can also be sub-classified by mechanism of activation, including: (a) nanoparticles act as photosensitizers themselves (such as quantum dots, zinc oxide and titanium dioxide nanoparticles), (b) surface plasmonic nanoparticles (such as gold nanoparticles), (c) self-illuminating nanoparticles, and (d) upconverting nanoparticles.

2.1. Tumor-specific Targeting

Targeted drug delivery is a promising strategy to further improve the specificity, efficacy and safety of photosensitizers. The use of nanoparticles as the drug-delivery system, based on passive or active targeting mechanism, may resolve the challenge of nonspecific photosensitizer accumulation.

2.1.1. Passive Targeting

Passive targeting relies on the fact that if nanoparticles circulate long enough in the blood stream, they have a high chance to accumulate preferentially in the highly vascularized tumor tissues. Due to the fast angiogenesis in malignant tissues, newly formed tumor vessels exhibit abnormal structures and morphologies with disorganized tissue architecture, enhanced vascular permeability, large microvascular fenestrations and absence of lymphatics, thus the opportunity for nanoparticles to accumulate in the tumor tissue through the leaky vasculature is much higher than they do in the normal tissues. This so-called "Enhanced Permeability and Retention" effect (EPR effect) provides the nanoparticles with passive targeting capability to tumor tissues.[43–45]

To achieve the long circulation and maintain better stability, nanoparticles often need to be further modified, e.g., immobilization of hydrophilic polyethylene glycol (PEG) onto the particle surface. [46] However, the increased stability of nanoparticles in aqueous environments may interfere their interactions with cells and decrease the efficacy in transferring photosensitizers to tumor cells.

2.1.2. Active Targeting

In contrast to passive targeting, active targeting can result in direct and specific localization of the photosensitizer to a particular site with increased PDT efficiency and selectivity. Active targeting generally encompasses the strategy to couple a specific entity to the nanoparticle surface for enhanced interaction with specific membrane markers on the target cells. A wide range of candidate molecules, such as monoclonal antibodies (MoAbs), aptamers, folate ligands, small peptides, glycoproteins, glycolipids, hyaluronic acid, *and the like*, can be used to achieve the active targeting purpose. [47]

Current challenges associated with active targeting include the elimination of unwanted immune reactions to the modified nanoparticles *in vivo* and the increase of the specificity for tumor cell recognition using cost-effective procedures and marker molecules. [43]

2.2. Nanoparticles as Passive carriers of Photosensitizers in PDT

The use of nanoparticles as drug carriers for PDT have increased in recent years, in which photosensitizers can be conjugated/adsorbed on the surface of nanoparticles or encapsulated in the nanomaterials to provide a higher therapeutic payload over free drugs. With the assistance of nanoparticles, hydrophobic photosensitizers can be transported through blood circulation and taken up efficiently by cells. In the meantime, the large surface area of nanoparticles allows for functionalization with specific cell-targeting biomolecules and ligands to further improve the specificity of drug delivery to targeted cells.

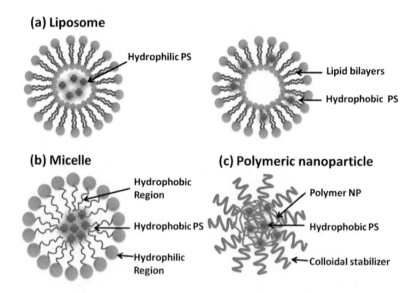

Figure 2. Nanoparticles as passive carriers of photosensitizers in PDT: (a) Liposome; (b) Micelle; (c) Polymeric nanoparticles.

2.2.1. Biodegradable Nanoparticles

2.2.1.1. Liposomes

Liposomes are artificially prepared spherical vesicles made from phospholipids and cholesterol. Liposomes are normally composed of bilayer phospholipids with a hydrophilic head and two hydrophobic tails, which enable them to entrap both hydrophilic and hydrophobic drugs. Hydrophilic photosensitizers are suspended in the aqueous interior of the liposomes, while hydrophobic photosensitizers can be trapped in the lipid bilayer (Figure 2a). Liposomes have thus far been the most intensively studied carrier system for photosensitizers. [48, 49] Recently, the liposomal benzoporphyrin derivative monoacid ring A (BPD-MA) (Visudyne®, QLT, Canada) has been approved in USA for the treatment of the wet form of age-related macular degenerescence. [48]

To prevent the short circulation time, irreversible disintegration and easy uptake by mononuclear phagocytic cells of unmodified liposomes, further modification of liposomes with passive or active targeting moieties is necessary. [40, 50] Modification of the nanoparticle surface with PEG or poly (ethylene oxide) (PEO) allows for longer plasma circulation. Conjugation with tumor-specific ligands for active targeting is another way to improve tumor selectivity with effective photosensitizer delivery. For example, Reshetov et al. compared the treatment efficacy and distribution characteristics of conventional photosensitizer temoporfin (meta-tetra[hydroxyphenyl]chlorin) (mTHPC) and its PEGylated liposomal formulations in PDT of tumor-grafted mice. Based on their results, PEGylated liposomal formulations provided a significant increase of blood-circulating liposomal mTHPC for up to 6 hours with liposomes remained intact, and also allowed for rapid accumulation of liposomal mTHPC in tumors by means of the EPR effect. [51] Gijsens et al. have demonstrated that a photosensitizer aluminum phthalocyanine tetrasulfonate (AlPcS4) encapsulated in a PEG-liposome (146 ± 23 nm) covalently bound to transferrin (Tf-Lip-AlPcS4) can efficiently photosensitize cancer cells that overexpress the transferrin receptor, such as Hela cells. In this study, the liposomes were prepared by repeated extrusion through the polycarbonate filter membranes with 100-nm pore size. They found their Tf-Lip-AlPcS4 nanoparticles caused 10 times more photocytotoxicity (IC50, 0.63 µM) than free AlPcS4 at a light dose of 45 kJ/m, which was the result of a high intracellular concentration of AlPCS4 (136.5 µM) in HeLa cells. [52]

In recognition of the fact that effective photosensitization in photodamage-responsible subcellular organs (e.g., mitochondria) can result in an induction of intensive phototoxicity, Takeuchi et al. have further modified their polycation liposomes (PCLs, 100 nm in diameter) with cetylated polyethylenimine (cetyl-PEI) for improved photosensitizer delivery. Polyethylenimine (PEI) is adopted as a cationic polymer and can facilitate the cytoplasmic delivery of BPD-MA through endocytic pathway into mitochondria with negative membrane potential. From their results, the PEI-modified PCLs not only resulted in an enhanced photosensitizer uptake level in human endothelial cell line ECV304 cells and human umbilical vein endothelial cells (HUVECs), but also delivered the photosensitizers into subcellular localization such as mitochondria, which led to further enhancement of PDT-induced cell destruction. [53]

2.2.1.2. Micelles

Micelles are closed monolayer particles with a hydrophobic core (e.g., fatty acid) and polar surface, or a polar core and hydrophobic surface (e.g., fatty acid surface) (Figure 2b). They have been widely used to entrap either hydrophobic or hydrophilic drugs in the core *via* polar-to-polar or nonpolar-to-nonpolar interactions. Meanwhile, tumor-targeting moieties such as integrin binding peptides can be coupled onto the micellar surface for active tumor targeting. [54, 55]

Polymeric micelles are emerging as an effective drug delivery system for hydrophobic photosensitizers in PDT. For instance, Li et al. compared the PDT efficacy of protoporphyrin

IX (PpIX) loaded micelles (methoxy poly (ethylene glycol)-b-poly (caprolactone) diblock copolymers, MePEG5000-b-PCL4100) and that of free PpIX. As-prepared spherical micelles (52.2 ± 6.4 nm) with a high PpIX-loading efficiency of 82.4% led to two-fold higher cellular uptake than that of free PpIX in RIF-1 cells, which consequently resulted in markedly increased photocytotoxicity upon light irradiation. [56]

In order to achieve favorable *in vivo* delivery and biodistribution of the photosensitizer of silicon phthalocyanine Pc 4 with high hydrophobicity, Master et al. have used the biocompatible poly(ethylene glycol)-polycaprolactone (PEG-PCL) nanoparticles as block copolymer micelles for Pc 4 delivery. Pc 4 was encapsulated within the micelle core by hydrophobic association with the PCL block with an encapsulation efficiency of 70%, while maintaining the micelle size under 100 nm. Micelle-delivered Pc 4 showed significant cytotoxicity on MCF-7c3 human breast cancer cells upon irradiation. [57]

Rijcken et al. used poly(ethylene glycol)-b-poly[N-(2-hydroxypropyl) methacrylamide-dilactate] micelles (mPEG-b-p(HPMAm-Lac2)) as novel delivery micelles for hydrophobic photosensitizer of solketal-substituted phthalocyanine (Si(sol)2Pc). Si(sol)2Pc could be loaded efficiently in the micelles up to a final concentration of 2 mg/mL without affecting the micellar size of approximately 75 nm. The Si(sol)2Pc-loaded micelles with a low loading showed a similar high photocytotoxicity as the free PS. [58]

2.2.1.3. Polymeric Nanoparticles

The use of polymeric nanoparticles as the drug delivery vehicles has the following promising advantages, including 1) the increase of photosensitizer delivery to target area with controlled release profile; 2) protection of the photosensitizers in a biological environment; 3) the possibility of loading multiple components such as targeting ligands and contrast agents to achieve tumor selectivity and/or diagnosis. [59, 60]

A variety of polymeric nanoparticles (Figure 2c) have recently been used for the delivery of PDT agents, for example, poly(D, L-lactide-co-glycolide) copolymers (PLGA), N-(2-hydroxypropyl)-methacrylamide (HPMA) copolymers, polyacrylamide (PAA), dendrimers, chitosan, *etc.* Photosensitizers such as porphyrins, chlorins, hypericin, phthalocyanines, methylene blue (MB), and 5-ALA have been loaded into such polymeric nanoparticles and investigated the potential in PDT.

The chemical composition and structure of polymers can be readily designed to accommodate drugs with various degrees of hydrophobicity, molecular weight and charge. [61] In addition, the surface properties, morphology, and composition of polymer matrices can be tuned with controlled degradation rates for kinetic release of photosensitizers. [62]

Fadel et al. prepared ZnPc-loaded PLGA nanoparticles (mean particle size of 374.3 nm) using the solvent emulsion evaporation method (SEEM) and investigated the *in vivo* photodynamic efficiency in tumor-bearing mice. Tumor-bearing mice injected with ZnPc nanoparticles exhibited significantly smaller mean tumor volume with delayed tumor growth and longer survival compared to those injected with free ZnPc during the time course of experiment, indicating that ZnPc-encapsulated-PLGA nanoparticles are effective for improving the photodynamic activity in target tissues. [63]

Jin et al. prepared the chitosan-based nanoparticles (CNPs) by self-assembling amphiphilic glycol chitosan-5β-cholanic acid conjugates in an aqueous solution and then encapsulating the water-insoluble photosensitizer of PpIX with high drug-loading efficiency (>90%) by using a dialysis method. The PpIX-encapsulated CNPs (PpIX-CNPs) (290 nm) exhibited enhanced tumor specificity and increased therapeutic efficacy compared to free PpIX in SCC7 tumor-bearing mice, with the potential as an effective drug delivery system for clinical PDT. [64]

Conjugation of photosensitizers to biocompatible water-soluble HPMA polymers reduces their dark toxicity and increases their accumulation in solid tumor tissues, resulting in high anticancer efficacy with PDT. From the *in vivo* study using human ovarian OVCAR-3 carcinoma-xenografted female athynmic mice, conjugation of photosensitizer of mesochlorin e6 (Mce6) into HPMA copolymers resulted in a maximum tumor uptake of 5.5% of the total administered dose, while in the case of free Mce6 it was less than 0.5%. With selective tumor accumulation, HPMA copolymer-Mce6 conjugate at a dose of 13.4 mg/kg (1.5 mg/kg of Mce6 equivalent) and light doses of 110 J/cm^2 at 12 and 18 h, respectively, resulted in significant suppression of the growth of OVCAR-3 tumors. [65]

The same group has also studied the synergism in anticancer effect toward human ovarian carcinoma OVCAR-3 cells by binary combination of free and HPMA copolymer-bound anticancer drugs (SOS thiophene) for chemotherapy and Mce6 for PDT. Sequential combinations of these therapeutics produced very strong synergism (nearly additivity) in the treatment of OVCAR-3 cells. Incorporation of targeting moieties, Fab (a widely used antibody fragment), into HPMA copolymer-drug conjugates results in specific delivery and enhanced internalization of the polymeric conjugate in OVCAR-3 cells *via* receptor-mediated endocytosis. [66]

Gupta et al. demonstrated the outstanding advantages of the multifunctional nanoplatforms based on PAA nanoparticles for cancer imaging and therapy. The non-toxic PAA nanoparticles (18-25 nm) drastically enhanced the uptake of ^{124}I-labeled photosensitizer of chlorophyll-a derivative by Colon26 tumors in BALB/c mice and showed a remarkable improvement for long-term tumor cure by PDT. More interestingly, this nanoplatform can also be applied for tumor-imaging purposes based on the PET/NIR fluorescence detection to achieve both PDT and diagnosis. [67]

Kojima et al. have developed the PEG-functionalized dendrimers as a drug-carrier candidate for PDT. Two PEG-functionalized dendrimers derived from poly(amido amine) (PAMAM) and poly(propylene imine) (PPI) dendrimers (PEG-PAMAM and PEG-PPI) were used to encapsulate rose bengal (RB) and protoporphyrin IX (PpIX). It was found that PEG-PPI held photosensitizers in a more stable manner than PEG-PAMAM because of their inner hydrophobicity. [68]

2.2.1.4. Stimuli-responsive Polymeric Nanoparticles

Encouraging evidence has demonstrated the potential use of stimuli-responsive polymeric nanoparticles for triggered release of photosensitizers. A variety of stimuli such as heat, light, pH, and target binding can be used as the trigger to increase the permeability of the nanoparticles, destabilize the phospholipid bilayer, and release the entrapped photosensitizers. [69–71]

For instance, poly(N-isopropylacrylamide) (PNIPAM) is a well-known thermo-responsive polymer with a volume phase transition temperature. He et al. investigated the PNIPAM-coated Fe$_3$O$_4$@SiO$_2$@CdTe multifunctional nanoparticles with photoluminescent, thermosensitive and magnetic properties as carriers to deliver water-soluble, fluorescent sulfonated Zn-phthalocyanine (ZnPcS) for PDT in Chinese hamster ovary (CHO) cells *in vitro* and zebra fish *in vivo*. The swollen PNIPAM at the temperatures lower than 32-34°C can encapsulate ZnPcS and then expel the drug upon shrinking at higher temperatures. ZnPcS-loaded nanoparticles were taken up by CHO cells at 27 °C, and then the release of ZnPcS from nanoparticles occurred at 37 °C with the diffusion of fluorescence in the cytoplasm as detected. Similar results were also found in the intestinal tract of zebra fish *in vivo* after intake of the nanoparticles. [72] However, some issues need to be addressed for practical applications of these nanoparticles. For example, it remains challenging to control the optimal temperature for corresponding response of the nanoparticles under the physiological conditions.

Solid tumor usually has a pH of ~6.8 and the endo/lysosomes experience even lower pH of 5.0-5.5. [73, 74] Ling et al. reported the use of multifunctional tumor pH-sensitive self-assembled nanoparticles for bimodal imaging and PDT treatment of resistant heterogeneous tumors. Ce6 grafted poly(ethylene glycol)-poly(β-benzyl-L-aspartate) (PEG-PBLA-Ce6) was synthesized to provide a platform ligand. Imidazole was then incorporated as an ionizable group to impart pH sensitivity to the tumor microenvironment. Two specific ligand derivatives on the basis of this platform were further engineered and cooperated with extremely small iron oxide nanoparticles (ESIONs) to form the final product, namely pH-sensitive magnetic nanogrenades (PMN) for self-assembly. These PMNs can readily target tumors *via* surface-charge switching triggered by the acidic tumor microenvironment, and are further disassembled into a highly active state in acidic subcellular compartments to turn on MR contrast, fluorescence and photodynamic therapeutic activity. After intravenous injection to HCT116 tumor-bearing nude mice, these PMNs resulted in pH-triggered generation of $^1O_2$ and thus enabled pH-dependent PDT to selectively kill cancer cells. [75]

Photo-activation is another attractive option for triggering photosensitizer release. Detailed mechanisms of light-triggered chemical changes in photo-reactive segments of these molecules are reviewed by Bisby et al. and Yavlovich et al. [76, 77] Roeder et al. have reported a method for enhanced PDT by applying dendrimer-photosensitizer complexes to bring multiple phototosensitizer moieties to the treatment location. Photosensitizer tetrapyrroles are covalently coupled to the peripheral bonding sites of dendrimers and can be separated from the dendrimers by light activation without the use of additional chemical agents. It is especially advantageous that the photosensitizer molecules bound to the dendrimer are not photoactive without light exposure and the photodynamic activity can be obtained momentarily upon exposure/activation. [78]

Collectively, all these studies suggest that encapsulation of photosensitizers in nanoparticles (liposomes/micelles/polymeric nanoparticles) can improve the therapeutic index of photosensitizers compared to their free format. The use of biodegradable nanoparticles as drug carriers can result in 1) prolonged circulation of photosensitizers, 2) targeted accumulation of photosensitizers in tumor site, 3) relatively lower drug concentration for system delivery, and 4) shorter incubation time for satisfactory photodynamic damages with minimally undesirable effects. With the proof of concept, there is a great need to translate the experimental advantages into clinical practice. Prior to the possible utility in clinical practice, further improvement of current biodegradable nanoparticle design should focus on the stability of polymer-based drug carriers, functional multilayer structures, and intelligent stimulation responsiveness, which can be realized in the physiological environment. A comprehensive evaluation of their physicochemical properties, pharmacokinetics, biodistribution, and biodegradability *in vivo* is necessary.

2.2.2. Non-Biodegradable Nanoparticles

Non-biodegradable nanoparticles can also be used as carriers to address the challenges with free photosensitizers. Among them, silica-based nanoparticles are the most widely studied and they have several advantages over organic nanoparticles. For instance, their particle size, shape, porosity, and monodispersibility can be exquisitely controlled during their preparation processes under ambient temperature conditions. Besides their compatibility in the biological systems and limited microbial attack, silica nanoparticles also display little swelling or porosity change with the pH change. In addition, the porous matrix of silica nanoparticles is permeable to photosensitizers, oxygen as well as $^1O_2$. Photosensitizers can be either noncovalently encapsulated inside or covalently conjugated on the surface of silica nanoparticles. However, noncovalent adsorption of photosensitizers into porous silica nanoparticles can result in drug leakage, while covalent bonding of the photosensitizers into silica nanoparticles may somehow affect the physicochemical properties of photosensitizers during the synthesis process. [79, 80]

Zhang et al. have reported a novel multifunctional core-shell nanocomposite structure that contains a nonporous dye-doped silica core and a mesoporous silica shell containing photosensitizer molecule of hematoporphyrin (HP). The mesoporous silica nanovehicle acts not only as a carrier for the photosensitizer but also as a nanoreactor to facilitate the photo-oxidation reaction. The efficiency of photo-oxidation within the core-shell hybrid nanoparticles was significantly improved in comparison to that with the homogeneous solution. Doping fluorescence dyes into the nonporous core endows the imaging capability. [81]

Guo et al. developed RB-decorated silica (SiO_2-NH_2-RB) nanoparticles to kill bacteria, such as methicillin-resistant Staphylococcus aureus (MRSA), with a high efficiency through the photodynamic action. The results showed that RB-decorated silica nanoparticles could inactivate the bacteria up to eight-order-of-magnitude reduction. Photosensitizers of such design should have a good potential as antimicrobial agents through a photodynamic mechanism. [82]

2.3. Active Participants

In addition to the benefits as passive carriers for photosensitizers, some nanostructures have intriguing physicochemical properties, such as unique optical properties, magnetic susceptibility, thermal or electrical conductivity, which introduce new features to improve various modalities of PDT.

2.3.1. Photosensitizing Nanoparticles

2.3.1.1. Quantum Dots

Quantum dots (QDs) are luminescent nanocrystals made out of semiconductor materials and they are small enough to display quantum mechanical properties and unique optical properties. QDs exhibit appealing features, such as high quantum yield, high photostability, and tunable size-dependent fluorescence emission spectra, enabling them for fluorescence resonance energy transfer and photodynamic therapy studies. QDs can transfer energy to surrounding O_2 under light irradiation, with consequent toxicity to cells (Figure 3a). [83, 84] Recent studies have explored their potential use as photosensitizers.

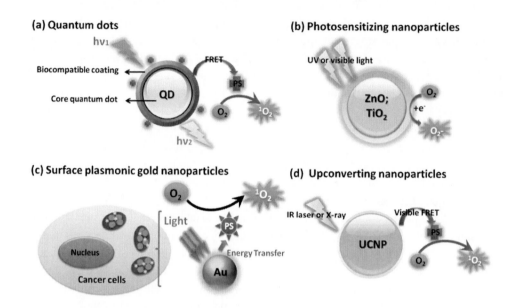

Figure 3. Nanoparticles as active participants in PDT: (a) Quantum dots; (b) Photosensitizing nanoparticles; (c) Surface plasmonic gold nanoparticles; (d) Upconverting nanoparticles.

Morosini et al. examined the potential of hydrophilic near-infrared emitting CdTe(S)-type QDs conjugated with folic acid as photosensitizers for PDT *in vitro*. As demonstrated, QDs at a concentration of 8 nM significantly enhanced the photodynamic efficiency with a light dose-dependent response. The folic acid appeared to be an optimal targeting ligand for selective delivery of QDs to folate receptor-alpha (FR-α)-overexpressing cancer cells. [85]

Markovic et al. have shown that electrochemically produced graphene quantum dots (GQD) irradiated with blue light (470 nm, 1W) can generate reactive oxygen species (e.g., $^1O_2$) and kill U251 human glioma cells through oxidative stress. Cell death regulated by photoexcited GQD is mediated by induction of oxidative stress and subsequent activation of both type I (apoptosis) and type II (autophagy) programmed cell death. [86] Ge et al. reported their study regarding the preparation of GQDs on a large scale using a simple hydrothermal method with polythiophenes as the precursors. The as-prepared GQDs exhibited a broad absorption band, a high $^1O_2$ generation yield (greater than 1.3), good aqueous dispersibility, and favorable biocompatibility. Both *in vitro* and *in vivo* studies have demonstrated the potential use of GQDs as the PDT agents, simultaneously allowing imaging and providing a highly efficient cancer therapy. [87]

Despite the successful use of QDs for PDT, QDs alone is somehow still inefficient to generate $^1O_2$ for desirable therapeutic effects. In this regard, attempts have been accordingly made to covalently conjugate photosensitizers to QDs *via* organic bridges. Part of the efforts are made to use QD as a Forster resonance energy transfer (FRET) pair for improving the excitation of a standard photosensitizer. Rakovich et al. synthesized the CdTe quantum dot-methylene blue (MB) hybrid as a novel photosensitizer for *in vitro* PDT of HepG2 and HeLa cancerous cells. Since there is a sufficient overlap between the CdTe nanocrystal emission and MB absorption bands, FRET occurs and causes an increased excitation of MB with enhanced ROS production and consequently improved cell killing efficiency compared to that of MB alone. [88]

However, the PS-QD conjugates usually have very low water solubility. Meanwhile, surface oxidation and subsequent leaching-out of heavy metal ions from the QD core cause inherent toxicity and remain a big challenge for their clinical translation. Surface modifications, e.g., PEG-ylation, can be used to reduce the cytotoxicity, however, the function of QDs may also be compromised. [89, 90]

2.3.1.2. Zinc Oxide and Titanium Dioxide Nanoparticles

Both ZnO and TiO_2 nanoparticles can produce ROS by electron transfer reactions involving oxygen and water upon light absorption (Figure 3b). The active species is thought to be mainly hydroxyl radical (HO·), but superoxide anion and $^1O_2$ are also produced. ROS generation after illumination with UV or visible light has been reported, but it is still unclear whether they could be utilized for PDT.

Ismail et al. showed that metal-doped zinc oxide nanoparticles (ZnO NPs) might induce anti-proliferative effect on adenocarcinoma HepG2 cells under UV-irradiation due to the generation of ROS, indicating the potential of ZnO NPs in clinical PDT. [91]

Fakhar-e-Alam et al. have synthesized porous ZnO NPs with a high surface to volume ratio on the tip of borosilicate glass capillaries and conjugated the particles with Photofrin for efficient intracellular drug delivery. The ZnO NPs could be excited intracellularly with 240 nm UV light, and the resultant 625 nm red light emission activated a chemical reaction of Photofrin that produced ROS. ZnO NPs exhibited synergistic cytotoxicity in A-549 cells under light exposure as compared to Photofrin alone, showing the potential of ZnO NPs in PDT application. [92] Besides the spherical structure, the same group has also studied the cytotoxic effects of other ZnO nanostructures such as ZnO nanowires conjugated with a photosensitizer (protoporphyrin IX). They observed that ZnO nanowires with a potent photosensitizer could induce ROS formation upon UV-A irradiation after uptake by human cancerous skin cells. [93] However, the biosafety of ZnO nanowires as drug delivery vehicles is still under debate. [94] Moreover, the light sources used for activating such nanoparticles are usually in the UV range, which has limited tissue penetration depth.

Zhang et al. prepared a TiO_2 nanoparticle/poly(ethylene glycol) double acrylates (PEGDA) hydrogel through *in situ* photopolymerization on tumor cells for PDT. TiO_2 nanorods with the diameter of ~5 nm and the length of ~25 nm in this system presented as effective photosensitizers for PDT and initiators for *in situ* formation of hydrogel under NIR irradiation. The hybrid hydrogel retained TiO_2 nanorods around the tumor cells to form a drug-loaded hydrogel shell. Under NIR irradiation a high concentration of $^1O_2$ accumulated around tumor cells and induced the apoptosis of tumor cells. Also, the hydrogel could reduce the side effects by preventing the migration of TiO_2 nanorods to normal tissue. [95]

2.3.1.3. Surface Plasmonic Nanoparticles

Certain noble metal nanoparticles exhibit unique physicochemical and optical properties such as the localized surface Plasmon resonance, which makes them intriguing not only as drug-delivery carriers but also as therapeutic agents for PDT. Among them, gold nanoparticles, in particular, hold great potentials due to their good biocompatibility and multi-functionalization capability for delivery of photosensitizers and cancer cell targeting.

Specifically, due to the surface Plasmon resonance properties, electromagnetic enhancement can be achieved upon light irradiation, in which the photonic energy absorbed onto the surface of Au NPs is amplified and then transferred to the neighboring photosensitizer molecule. Therefore, while serving as a carrier for photosensitizer, Au NPs can be used as an active enhancer in PDT, and more photosensitizer molecules can be activated with the presence of Au NPs, and subsequently the formation of singlet oxygen species can be enhanced to cause more cell death (Figure 3c). In our previous study, elevated formation of reactive oxygen species (ROS) was detected on fibrosarcoma tumor cells treated with 5-aminolevulinic acid (5-ALA)-conjugated Au NPs, leading to 50% more cell death compared to those treated with 5-ALA alone. [96] The convergence of experimental findings and theoretical simulation on size-dependent ROS formation and plasmonic enhancement suggests that elevated generation of ROS in the presence of Au NPs is attributed to highly localized plasmonic resonance fields on Au NP surface, which increases with particle size [97] and can be further enhanced by intracellular gold nanoaggregates formation. [98] Following the similar mechanism, other gold nanostructures such as nanorods and nanoshells can also be used in PDT to enhance ROS formation.

Wang et al. conjugated rose bengal (RB) molecules with gold nanorods (GNRs) (average diameter and length are 13 ± 2 nm and 52 ± 4 nm, respectively), which exhibited efficient singlet oxygen generation when illuminated by 532 nm green light and high photothermal efficiency under 810 nm near-infrared (NIR) irradiation. Significant anticancer effects were observed from the RB-GNRs during combined photothermal and photodynamic therapy, as confirmed *in vitro* and *in vivo* using hamster cheek pouch as the animal model. [99]

Kah et al. reported their study about the use of gold nanoshells (a silica core radius of 81 nm and gold shell thickness of 23 nm) conjugated to anti-epidermal growth factor receptor as a photothermal agent and PDT using hypericin as the photosensitizer, which proved to be an effective treatment strategy. Compared to PDT and PTT alone that can reduce cell viability to 30.9% and 44.0% respectively, a combined treatment regime under a single irradiation (light dose of 1.44 J/cm^2) can further reduce the cell viability to 17.5%. [100]

Clearly, gold nanostructures have demonstrated not only as extraordinary carriers for delivery of therapeutics with better targeting and intracellular trafficking, but also as efficient radiosensitizer, providing enhanced SPR effect or thermal effects with appropriate light irradiation. Despite the negligible cytotoxicity, a judicious choice of the size and functionalization of the gold nanostructures is a prerequisite for their use in various biomedical applications. Future efforts are needed to design and functionalize gold nanostructures with enhanced bioavailability, less immunogenicity and high system retention *in vivo*. [101]

2.3.1.4. Self-illuminating Nanoparticles

When the nanoparticles have persistent luminescence, instead of using light as irradiating source, scintillation luminescence can emit from the nanoparticles upon exposure to ionizing radiation such as X-rays, and activate the attached photosensitizers to produce singlet oxygen. These so-called self-illuminating nanoparticles can be used for PDT treatment with the combination of radiation therapy of cancer. For example, BaFBr:Eu2+:Mn2+ nanoparticles excited by X rays have three emission bands, peaking at approximately 400, 500 and 640 nm, which is well matched to the absorption spectrum of hematoporphyrin. [102] Compared to the conventional radiation therapy, lower dose of radiation may be sufficient for PDT application.

However, direct application of these self-illuminating nanoparticles in biological systems has not yet been reported. [102]

2.3.1.5. Upconverting Nanoparticles

Upconversion (UC) refers to a family of nonlinear optical processes in which the sequential absorption of two or more photons leads to the emission of light at shorter wavelength than the excitation wavelength (anti-Stokes-type emission). [40] Upconverting nanoparticles (UCN) are such a type of nanometer-sized composites that can generate higher energy light (shorter wavelength) from lower energy radiation (longer wavelength), usually near-infrared (NIR) or infrared (IR) (Figure 3d). [103]

The UCN themselves are unable to generate $^1O_2$ from dissolved oxygen. Nevertheless, with an appropriate photosensitizer attached, and if the excitation band of the photosensitizer is matching the emission of UCN, the UCN can serve as nanotransducer to activate photosensitizer under low energy light irradiation. This phenomenon owns particular advantages in extending PDT to deep tumor sites, that is, several centimeters below the skin/mucosal surface, as the excitation light in NIR range is known to penetrate human tissues deeply. [21, 104]

UCN can be synthesized using several different ionic materials—usually rare earth ions like lanthanides and actinides-doped in a suitable crystalline matrix. Sodium yttrium fluoride (NaYF4) is being increasingly used as the core material of choice for UCNs with biological applications.

In a recent review, Wang et al. summarized the latest progress regarding the applications of UCNs for PDT. [104] Guo et al. studied the photodynamic effect of UCNs loaded with photosensitizer zinc (II)-phthalocyanine on murine bladder cancer cells (MB49). Mesoporous silica was coated onto NaYF4 upconversion nanocrystals to form a core-shell structure and then photosensitizer zinc (II)-phthalocyanine was loaded into the porous silica. The nanoparticles displayed a uniform spherical shape with an average diameter of about 50 nm and showed good dispersibility in water. Upon irradiation with 980-nm NIR light, their efficiency in activating the loaded zinc (II)-phthalocyanine to generate $^1O_2$ was confirmed in live cells. A laser power at 0.5 W and an irradiation time of 5 min were needed to induce significant cell death. [105]

In another report, Shan et al. increased the loading ratio of meso-tetraphenyl porphine photosensitizer molecules on NaYF4:Yb3+, Er3+ UCNs to be about 10 wt. % by encapsulating 100 nm UCNs and photosensitizers in biocompatible poly(ethylene gly-col-block-(DL)lactic acid) (PEG-b-PLA) block copolymers via the Flash NanoPrecipitation (FNP) process. A sterically stabilizing PEG layer on the composite nanoparticle surface prevents nanoparticle aggregation and ensures nanoparticle stability. The composite nanoparticles were shown to exhibit low dark toxicity and efficient HeLa cervical cancer cell-killing activity (75% cell death) upon NIR excitation by 980-nm irradiation at 134 W/cm^2 for 45 min. [106]

CONCLUSION AND FUTURE DIRECTIONS

PDT has been around for the past 100 years and has been an experimental clinical modality for the past two decades. Overall, PDT has the potential of being a palliative therapy or a primary therapy, depending on the specific indications. In the future, it is likely that PDT will continue to be used as a stand-alone modality or in combination with other strategies such as chemotherapy, surgery, or radiotherapy. Researchers are now investigating the ability to improve PDT including the development of new photosensitizers and the optimization of PDT protocols such as fractionation of light. The advent and advancement of nanotechnology, though still on its early stage, has also introduced many potentially exciting and revolutionary solutions to address the unmet challenges confronting with current PDT. In particular, the high surface/volume ratios, deep tissue penetration, versatile surface chemistry for modification, and distinct optical and magnetic properties have empowered various nanoparticles with potentials to enhance the efficacy and improve the specificity of PDT. The use of nanostructures as delivery vehicles for photosensitizers in PDT can improve the overall pharmacokinetics and biodistribution of traditional photosensitizer drugs, while significantly reducing the unwanted side effects. Meanwhile, these nanostructures can also be modified with chemical and/or biochemical moieties, which bind specifically to the targeted tissues for better confinement of the treatment to the diseased tissues. Besides their function for drug carrier and targeting capability, some nanostructures themselves can act as active reagents during photodynamic reaction as a result of their inherent optical and dielectric properties, magnetic susceptibility, thermal or electrical conductivity.

Along with the exploration of those advantageous properties, more attention needs to be paid to their biodistribution and biosafety prior to clinical applications of nanoparticles. The bulk properties of materials with known interaction profile with biological system cannot be simply translated to the materials on the nanoscale. As a matter of fact, the small size of nanoparticles allows them to penetrate into tissue and accumulate inside the cells, and the large surface area would lead to more interactions between nanoparticles and cells as well as the intracellular organelles. Nanoparticles have much larger surface area to unit mass ratio, which in some cases may lead to greater proinflammatory effects. [107, 108] The cellular response to nanomaterials is often dependent on the concentration of nanomaterials and is related to other physicochemical properties such as size and geometries, further complicating the studies on the interaction between biological system and nanoparticles. To this end, the systematic studies on the interaction between nanoparticles and biological system as well as comprehensive understanding of 1) the cellular uptake mechanism and intracellular destination, 2) biological distribution and clearance, and 3) short- and long-term toxicity of nanomaterials, can help to better design the PDT strategy.

In addition, insightful understanding of the underlying mechanism between light and nanoparticle interactions will also formulate the basis to develop new photodynamic systems. As many nanoparticles can potentially be used as antenna systems or even as light sources themselves to exert their photosensitizing action for phototherapeutic applications, more detailed studies on their physicochemical properties upon different light irradiation are necessary to utilize the full potential of those functional nanoparticles.

REFERENCES

[1] Ackroyd R, Kelty C, Brown N, Reed M. The history of photodetection and photodynamic therapy. Photochem. Photobiol. 2001;74(5):656–69.

[2] Dougherty TJ, Gomer CJ, Henderson BW, et al. Photodynamic therapy. *J. Natl. Cancer Inst.* 1998;90(12):889–905.

[3] Yang Y, Wang H. Perspectives of nanotechnology in minimally invasive therapy of breast cancer. *J. Healthc. Eng.* 2013;4(1):67–86.

[4] Yang Y, Wang H. Applications of nanomaterials for cancer treatment: recent patents review. *Recent Patents Nanomed.* 2013, 3(2): 75–82.

[5] Agostinis P, Berg K, Cengel KA, et al. Photodynamic therapy of cancer: an update. *CA Cancer J Clin.* 2011, 61(4): 250–81.

[6] Huang Z. A review of progress in clinical photodynamic therapy. *Technol. Cancer Res. Treat.* 2005;4(3):283–93.

[7] Dhaneshwar S, Patil K, Bulbule M, et al. Photodynamic Therapy for Cancer. *Int. J. Pharm. Sci. Rev. Res.* 2014;27(20):125–141.

[8] Usuda J, Kato H, Okunaka T, et al. Photodynamic therapy (PDT) for lung cancers. *J. Thorac. Oncol.* 2006;1(5):489–93.

[9] Dolmans DEJGJ, Fukumura D, Jain RK. Photodynamic therapy for cancer. *Nat. Rev. Cancer.* 2003;3(5):380–7.

[10] Sibata CH, Colussi VC, Oleinick NL, Kinsella TJ. Photodynamic therapy: a new concept in medical treatment. *Brazilian J. Med. Biol. Res.* 2000;33(8):869–880.

[11] Josefsen LB, Boyle RW. Unique diagnostic and therapeutic roles of porphyrins and phthalocyanines in photodynamic therapy, imaging and theranostics. *Theranostics.* 2012;2(9):916–66.

[12] Josefsen LB, Boyle RW. Photodynamic therapy and the development of metal-based photosensitisers. *Met. Based. Drugs.* 2008;2008:276109.

[13] Wachowska M, Muchowicz A, Firczuk M, et al. Aminolevulinic acid (ala) as a prodrug in photodynamic therapy of cancer. *Molecules.* 2011;16(5):4140–4164.

[14] Monge-fuentes V, Muehlmann LA, Azevedo RB De. Perspectives on the application of nanotechnology in photodynamic therapy for the treatment of melanoma. *Nano Rev.* 2014;1(5): 24381.

[15] Master A, Livingston M, Gupta A Sen. Photodynamic nanomedicine in the treatment of solid tumors: perspectives and challenges. *J.Control Release.* 2014;168(1):88–102.

[16] Pushpan SK, Venkatraman S, Anand VG, et al. Porphyrins in photodynamic therapy - a search for ideal photosensitizers. *Curr. Med. Chem. Anticancer. Agents.* 2002; 2(2):187–207.

[17] Brancaleon L, Moseley H. Laser and non-laser light sources for photodynamic therapy. *Lasers Med. Sci.* 2002;17:173–186.

[18] Clark C, Bryden a, Dawe R, et al. Topical 5-aminolaevulinic acid photodynamic therapy for cutaneous lesions: outcome and comparison of light sources. *Photodermatol. Photoimmunol. Photomed.* 2003;19(3):134–41.

[19] Hörfelt C, Stenquist B, Larkö O, Faergemann J, Wennberg A-M. Photodynamic therapy for acne vulgaris: a pilot study of the dose-response and mechanism of action. *Acta Derm. Venereol.* 2007;87(4):325–9.

[20] Weissleder R. A clearer vision for in vivo imaging. *Nat. Biotechnol.* 2001;19(4):316–7.

[21] Idris NM, Gnanasammandhan MK, Zhang J, et al. In vivo photodynamic therapy using upconversion nanoparticles as remote-controlled nanotransducers. *Nat. Med.* 2012;18(10):1580–5.

[22] Santosa V, Limantara L. Review photodynamic therapy : new light in medicine world. *Indo. J. Chem.* 2008;8(2):279–291.

[23] Huang Z, Xu H, Meyers AD, et al. Photodynamic therapy for treatment of solid tumors-potential and technical challenges. *Technol Cancer Res Treat.* 2008;7(4):309–320.

[24] Hasan T, Moor ACE, Ortel B. Photodynamic therapy of cancer cancer medicine. 2000. *Hamilton: B.C. Decker Inc*; 489–502.502 *Holland JF, Frei E* (eds).

[25] Castano AP, Demidova TN, Hamblin MR. Mechanisms in photodynamic therapy: part one-photosensitizers, photochemistry and cellular localization Ana. *Photodiagnosis Photodyn Ther.* 2004;1(4):279–293.

[26] Wilson BC, Patterson MS. The physics, biophysics and technology of photodynamic therapy. *Phys. Med. Biol.* 2008;53(9):R61–109.

[27] Castano AP, Mroz P, Hamblin MR. Photodynamic therapy and anti-tumour immunity Ana. *Nat Rev Cancer.* 2010;6(7):535–545.

[28] Mroz P, Yaroslavsky A, Kharkwal GB, et al. Cell death pathways in photodynamic therapy of cancer. *Cancers (Basel).* 2011;3(2):2516–39.

[29] Oleinick NL, Morris RL, Belichenko I. The role of apoptosis in response to photodynamic therapy: what, where, why, and how. *Photochem. Photobiol. Sci.* 2002;1(1):1–21.

[30] Odeh AM, Craik JD, Ezzeddine R, et al. Targeting mitochondria by Zn(II)N-alkylpyridylporphyrins: the impact of compound sub-mitochondrial partition on cell respiration and overall photodynamic efficacy. *PLoS One.* 2014;9(9):e108238.

[31] Rosenkranz AA, Jans DA, Sobolev AS. Targeted intracellular delivery of photosensitizers to enhance photodynamic efficiency. *Immunol. Cell Biol.* 2000;78(4):452–64.

[32] Wilson BC, Olivo M, Singh G. Subcellular localization of Photofrin and aminolevulinic acid and photodynamic cross-resistance in vitro in radiation-induced fibrosarcoma cells sensitive or resistant to photofrin-mediated photodynamic therapy. *Photochem. Photobiol.* 1997;65(1):166–76.

[33] Hopper C. Photodynamic therapy: a clinical reality in the treatment of cancer. *Lancet Oncol.* 2000;1(4):212–219.

[34] Svensson J, Johansson A, Gräfe S, et al. Tumor selectivity at short times following systemic administration of a liposomal temoporfin formulation in a murine tumor model. *Photochem. Photobiol.* 2007;83(5):1211–9.

[35] Petersen BT, Chuttani R, Croffie J, et al. Photodynamic therapy for gastrointestinal disease. *Gastrointest. Endosc.* 2006;63(7):927–32.

[36] Van den Bergh H. On the evolution of some endoscopic light delivery systems for photodynamic therapy. *Endoscopy.* 1998;30(4):392–407.

[37] Allison RR, Downie GH, Cuenca R, et al. Photosensitizers in clinical PDT. *Photodiagnosis Photodyn. Ther.* 2004;1(1):27–42.

[38]   Wang A, Long L, Zhang C. Synthesis and properties of photo-activable phthalocyanines: a brief overview. *J. Incl. Phenom. Macrocycl. Chem.* 2011;71(1-2):1–24.

[39]   Chatterjee DK, Fong LS, Zhang Y. Nanoparticles in photodynamic therapy: an emerging paradigm. *Adv. Drug Deliv. Rev.* 2008;60(15):1627–37.

[40]   Huang Y-Y, Sharma SK, Dai T, et al. Can nanotechnology potentiate photodynamic therapy? *Nanotechnol. Rev.* 2012;1(2):111–146.

[41]   Allison RR, Mota HC, Bagnato VS, et al. Bio-nanotechnology and photodynamic therapy--state of the art review. *Photodiagnosis Photodyn. Ther.* 2008;5(1):19–28.

[42]   Zhang L, Gu FX, Chan JM, et al. Nanoparticles in medicine: therapeutic applications and developments. 2008;83(5):761–769.

[43]   Yu MK, Park J, Jon S. Targeting strategies for multifunctional nanoparticles in cancer imaging and therapy. *Theranostics.* 2012; 2(1):3–44.

[44]   Ruoslahti E, Bhatia SN, Sailor MJ. Targeting of drugs and nanoparticles to tumors. *J. Cell Biol.* 2010;188(6):759–68.

[45]   Danhier F, Feron O, Préat V. To exploit the tumor microenvironment: Passive and active tumor targeting of nanocarriers for anti-cancer drug delivery. *J. Control. Release.* 2010;148(2):135–46.

[46]   Jokerst J V, Lobovkina T, Zare RN, Gambhir SS. Nanoparticle PEGylation for imaging and therapy. *Nanomedicine (Lond).* 2012;6(4):715–728.

[47]   Olivo M, Bhuvaneswari R, Lucky SS, Dendukuri N, Soo-Ping Thong P. Targeted therapy of cancer using photodynamic therapy in combination with multi-faceted anti-tumor modalities. *Pharmaceuticals.* 2010;3(5):1507–1529.

[48]   Konan YN, Gurny R, Allémann E. State of the art in the delivery of photosensitizers for photodynamic therapy. *J. Photochem. Photobiol. B.* 2002;66(2):89–106.

[49]   Derycke AS, de Witte PA. Liposomes for photodynamic therapy. *Adv. Drug Deliv. Rev.* 2004;56(1):17–30.

[50]   Schiener M, Hossann M, Viola JR, et al. Nanomedicine-based strategies for treatment of atherosclerosis. *Trends Mol. Med.* 2014;20(5):271–81.

[51]   Reshetov V, Lassalle H-P, François A, et al. Photodynamic therapy with conventional and PEGylated liposomal formulations of mTHPC (temoporfin): comparison of treatment efficacy and distribution characteristics in vivo. *Int. J. Nanomedicine.* 2013;8:3817–31.

[52]   Gijsens A, Derycke A, Missiaen L, et al. Targeting of the photocytotoxic compound AlPcS4 to Hela cells by transferrin conjugated PEG-liposomes. *Int. J. Cancer.* 2002;101(1):78–85.

[53]   Takeuchi Y, Ichikawa K, Yonezawa S, et al. Intracellular target for photosensitization in cancer antiangiogenic photodynamic therapy mediated by polycation liposome. *J. Control. Release.* 2004;97(2):231–40.

[54]   Vannostrum C. Polymeric micelles to deliver photosensitizers for photodynamic therapy. *Adv. Drug Deliv. Rev.* 2004;56(1):9–16.

[55]   Gibot L, Lemelle A, Till U, et al. Polymeric micelles encapsulating photosensitizer: structure/photodynamic therapy efficiency relation. *Biomacromolecules.* 2014;15(4):1443–55.

[56] Li B, Moriyama EH, Li F, et al. Diblock copolymer micelles deliver hydrophobic protoporphyrin IX for photodynamic therapy. *Photochem. Photobiol.* 2007;83(6):1505–12.

[57] Master AM, Rodriguez ME, Kenney ME, et al. Delivery of the Photosensitizer Pc 4 in PEG - PCL Micelles for In Vitro PDT Studies. 2010;99(5):2386–2398.

[58] Rijcken CJF, Hofman J-W, van Zeeland F, et al. Photosensitiser-loaded biodegradable polymeric micelles: preparation, characterisation and in vitro PDT efficacy. *J. Control. Release.* 2007;124(3):144–53.

[59] Kim H, Mun S, Choi Y. Photosensitizer-conjugated polymeric nanoparticles for redox-responsive fluorescence imaging and photodynamic therapy. *J. Mater. Chem. B.* 2013;1(4):429.

[60] Grimland JL, Wu C, Ramoutar RR, et al. Photosensitizer-doped conjugated polymer nanoparticles with high cross-sections for one- and two-photon excitation. *Nanoscale.* 2011;3(4):1451–5.

[61] Kamaly N, Xiao Z, Valencia PM, et al. Targeted polymeric therapeutic nanoparticles: design, development and clinical translation. *Chem. Soc. Rev.* 2012;41(7):2971–3010.

[62] Wang S, Gao R, Zhou F, et al. Nanomaterials and singlet oxygen photosensitizers: potential applications in photodynamic therapy. *J. Mater. Chem.* 2004;14(4):487.

[63] Fadel M, Kassab K, Fadeel DA. Zinc phthalocyanine-loaded PLGA biodegradable nanoparticles for photodynamic therapy in tumor-bearing mice. *Lasers Med. Sci.* 2010;25(2):283–72.

[64] Lee SJ, Park K, Oh Y-K, et al. Tumor specificity and therapeutic efficacy of photosensitizer-encapsulated glycol chitosan-based nanoparticles in tumor-bearing mice. *Biomaterials.* 2009;30(15):2929–39.

[65] Shiah JG, Sun Y, Peterson CM, et al. Antitumor activity of N-(2-hydroxypropyl) methacrylamide copolymer-Mesochlorine e6 and adriamycin conjugates in combination treatments. *Clin. Cancer Res.* 2000;6(3):1008–15.

[66] Hongrapipat J, Kopec P. articles Combination chemotherapy and photodynamic therapy with fab′ fragment targeted HPMA copolymer conjugates in human ovarian carcinoma cells. 2008;3(5):351–362.

[67] Gupta A, Wang S, Marko A, et al. Polyacrylamide-based biocompatible nanoplatform enhances the tumor uptake, PET/fluorescence imaging and anticancer activity of a chlorophyll analog. *Theranostics.* 2014;4(6):614–28.

[68] Kojima C, Toi Y, Harada A, et al. Preparation of poly(ethylene glycol)-attached dendrimers encapsulating photosensitizers for application to photodynamic therapy. *Bioconjug. Chem.* 2007;18(3):663–70.

[69] Moses B. Emerging Strategies for controlling drug release by using visible/near IR light. *Med. Chem. (Los. Angeles).* 2013;03(02):192–198.

[70] You J-O, Almeda D, Ye GJ, et al. Bioresponsive matrices in drug delivery. *J. Biol. Eng.* 2010;4(1):15.

[71] Fomina N, Sankaranarayanan J, Almutairi A. Photochemical mechanisms of light-triggered release from nanocarriers. *Adv. Drug Deliv. Rev.* 2012;64(11):1005–20.

[72] He J, Chen J-Y, Wang P, et al. Poly(N -isopropylacrylamide)-coated thermo-responsive nanoparticles for controlled delivery of sulfonated Zn-phthalocyanine in Chinese hamster ovary cells in vitro and zebra fish in vivo. *Nanotechnology.* 2007;18(41):415101.

[73] Xu W, Ling P, Zhang T. Polymeric micelles, a promising drug delivery system to enhance bioavailability of poorly water-soluble drugs. *J. Drug Deliv.* 2013;2013:340315.

[74] Li Y, Wang J, Wientjes MG, Au JL-S. Delivery of nanomedicines to extracellular and intracellular compartments of a solid tumor. *Adv. Drug Deliv. Rev.* 2012;64(1):29–39.

[75] Ling D, Park W, Park S-J, et al. Multifunctional tumor pH-sensitive self-assembled nanoparticles for bimodal imaging and treatment of resistant heterogeneous tumors. *J. Am. Chem. Soc.* 2014;136(15):5647–55.

[76] Yavlovich A, Smith B, Gupta K, et al. Light-sensitive lipid-based nanoparticles for drug delivery: design principles and future considerations for biological applications. *Mol Membr Biol.* 2010;27(7):364–381.

[77] Bisby RH, Mead C, Mitchell AC, et al. Fast laser-induced solute release from liposomes sensitized with photochromic lipid: effects of temperature, lipid host, and sensitizer concentration. *Biochem. Biophys. Res. Commun.* 1999;262(2):406–10.

[78] Roeder B, Hackbarth S, Woehlecke G. Dendrimer-photosensitizer complexes for medical applications. WO2001008704 A2, 2001.

[79] Couleaud P, Morosini V, Frochot C, et al. Silica-based nanoparticles for photodynamic therapy applications. *Nanoscale.* 2010;2(7):1057.

[80] Tang L, Cheng J. Nonporous silica nanoparticles for nanomedicine application. *Nano Today.* 2013;8(3):290–312.

[81] Zhang R, Wu C, Tong L, et al. Multifunctional core-shell nanoparticles as highly efficient imaging and photosensitizing agents. *Langmuir.* 2009;25(17):10153–8.

[82] Guo Y, Rogelj S, Zhang P. Rose Bengal-decorated silica nanoparticles as photosensitizers for inactivation of gram-positive bacteria. *Nanotechnology.* 2010;21(6):065102.

[83] Juzenas P, Chen W, Sun Y-P, et al. Quantum dots and nanoparticles for photodynamic and radiation therapies of cancer. *Adv Drug Deliv Rev.* 2009;60(15):1600–1614.

[84] Malik P, Gulia S, Kakkar R. Quantum dots for diagnosis of cancers. *Adv. Mat. Lett.* 2013;4(11):811–822.

[85] Morosini V, Bastogne T, Frochot C, et al. Quantum dot-folic acid conjugates as potential photosensitizers in photodynamic therapy of cancer. *Photochem. Photobiol. Sci.* 2011;10(5):842–51.

[86] Markovic ZM, Ristic BZ, Arsikin KM, et al. Graphene quantum dots as autophagy-inducing photodynamic agents. *Biomaterials.* 2012;33(29):7084–92.

[87] Ge J, Lan M, Zhou B, et al. A graphene quantum dot photodynamic therapy agent with high singlet oxygen generation. *Nat. Commun.* 2014;5:1–8.

[88] Rakovich A, Savateeva D, Rakovich T, et al. CdTe Quantum Dot/Dye Hybrid System as Photosensitizer for Photodynamic Therapy. *Nanoscale Res. Lett.* 2010;5(4):753–60.

[89] Ho Y-P, Leong KW. Quantum dot-based theranostics. *Nanoscale.* 2010;2(1):60–8.

[90] Yildirimer L, Thanh NTK, Loizidou M, Seifalian AM. Toxicology and clinical potential of nanoparticles. *Nano Today.* 2011;6(6):585–607.

[91] Ismail AFM, Ali MM, Ismail LFM. Photodynamic therapy mediated antiproliferative activity of some metal-doped ZnO nanoparticles in human liver adenocarcinoma HepG2 cells under UV irradiation. *J. Photochem. Photobiol. B.* 2014;138:99–108.

[92]   Fakhar-e-Alam M, Ali SMU, Ibupoto ZH, et al. Sensitivity of A-549 human lung cancer cells to nanoporous zinc oxide conjugated with Photofrin. *Lasers Med. Sci.* 2012;27(3):607–14.

[93]   Fakhar-e-Alam M, Kishwar S, Willander M. Photodynamic effects of zinc oxide nanowires in skin cancer and fibroblast. *Lasers Med. Sci.* 2014;29(3):1189–94.

[94]   Li Z, Yang R, Yu M, et al. Cellular level biocompatibility and biosafety of ZnO nanowires. *J. Phys. Chem. C.* 2008;112(51):20114–20117.

[95]   Zhang H, Shi R, Xie A, et al. Novel TiO2/PEGDA hybrid hydrogel prepared in situ on tumor cells for effective photodynamic therapy. *ACS Appl. Mater. Interfaces.* 2013;5(23):12317–22.

[96]   Oo MKK, Yang X, Du H, et al. 5-aminolevulinic acid-conjugated gold nanoparticles for photodynamic therapy of cancer. *Nanomedicine.* 2008;3(6):777–86.

[97]   Oo MKK, Yang Y, Hu Y, et al. Gold nanoparticle-enhanced and size-dependent generation of reactive oxygen species from protoporphyrin IX. *ACS Nano.* 2012;6(3):1939–47.

[98]   Yang Y, Hu Y, Du H, et al. Intracellular gold nanoparticle aggregation and their potential applications in photodynamic therapy. *Chem. Commun. (Camb).* 2014;50(55):7287–90.

[99]   Wang B, Wang J-H, Liu Q, et al. Rose-bengal-conjugated gold nanorods for in vivo photodynamic and photothermal oral cancer therapies. *Biomaterials.* 2014;35(6):1954–66.

[100] Kah JCY, Wan RCY, Wong KY, et al. Combinatorial treatment of photothermal therapy using gold nanoshells with conventional photodynamic therapy to improve treatment efficacy: an in vitro study. *Lasers Surg. Med.* 2008;40(8):584–9.

[101] Tiwari P, Vig K, Dennis V, Singh S. Functionalized Gold Nanoparticles and Their Biomedical Applications. *Nanomaterials.* 2011;1(1):31–63.

[102] Chen W, Zhang J. Using nanoparticles to enable simultaneous radiation and photodynamic therapies for cancer treatment. *J. Nanosci. Nanotechnol.* 2006;6(4):1159–66.

[103] Idris NM, Jayakumar MKG, Bansal A, Zhang Y. Upconversion nanoparticles as versatile light nanotransducers for photoactivation applications. *Chem. Soc. Rev.* 2014.

[104] Wang C, Cheng L, Liu Z. Upconversion nanoparticles for photodynamic therapy and other cancer therapeutics. *Theranostics.* 2013;3(5):317–30.

[105] Guo H, Qian H, Idris NM, Zhang Y. Singlet oxygen-induced apoptosis of cancer cells using upconversion fluorescent nanoparticles as a carrier of photosensitizer. *Nanomedicine.* 2010;6(3):486–95.

[106] Shan J, Budijono SJ, Hu G, et al. Pegylated composite nanoparticles containing upconverting phosphors and meso-tetraphenyl porphine (TPP) for photodynamic therapy. *Adv. Funct. Mater.* 2011;21(13):2488–2495.

[107] Buzea C, Pacheco II, Robbie K. Nanomaterials and nanoparticles: sources and toxicity. *Biointerphases.* 2007;2(4):MR17–71.

[108] De Jong WH, Borm PJA. Drug delivery and nanoparticles:applications and hazards. *Int. J. Nanomedicine.* 2008;3(2):133–49.

In: Photodynamic Therapy
Editor: Adrian G. Hugo

ISBN: 978-1-63463-857-9
© 2015 Nova Science Publishers, Inc.

Chapter 3

THE MECHANISM OF ACTION OF TOPICAL DERMATOLOGICAL PHOTODYNAMIC THERAPY

Alison Curnow and Jessica Tyrrell*

European Centre for Environment and Human Health, University of Exeter, UK

ABSTRACT

Evidence indicates that good clinical outcomes and excellent cosmesis can be achieved with topical dermatological photodynamic therapy (PDT) when treating licensed superficial malignant and premalignant lesions with protoporphyrin IX (PpIX) precursors. Topical dermatological PDT protocols have been standardised for clinical practice to good effect but the mechanism of action underlying the photodynamic process is complex and opportunities still exist to further improve outcomes and widen the application of this modality.

By providing copious amounts of PpIX precursors exogenously it is possible to manipulate the innate capacity of neoplastic cells to synthesise and accumulate PpIX more rapidly than their surrounding normal cells. This naturally occurring photosensitiser (PpIX) can then be activated by red light of 635 nm to produce (in the presence of molecular oxygen) necrosis and apoptosis via Type I and II photochemical reactions. Non-invasive monitoring of PpIX fluorescence and oxygen saturation during clinical PDT of licensed dermatological lesions has provided increased understanding of this process *in situ*, thus identifying opportunities for further improvement.

INTRODUCTION

Photodynamic therapy (PDT) requires three key components for a successful clinical effect – a photosensitiser, activating light of a specific wavelength and molecular oxygen [1]. When combined concurrently in sufficient amounts these components result in the production of reactive oxygen species (ROS) and oxidative stress [2]. The absence of any one of the

---

* Corresponding author. University or Exeter Medical School, Knowledge Spa, Royal Cornwall Hospital, Truro, Cornwall, TR1 3HD, Tel: +44 (0)1872 256432. E-mails: a.curnow@exeter.ac.uk and j.tyrrell@exeter.ac.uk.

three components prevents the formation of ROS and thus tissue ablation [3]. This intricate process directly and indirectly damages cellular components leading to cell death through necrosis, apoptosis and/or autophagic mechanisms depending on the type of photosensitiser employed, its subcellular localisation as well as the particular dose parameters utilised [1, 4-5].

Many different types of photosensitising agents have been investigated for a variety of different clinical applications [6-8]. However within dermatology, protoporphyrin IX (PpIX)-induced PDT is most commonly utilised as topical method of localised ablation of certain non-melanoma skin cancers and precancers [9]. This form of PDT was first introduced experimentally by Malik and Lugaci in 1987 [10], with the first clinical treatments reported by Kennedy and co-workers in 1990 [11]. This approach has a number of advantages over the other photosensitising agents currently available for clinical PDT, including topical (rather than systemic) administration and reduced duration cutaneous photosensitivity, which is also limited to the treatment site with dermatological PpIX-PDT. Within a clinical setting topical PpIX-PDT now involves the application of a cream formulation containing a PpIX precursor – usually aminolaevulinic acid (ALA) or its methyl ester (MAL) – to the area to be treated. The area is then covered with a light-occluding dressing for a number of hours (usually 3 h) during which time the precursor is absorbed into the lesion and biochemically converted relatively rapidly by the diseased cells into the natural photosensitiser PpIX via haem biosynthesis. ALA or MAL applied in this way act as substrates for the production of haem and its precursors whilst avoiding the negative feedback loop that haem has on its own production.

The intermediate immediately preceding haem in the haem biosynthesis pathway is PpIX and this accumulates following ALA or MAL administration because the last step of haem biosynthesis (the insertion of ferrous iron into the porphyrin ring of PpIX by ferrochelatase to form haem) [12] is relatively slow and is in fact the secondary rate limiting step of the pathway (the primary rate limiting step being the formation of ALA by ALA synthase which is bypassed by exogenous ALA/MAL administration). Furthermore the accumulation of PpIX occurs more rapidly within (pre)cancerous lesions/cells due to their disrupted stratum corneum (facilitating better cream absorption), upregulation of the haem biosynthesis pathway within diseased cells that have greater metabolic demands as well as alterations in the expression of the porphobilinogen deaminase and ferrochelatase enzymes within the haem biosynthesis pathway [2, 4]. These factors in combination result in a window of opportunity for therapeutic light delivery (around 3 hours following cream, application), where PpIX is preferentially accumulated within the target diseased cells and as a result the surrounding normal cells are relatively spared by this localised ablative therapy [4].

Once PpIX accumulation has occurred within the tumour cells in this manner, visible light matching both the absorption spectrum of the photosensitiser (PpIX) and the optimum wavelength for tissue transmission is applied to the tumour. Normally 635 nm is utilised for all but the most superficial dermatological lesions (frequently delivered using a LED array) [13] because although PpIX is activated by several wavelengths of light (with most intense absorbance occurring at 410 nm), a longer wavelength of light (635 nm) increases efficacy because light penetration of the tissue is increased despite lower absorbance [14]. PpIX absorbs energy from the light and enters a higher singlet energy state. This absorbed energy is then either released as fluorescence as the photosensitiser returns to the ground state or is transferred via intersystem crossing to the longer lived triplet state allowing more opportunity for energy to be transferred to nearby molecules in the cell. This transfer of energy from the triplet state can occur via Type I or Type II reactions. Type II reactions involve the transfer of energy to oxygen to form singlet oxygen and this type of reaction is thought to predominate initially within the PpIX-PDT process [15]. Singlet oxygen can however subsequently transfer energy to other molecules resulting in the production of ROS cascades. If enough damage is produced, cell death can result [16]. Due to its multiple valences, iron can play an important role in these processes [17] and has the potential to increase cytotoxicity from PDT. Iron is important in the generation of the hydroxyl radical as well as in lipid peroxidation [18]. Singlet oxygen generated by PpIX-induced PDT can itself react with oxygen to generate superoxide. Superoxide is fairly stable under physiological conditions and does not readily react with other biomolecules, but its ability to generate further, more reactive ROS, makes it toxic. Superoxide is dismutated by superoxide dismutase within cells to form hydrogen peroxide, which readily diffuses through membranes (due to its uncharged nature and poor reactivity). Hydrogen peroxide is detoxified via catalase to produce water and oxygen. However if hydrogen peroxide comes into contact with metal ions (especially in the ferrous Fe^{2+} form) then the highly reactive hydroxyl radical can be formed via Fenton reactions and this can lead to damage to cellular proteins, lipids and DNA [19]. The level of cellular free iron is therefore tightly controlled by homeostatic iron regulatory proteins (IRPs) which can either act by up regulating the iron-sequestering protein ferritin or by up regulating transferrin receptor synthesis [20].

Direct killing of tumour cells in PDT has been shown to occur by both necrosis and apoptosis [21]. Necrosis results from photodamage to vital subcellular components leading to a loss of cellular function and uncontrolled cell death. In addition activation of the photosensitiser can also result in damage to the tumour vasculature. This can reduce the blood supply to the tumour resulting in hypoxia and starvation of the cells but it thought to be a lesser route of damage with PpIX-PDT. There is also evidence that autophagy (the degradation of cellular components internally) occurs following PDT [22-23]. This process, like apoptosis, is tightly controlled and depending on the level of damage, autophagy can lead to cell repair and survival or the induction of apoptosis. PDT in tumour cells has been demonstrated to result in an immediate/early form of apoptosis which occurs within 30-60 minutes of irradiation [24]. Apoptosis has two major pathways (extrinsic and intrinsic) and both can be triggered by PDT. The extrinsic pathway involves cell death ligands on the cell surface and the formation of a death-inducing signal complex on the cell membrane resulting in activation of the initiator caspase-8 [25]. This pathway is thought to be activated during PDT with photosensitisers that preferentially accumulate in the cell membrane. In PpIX-induced PDT the intrinsic pathway is thought to be more important due to PpIX localisation within mitochondria [26]. Damage to mitochondria or loss of the mitochondrial membrane potential, which may occur during PDT, may lead to an excessive release of ROS into the cytoplasm. These ROS as well as causing direct damage, may also change the redox state of the cell and initiate/modulate ROS sensitive signalling cascades in turn inducing secondary cellular damage.

Clinically, substantial subsets of skin tumours exist which are relatively difficult to treat with conventional therapies such as surgery and cryotherapy because of their size, location or number within an area of field change [27]. PDT can be advantageous in these situations and is associated with excellent cosmesis making it a particularly attractive treatment option for cosmetically conspicuous sites [28]. Standardised topical PpIX-PDT protocols utilising both

ALA (Ameluz, Spirit Healthcare, UK) and MAL (Metvix®, Galderma, UK) have been implemented within dermatology to good effect when the disease remains superficial [29] but improvement is required to treat thicker or acrally located conditions [30]. Furthermore PDT negates several other issues that commonly arise in the standard treatment of these indications, including lesion size and multiplicity as well as also resulting in a better cosmetic outcome [31].

Non-melanoma skin cancers (NMSC) and associated precancerous lesions originate from non-melanocytic cell types within the epidermis and are the most common malignancy in Caucasians [32]. In the United States more than one third of all adult cancers are NMSC, with between 900,000 to 1,200,000 new cases occurring per year [3]. Worldwide incidence is steadily increasing at a rate of 3 % − 8 % each year [33]. Although these cancers rarely metastasise, when left untreated they can cause extensive local damage to the skin and often disfigure the patient (due to their frequently prominent localisation in sun exposed areas). The treatment of NMSC and the associated precancerous lesions therefore places a huge burden on health services. Topical PDT with the application of a prodrug (aminolaevulinic acid, ALA or its methyl ester MAL) has therefore found a niche in the treatment of dermatological conditions, especially in treating NMSC and other precancerous skin lesions (e.g. basal cell carcinoma (BCC), Bowen's disease (BD) and actinic keratosis (AK)), which are all licensed indications in the UK [27]. High complete response rates are observed when treating these lesions with topical PDT and these are comparable to the standard treatment modalities of cryosurgery and surgical excision [32, 34-40]. PDT has several advantages over standard treatment for NMSC and precancerous lesions, particularly in terms of improved cosmetic outcome and the ability to easily treat large or multiple lesions, which present a greater challenge for more conventional treatments [34-38].

PpIX exhibits characteristic fluorescent properties and therefore fluorescence can be used as a diagnostic tool. PpIX exhibits red fluorescence (peak wavelengths at 635 nm and 700 nm) when excited by blue light (wavelength 410 nm) and therefore cells accumulating PpIX can be identified [41-42]. Fluorescence diagnosis in ALA-PDT can aid the identification of pre-cancerous lesions and ensure the whole lesion is properly removed during tumour excision [43-44]. The fluorescent properties of PpIX can also be exploited to follow the changes in PpIX concentration within the skin during PDT. Previously clinical changes in photosensitiser concentration during ALA or MAL induced PDT have been poorly understood. It is known that increasing photosensitiser levels in the treatment area results in better clinical outcomes when ALA is employed as the prodrug [4]. However, the ability to follow the level of PpIX within lesions throughout PDT has to date been limited by the poor reproducibility of results and numerous factors influencing fluorescence detection [31, 45]. Many parameters including tissue autofluorescence, tissue detector geometry and the absorbing and scattering properties of tissue contribute to quantification errors [46]. Previous investigations into the accumulation of PpIX due to the exogenous application of ALA or MAL have utilised invasive techniques to determine the presence and concentration of the photosensitiser within the tissues. Chemical extraction from tissues followed by high performance liquid chromatography analysis (HPLC) indicated that PpIX was the predominant porphyrin present in tumour tissue treated with ALA [47-48]. This invasive technique does not enable the photosensitizer to be followed during real-time however, it simply provides information about the concentration of the photosensitizer at one specific point following the process being terminated. It therefore has limited practical application in real-time monitoring in the clinical environment.

Whilst it is possible to conduct fluorescence imaging with a number of different setups [49] including non-commercial 'home made' systems (which are commonly used in pre-clinical and clinical PDT monitoring) [50-53] a commercially available piece of equipment (Dyaderm, Biocam, Germany) was selected here as it could be purchased internationally in a standardised format and was already utilised by several groups for photodiagnosis of skin lesions [54-55]. This is important as the majority of dermatology clinics conducting PDT treatments do not have the facilities or expertise to develop their own fluorescence imaging equipment and may simply want to be able to buy a piece of equipment for this dual purpose of fluorescence diagnosis and fluorescence monitoring or indeed use an existing piece of fluorescence diagnosis equipment for this extended use (fluorescence monitoring). Following extensive validation the Dyaderm system was considered to be capable of monitoring changes in PpIX during real-time MAL-PDT [56]. Whilst numerous factors hinder reproducibility in fluorescence imaging, it was shown that consistent application resulted in reproducible images been acquired of normal human skin [56]. This fluorescence imaging system was therefore employed to acquire colour and fluorescent images simultaneously and non-invasively to follow changes in PpIX levels in lesional and non-lesional skin during various time points of clinical PDT, following validation with an *in vitro* fluorescence standard. PpIX fluorescence accumulation and dissipation was therefore monitored in real-time during MAL-PDT treatment of licensed indications (AK, BD and sBCC) occurring within the Dermatology PDT Clinic at Royal Cornwall Hospital (Truro, UK). Investigations of this nature within the clinical setting are currently limited as monitoring PpIX fluorescence during real-time PDT treatment is not trivial, although clinically photobleaching has previously been monitored during ALA-PDT of superficial basal cell carcinomas at a variety of different fluence rates [57]. Previous *in vivo* studies have also indicated a positive correlation between PpIX photobleaching and cellular damage, indicating that greater photobleaching enhances the efficacy of the treatment [50, 58-59]. It is important to establish the clinical relationship between photobleaching and light fluence as it may further elucidate the mechanism of action of topical dermatological PDT or alternatively aid treatment enhancement in the future by highlighting when treatment is limited when utilising the current standard licensed protocol.

In addition to fluorescence imaging of PpIX levels during topical PpIX-PDT, tissue oxygenation, perfusion and patients' perception of pain have also been monitored here. The major adverse effect of MAL-PDT is known to be the pain that can be experienced by patients during light irradiation. This is localised to the treatment area but has been described as a burning, stinging or prickling sensation [3, 38, 58, 60]. It is proposed that this pain is the consequence of nerve stimulation/damage by the ROS produced on irradiation although this process is not well understood and remains uncertain [61]. Pain during PDT can be related to location, size and histological type of the lesion [62-64] as well as PpIX photobleaching and fluence rate [51, 65]. Pain reduction strategies include topical anaesthetics (e.g. Ametop which has limited efficacy [66]), nerve blocks (effective and not thought to alter clinical outcome, but usually only used for extensive treatment areas [67-68]), air cooling devices (ACD - which produce air at a temperature of -35°C to rapidly cool the treatment area) and water sprays. Water sprays and ACD devices tend to be preferred clinically due to the ease of application during nurse-led treatment delivery [58]. Previous studies have indicated that the application of an ACD during treatment does not alter treatment efficacy but significantly reduces the pain experienced during PDT treatment [69], although it is not as effective as a nerve block [70].

The critical importance of a plentiful oxygen supply during PDT (for ROS production on light activation of the photosensitiser) has long been recognised [71-73] with studies demonstrating that tumours with pre-existing hypoxia or tumours that develop hypoxia during PDT only respond with limited efficacy to PDT [74-76]. Monitoring tissue oxygenation during and after PDT therefore has the potential to enhance our understanding of the basic physiological mechanisms involved during light irradiation as well the potential to predict effectiveness as the cytotoxic effect of PDT is partly dependent on the availability of oxygen [14, 77]. Many studies (undertaken in animal models in all but one case) have utilised a variety of different techniques to monitor oxygen saturation (or the partial pressure of oxygen, pO_2) in the tissue before, during and after the light irradiation phase of PDT. Significant changes in oxygenation have been observed to occur during and after PDT, with markedly different responses noted for the different photosensitisers employed [74-75, 78-80]. A rapid decline in pO_2 immediately on the initiation of light treatment was also noted in a number of studies [76, 79, 81-82]. This rapid depletion in oxygen is attributed to the photochemical consumption of oxygen and damage to the microvasculature reducing the capacity of the circulation to replenish the tissue with oxygen [78, 83]. A steep decline in pO_2 was noted immediately after commencing light treatment in mouse and rat models treated with PpIX mediated-PDT where aminolaevulinic acid (ALA) was utilised as the topical pro-drug [79, 84], although evidence is conflicting as other studies have observed large increases in tumour oxygenation during ALA-PDT [80]. The clinical study undertaken with ALA-PDT, monitored eight nodular BCC lesions, indicating 5-20% reductions in haemoglobin saturation, which were highly dependent on the fibre position [85].

Investigations of perfusion during PpIX mediated PDT have not demonstrated unified alterations, with fluence and fluence rate influencing the perfusion alterations. Increased perfusion within BCC lesions has been observed following ALA-PDT [86], although alternative clinical studies have indicated no immediate perfusion alterations during either ALA or MAL-PDT and significant reductions in perfusion during high fluence ALA-PDT (100 Jcm^{-2}) have been observed in pre-clinical [87] and clinical studies [88]. It is therefore clear that all these parameters are both of interest and in need of further investigation when trying to further elucidate the detailed mechanism of action of topical dermatological PDT undertaken with PpIX precursors.

MATERIALS AND METHODS

Fluorescence Imaging System

A commercially available non-invasive fluorescence imaging system (Dyaderm, Biocam, Germany) was utilised to monitor PpIX fluorescence during routine dermatological MAL-PDT. The system consisted of a Xenon flash light source that has a custom bandpass filter (370-440 nm) that alternated between white and blue light (370-440 nm) and a 12-bit Sony charge coupled device (CCD) camera combined in one adjustable arm coupled to a Pentium

IV computer equipped with custom-made image capturing software (Dyaderm Pro v2, Biocam, Germany).

Seven light pulses per second were released from the camera to the area of interest, and the returning light was collected by the CCD camera (exposure time 100 µs) which utilised a special Schott GG 455 longpass filter to exclude the excitation light (370-440 nm). The light source had a low irradiance (3–5 mWcm^{-2}) and a short exposure time to minimise ROS production during light irradiation. Previous investigations within our group have shown no significant alterations in PpIX fluorescence when sequential measurements were acquired (data not shown). The red pixels of the CCD camera (spectral sensitivity of which at 630 nm is between 85% and 90%) were used to generate a fluorescence image from the red spectrum fluorescence emitted from the excited PpIX. In this way, a normal coloured image (from the white light) and a fluorescence image (from the blue light 370-440 nm) were simultaneously collected and processed by the system in real time. The images acquired were magnified by a factor of three. The software computed a "PpIX filtered" image which corrected for the heterogeneity due to imperfections in the excitation light and the natural curvature of the object imaged by combining the red and green fluorescence images. As PpIX is not the sole fluorophore within the skin to be activated by blue light (lipopigments and flavins both emit light in the green spectrum when excited with blue light), the autofluorescence was also recorded by the camera. This enabled changes in autofluorescence to be considered during real time MAL-PDT and these measurements were subtracted from the PpIX image produced to ensure the sole changes recorded resulted from changes in the concentration of the porphyrins of interest. To ensure the stability of the camera a synthetic PpIX fluorescence standard (Biocam, Germany) was imaged on each clinic day to ensure the continuity of the system.

Standard PDT Treatment and Imaging Protocol

All patients attending for their first routine MAL-PDT appointment for licensed indications (AK and biopsy proven BD and sBCC) at the Dermatology Department, Royal Cornwall Hospital (Truro, UK) were informed (both verbally and in writing) about this ethically approved study (Cornwall and Plymouth Research Ethics Committee) before giving written consent if they wanted to take part. This study was therefore, a non-interventional, non-randomised, observational study. All the lesions included were dermatological indications (AK, BD and BCC) for which MAL-PDT has been approved in the UK [27, 89]. The majority of BCC and BD lesions were biopsied prior to referral for MAL-PDT treatment; in contrast AK lesions were referred at the Consultant Dermatologist's discretion. The BCC lesions monitored were all histologically considered to be superficial (less than 0.5 mm thick) in nature following clinical observation and biopsy. Patients' lesion(s) were imaged at both their first and second clinic visits if they received more than one PDT treatment.

All patients were treated as for a normal MAL-PDT clinic. Any crust overlying the lesion prior to treatment was gently removed with curettage. The topical pro-drug MAL (commercially available as Metvix®, 160 mg/g MAL, Galderma, UK) was then applied to the lesion at approximately 1 mm thickness, with a 5 mm border. The lesion was then covered with an occlusive dressing for the three hour application period. Any excess MAL was then wiped away and the lesion irradiated with a standard light protocol (Aktilite, Photocure,

Norway, 635 +/- 5 nm, 37 Jcm^{-2}, 80 mWcm^{-2}, positioned 5-8 cm above the lesion positioned by the specialist nurse practitioner). Lesions were covered with a dressing to prevent any subsequent light exposure as the area was photosensitive for approximately 24 hours.

The patients' lesion was normally imaged at three distinct time points during the treatment process; prior to the application of MAL, after the three hour application of MAL and immediately following light irradiation. Only one lesion was imaged per patient to increase statistical power. All images were taken in accordance with our previously derived standardised operating procedure which enabled reproducible images to be acquired by limiting the other factors potentially altering image acquisition [56]. To enable the identical region to be imaged the position of the camera was marked on the patients' skin to enable replacement of the camera in the same place.

When considering PpIX fluorescence during light delivery in more detail, in addition to the three standard monitoring points described above, an extra fluorescence image was recorded at the half way stage of light irradiation or alternatively, every minute for the first half of light treatment. The images acquired during light irradiation required the treatment light to be paused prior to image acquisition as the camera could not be placed appropriately with the light in position and the wavelength of treatment light would alter the images acquired with the imaging system. Following image acquisition the light was repositioned and restarted. The light was never paused for more than sixty seconds.

Details including the patients age, gender, lesion type, location and size were all recorded prior to commencement of imaging and if the air cooling device (SmartCool, Cynosure UK Ltd, UK, which produces air at -35 °C via a hand-held nozzle to a local area as directed) available for pain relief during light delivery was utilised, this was also noted. The lesions were treated as per the National Institute of Clinical Excellence (NICE) guidelines [90] however due to clinic arrangements within the department, the second PDT treatment was conducted nine days following the first. Some superficial AK patients only received (as recommended) a single PDT treatment. When patients attended the clinic for a second treatment, images were acquired and analysed in exactly the same manner. When the treatment was complete the images were exported for further image analysis. All patients were routinely invited to attend an outpatient clinic three months after their last PDT treatment for examination by a Consultant Dermatologist.

Fluorescence Imaging Data Analysis

The images were exported as Bitmaps (640*512 pixels - to avoid data loss) and analysed in NIH ImageJ software (http://rsb.info.nih.gov/ij/). The images were analysed from the same point within the lesion, as previous studies indicated that this lowered the coefficient of variance (data not shown) and the mean grayscale values recorded for each time point, enabling quantitative analysis of PpIX levels. These data were analysed for statistical significance via either the repeated measures ANOVA or the paired student's t-test, comparing and contrasting the fluorescence changes observed during the first and second PDT treatment cycles, the distribution of the photosensitiser and any possible relationships between changes in accumulation/dissipation and patient gender, patient age and lesion size. However, our studies have indicated (data not shown) that patient gender and age do not appear to contribute significantly to the changes in PpIX levels observed. Fluorescence distribution was also monitored in all lesions by measuring the grayscale values at fourteen locations spiralling out from the lesion centre.

Clinical Outcome Analysis

All patients attended an outpatient clinic three months after their last PDT treatment and the lesions were visually assessed by a Consultant Dermatologist who was blinded to the fluorescence imaging results. The outcome reported was based on the initial assessment of the lesion entered in the notes, which included details of the lesion size and an image of the lesion prior to treatment. If no clinical evidence of the tumour remained at three months then the lesions were considered to have undergone complete clinical clearance. Lesions that were observed to have decreased in size but where (pre)cancerous cells clearly remained were reported to have undergone a partial clearance. Lesions which remained unaltered following the one or two PDT treatments they had received were reported as no clearance.

The clinical outcomes recorded were related to the image analysis data in particular the total PpIX fluorescence recorded after the three hour MAL application and the percentage change in fluorescence intensity observed during light irradiation. For each patient the total fluorescence after the three hour application of MAL was noted and the percentage change in fluorescence during light irradiation was calculated. The values were then allotted to the appropriate group (i.e. complete, partial or no clearance) and the median values of the outcome group calculated. The analysis looked initially at the first and second MAL-PDT treatments separately and then these data were combined. These non-parametric data were analysed using the Mann Whitney U test to compare the percentage changes in fluorescence during light irradiation or total PpIX fluorescence after the three hour MAL application observed in lesions undergoing complete, partial and no clearance. Due to the low number of patients undergoing no clearance statistical analysis was only conducted between the complete and partial clearance groups. The z-test for two proportions was utilised to compare the percentage of patients within the complete and partial clearance groups that underwent a greater than 40%, 50% and 60% fluorescence change in PpIX. It should be noted that this non-interventional, non-randomised, observational study of routine dermatological MAL-PDT practice was not powered in advance as no idea of the size of change in fluorescence intensity that might be observed during clinical light irradiation was previously known or indeed how this may be related (if at all) to the clinical outcome observed at three months.

The data set collected to consider the effect of utilising the air cooling device was analysed for normality and on the basis that these data were normally distributed, parametric statistical analysis was conducted. Comparisons of PpIX accumulation and destruction between the two groups were compared utilizing an unpaired Student's t-test. Within the groups PpIX accumulation and destruction were compared with a paired Student's t-test. The non-parametric clearance data were compared with a Chi-squared test.

Fluorescence/Clinical Outcome Patient Numbers and Demographics

For the initial PpIX fluorescence studies, seventy-five patients (twenty five of each lesion type) undergoing standard MAL-PDT for licensed dermatological applications were recruited and monitored for each of their two PDT treatments (42 males and 33 females; age ranging from 46 to 98 years, mean age = 77 years), so that the PpIX fluorescence accumulation and dissipation throughout the PDT treatment process could be observed and compared between the different lesion types investigated (25 AK, 25 BD and 25 sBCC).

When considering any potential relationship between the PpIX fluorescence observations made during PDT treatment and subsequent clinical outcome at 3 months, one hundred patients were recruited (with only one lesion being monitored in each patient to limit statistical error). There was an approximately equal split in terms of the three licensed lesions (37 AK, 29 BD and 34 sBCC) and patient gender (56 males and 44 females), with the age of the patient ranging from 45 – 96 years, with an average of 77 years. The majority of patients (84 patients) received two treatments, nine days apart, to the individual lesions as per the NICE clinical guidelines [90] with the exception being superficial AK (16 patients) which only received (as recommended) a single PDT treatment.

The potential effect of the utilisation of the air cooling device (ACD) on PpIX fluorescence and subsequent clinical outcome at 3 months was elucidated by considering all patients attending clinic for standard MAL-PDT treatment to licensed indications (AK, BD and sBCC) from the 1st June 2008 until the 1st June 2009. One hundred patients (58 males and 42 females) were included within this study, with one lesion investigated per patient. The 100 lesions investigated were broken down as follows into histologically distinct lesion types; 39 AK (21 ACD, 18 No ACD), 29 sBCC (10 ACD, 19 No ACD) and 32 BD (19 ACD and 13 No ACD). These data were compared from the first fifty patients who utilised the ACD throughout irradiation and the first fifty patients not requiring any pain relief (i.e. every patient who consented for non-invasive monitoring was imaged routinely irrespective of the type of pain relief (if any) they subsequently opted for, but data was only analysed for the first fifty patients which fitted each criterion).

The influence of anatomical lesion location (including acral and non-acral sites) on PpIX fluorescence and clinical outcome at 3 months was investigated in the licensed indications (AK, BD and sBCC) treated with MAL-PDT within patients recruited at our clinic between January 2008 – December 2009. A total of two hundred patients (112 males and 88 females; age range 42-98, average = 73 years) were recruited and one lesion was monitored in each patient to limit statistical error. There was an approximately equal split in terms of the lesion localisation (104 non-acral and 96 acral, with acral defined as of, relating to, or affecting peripheral parts, such as limbs, fingers or ears) and these were further subdivided into the histologically distinct lesions (83 AK (with individual lesions monitored) (52 non-acral and 31 acral), 75 BD (21 non-acral and 54 acral) and 42 sBCC (31 non-acral and 11 acral).

For the study considering PpIX fluorescence during light delivery in more detail, fifty patients (24 males and 26 females; mean age = 73 +/- 7 years) were recruited with licensed dermatological lesions, which were due to be treated with MAL-PDT. Forty patients (17 males and 23 females; mean age = 73 +/- 8 years; 12 AK, 15 BD and 13 sBCC) were monitored at four distinct time points during treatment; prior to the application of MAL, after the three hour MAL application, at the half way stage of light irradiation and after the completion of light treatment. The remaining ten patients (7 males and 3 females; mean age = 77 +/- 8 years; 8 AK and 2 sBCC) were monitored in the same manner except during light irradiation where an image was acquired every minute for the first half of light treatment. The fluorescence changes observed during MAL-PDT were statistically analysed with a repeated measures one-way ANOVA. Direct comparison of the changes in PpIX fluorescence during light irradiation were monitored with either paired t-tests or the repeated measures one-way ANOVA. Regression analysis of the ten patients periodically monitored involved least squares linear regression and exponential decay analysis. Comparison of the photobleaching rate for complete and partial responders utilised an unpaired t-test.

Histological Assessment of Depth of PpIX Fluorescence

In an observer blinded pilot study of a single application of topical MAL to nBCC tumours, patients with a single clinically diagnosed nBCC were included into each of the five study groups (0, 30, 60, 120 or 180 minutes MAL cream application) in strict order of recruitment. All patients were recruited at the Dermatology Department, Royal Cornwall Hospital (Truro, UK) and were informed (both verbally and in writing) about this ethically approved study (Cornwall and Plymouth Research Ethics Committee) before giving written consent if they wanted to take part.

MAL cream containing 160 mg/g methyl aminolevulinate (Metvix®, Galderma, UK) was applied 1 mm thick to the nBCCs with a 5 mm margin before being covered with a sterile dressing (Tegaderm®, 3M) followed by a light occlusive dressing (Mepore®). Tumours were excised at 0, 30, 60, 120 or 180 minutes following MAL application (depending on recruitment group) and the specimens immediately transported to the histopathology department in light occluding transport bags at room temperature to avoid possible photobleaching of any PpIX present in the tumours. Prior to freezing the excised tissue was measured and processed for light microscopy by a trained dermatopathologist. Only specimens found to be nodular BCC and less than 2 mm thick on histology could be included in the study. Sectioning was carried out rapidly in a darkened room, to minimise light exposure. Sections were then mounted on an appropriate sized cork base with Optimal Cutting Temperature (OCT) mounting fluid (Tissue-Tek®, Zoeterwoude, Netherlands),and then snap frozen using chlorodifluromethane (Cryospray 22, Bright Instruments Co Ltd, Cambs, UK). After freezing sections were placed into universal containers and temporarily stored in liquid nitrogen before being transported to a -70 °C freezer for longer term storage.

On the day of imaging, frozen sections were removed from storage and transported in a dark flask of liquid nitrogen to the cryostat (Bright, OFT5000) for cutting. The cork embedded tissue was then mounted onto a cryostat chuck using OCT mounting fluid and allowed to equilibrate with the cryostat operating temperature (~ -35 °C). Once equilibrated 10 µm thick serial sections were cut from the tissue and mounted onto glass microscope slides using the Bright 5040 rotary microtome housed in the cryostat. The specimens showing the maximum depth of tumour were used for fluorescence microscopy. One section was then stained using haematoxylin and eosin. The remaining sections were coved in a tray and transported to the fluorescence microscope (Olympus BX51, Olympus, UK), which was connected to a CCD camera (Olympus DP70, Olympus, UK) and attached to a computer for capture and analysis of the acquired images. Sections were excited with light filtered between 385 nm and 425 nm (XF1008 (405DF40) filter (Omega Optical Incorporated; available from Glen Spectra, Middlesex, UK). The resultant fluorescence was filtered between 615 nm and 645 nm (XF3028 (630DF30) filter (Omega Optical Incorporated; available from Glen Spectra, Middlesex, UK). These filters were housed in a filter block with a XF2040 (435DRLP) dichroic mirror (Omega Optical Incorporated; available from Glen Spectra,

Middlesex, UK). The suitability of these filter ranges for the detection of PpIX had previously been determined in preliminary experiments using both presynthesised PpIX and PpIX produced from MAL treated cells. Images were captured at a magnification of x20 using the Olympus DP70 camera and analySIS® imaging software. The microscope light shutter was opened and an image simultaneously taken with an exposure time of 20 seconds. During this exposure all external light sources were removed and the lighting levels kept to a minimum. Haematoxylin and eosin sections were imaged using unfiltered visible light and the automatic camera settings of the analySIS® software control panel (exposure time < 1 second). A measurement was taken of the depth of fluorescence from the surface epithelium to the maximal depth within the tumour and this figure was compared with the maximum tumour depth using the H and E section for guidance. This gave a relative depth of fluorescence in each tumour, at each time interval. Fluorescence intensity was not calculated in this study.

Effect of Iron Chelation on Histological and Clinical Outcome

A parallel, open, dose-escalating, pilot study was conducted by two centres: Royal Cornwall Hospital, Truro and Forth Valley Dermatology Centre (Stirling and Falkirk Royal Infirmary). Full ethical approval was obtained for the study and the Declaration of Helsinki protocols were followed. The patients were recruited from the standard outpatient clinic. Thirty six patients (23 males and 13 females) participated in the study, with a mean age of 72 years (range: 32-88 years). This number was chosen to establish the safety of this modified formulation. Each patient had a solitary, previously untreated, nodular BCC. Twenty lesions were located on the face or neck, seven on the limbs and nine on the trunk and back. Each lesion had a minimum diameter of 5 mm and a maximum diameter of 20 mm. Patients under the age of 18 and pregnant women were excluded from the study. Patients within the child-bearing years were only included if they were able to use adequate contraceptive measures. Patients taking photoactive drugs were excluded. After written informed consent was obtained, a 3 mm punch biopsy was taken from the area within the lesion which appeared clinically to be the thickest. A 5.0 Vicryl rapide suture was used to close the biopsy site. Histology was performed on each specimen including Breslow thickness and two weeks later patients were allocated into one of the following groups in strict order of recruitment at each centre.

Six patients (3 per centre in parallel) were treated in each treatment group as follows: i) 20% ALA alone (0% CP94), ii) 20% ALA + 5% CP94, iii) 20% ALA + 10% CP94, iv) 20% ALA + 20% CP94, v) 20% ALA + 40% CP94 and vi) 40% CP94 alone (0% ALA).

The lesions were digitally photographed and measured using skin landmarks to help isolate the exact area for future excision. Each lesion received one application of topical ALA (20% ALA w/w in Unguentum Merck cream base, Crawfords Pharmaceuticals, UK) +/- the various doses of the iron chelator CP94 w/w depending on the treatment group. The various concentrations of ALA with CP94 were made up in the pharmacy of each hospital under strict protocol, no more than 1 hour prior to application to the lesion. No prior lesion preparation was performed and approximately 2 mm thickness of the cream was applied to the whole lesion and a 5 mm rim of surrounding normal skin, using a wooden spatula. The lesion was then covered with an occlusive dressing (Tegaderm®, 3M, Loughborough, UK) followed by a light occlusive Mepore® dressing as per the standard protocol for ALA-PDT. Six hours following application of the cream, the lesion was illuminated by a filtered narrow-band (630 nm +/-15 nm) red xenon light source (Photo Therapeutics Limited, UK, 100 J/cm^2, <130 mW/cm^2). Six hours is the standard preillumination interval for ALA-PDT for BCC up to 2 mm thick [91]. This activating red light was delivered, in a continuous manner to the entire lesion and to at least a 5 mm margin of adjacent skin. The treatment regime employed, apart from the incorporation of the CP94, was therefore the same as our standard dermatological ALA-PDT protocol. In all cases, at 6 weeks following the single PDT treatment, clinical response rate was assessed and surgical excision of the whole treatment site was undertaken for histology. Previous photographs, skin landmarks and precise measurements were used to ensure exact excision margins. Histolological examination was carried out on each specimen by the one dermatopathologist at each centre, using transverse bread slice histological examination and maximum Breslow thickness of the tumour was measured. The dermatopathologists were blinded in that they received the specimens without knowledge of the treatments received.

In an extension to the above investigation, a further clinical pilot study of MAL-induced-PpIX enhancement by CP94 was undertaken at Royal Cornwall Hospital (Truro, UK) alone. Full ethical approval was obtained for the study and the Declaration of Helsinki protocols were followed. The patients were recruited from the standard outpatient clinic. Twelve patients participated in the study (4 males and 8 females), with a mean age of 79 years (range: 54-93 years). This number was chosen to establish the safety of this modified MAL (Metvix®, Galderma, UK) formulation. All procedures were conducted as outlined above except three patients were recruited into the following treatment groups: i) MAL alone (0% CP94); ii) MAL + 20% CP94, iii) MAL + 30% CP94 and iv) MAL + 40% CP94.

Each lesion therefore received one application of topical Metvix® (Galderma, UK) +/- the various doses of CP94 (depending on treatment group). Three hours following application of the cream, the lesions were illuminated with an Aktilite (Galderma, UK) LED light array (37 J/cm^2, 635 nm +/- 2 nm). This activating red light was delivered in a continuous manner to the entire lesion and to at least a 5 mm margin of adjacent skin. The treatment regime employed, apart from the incorporation of CP94, was therefore the same as our standard dermatological MAL-PDT protocol. Once more, 6 weeks following the single PDT treatment, clinical response rate was assessed and surgical excision of the whole treatment site was undertaken for histology.

Effect of Wavelength on PDT Effect *In Vivo*

ALA powder (ALA.HCl, 99% purity, DUSA Pharmaceuticals, Inc., New York, USA) was dissolved in physiological strength phosphate-buffered saline (PBS, pH 2.8) and administered intravenously (with a concentration of 50 mg/ml and a maximum volume of 0.2 ml) to normal, female, Wistar rats (120 - 200 g; supplied by the Imperial Cancer Research Fund, London, UK) 75 minutes prior to surgery. The animals were anaesthetised for all parts of the procedure using inhaled halothane (ICI Pharmaceuticals, Cheshire, UK) and analgesia was administered subcutaneously following surgery (Buprenorphine hydrochloride, Reckitt & Colman Products Ltd, Hull, UK). The colon was accessed for PDT via a laparotomy. The light source was either a pulsed (12 kHz) copper vapour pumped dye laser (Oxford Lasers, Oxford, UK) tuned to 635 nm (+/- 1-2 nm) or a laser diode (Diomed Ltd, Cambridge, UK) set at 628 nm (+/- 1-2 nm). A total energy of 100 J was delivered via a 200 μm plane cleaved optical fibre (output power, 100 mW) passed through the anti-mesenteric colon wall (approximately 1 cm distal to the caecum) so that it just touched the mucosa of the opposite side (area of contact = 0.03 mm^2). The rest of the abdominal viscera were shielded from forward light scatter by a piece of opaque paper positioned so that it did not touch the colon, or affect its light distribution. This is a model that we have used many times successfully in the past [92-93]. The light fluence where the fibre touches the tissue is very high (320 W/cm^2) but no thermal effect was observed in the light only control group. As the light fluence falls off rapidly with increasing distance along the colon wall from the fibre tip, measuring the diameter of the zone of necrosis in the wall of the colon is a convenient way of comparing the efficacy of PDT necrosis with different treatment parameters.

All animals were recovered following surgery and killed after three days, as mucosal damage is maximal at this time [94]. The treated area of colon was excised, cut longitudinally and flattened out so that the lesion produced by the treatment could be determined macroscopically by measuring the minimum (a) and maximum (b) perpendicular diameters of the lesion with a micrometer. These values were then used to calculate the area of necrosis using the formula πab/4, as the lesions produced were approximately elliptical. All appropriate drug only and light only control groups were also conducted. Representative specimens were fixed in formalin, sectioned and stained with haematoxylin and eosin, so that conventional light microscopy could confirm the macroscopic findings. This endpoint enabled a direct comparison of the treatment groups so that the most effective regime (the one which produced the most necrosis) could be determined. The experimental data of Messmann et al. [93] was also included on the figure, so that further comparisons could be made whilst using each set of experimental parameters and the copper vapour laser tuned to 630 nm. Statistical analysis between the means of the different treatment groups was conducted using unpaired student t-tests. Error bars were determined by the standard error of the mean.

Perfusion and Oxygen Saturation during Dermatological PDT

Fifty-five patients (20 males and 35 females; mean age = 70 +/- 10 years) were recruited at Royal Cornwall Hospital, Truro with a variety of licensed indications (24 AK, 14 BD and 17 sBCC) localised at both acral and non-acral sites (22 acral and 33 non-acral) for standard MAL-PDT treatment. The average surface area of the lesion was 35 mm^2 +/- 9 mm^2.

Each lesion was imaged for fluorescence at four distinct time points during treatment; i) prior to the application of MAL, ii) after the three hour application of MAL, iii) during light irradiation either after 1 minute (4.75 Jcm^{-2}; 10 patients - 5 males and 5 females, mean age = 75 +/- 4 years; 3 AK, 3 BD and 4 sBCC) or alternatively at the half way stage (18.5 Jcm^{-2}) during treatment (45 patients (based on previous studies where statistical significance was demonstrated at 90 % power at $p < 0.001$ [95]) - 15 males and 30 females, mean age = 69 +/- 11 years; 12 AK, 7 BD and 6 sBCC) and iv) following the completion of light treatment (37 Jcm^{-2}).

In addition to this fluorescence imaging, the mean blood oxygen saturation (SmbO$_2$ - percentage of haemoglobin carrying oxygen, averaged across all the microvessels in the volume of skin studied) of the tissue was monitored prior to, during (10 patients - 5 males and 5 females, mean age = 75 +/- 4 years; 3 AK, 3 BD and 4 sBCC) at 4.75 Jcm^{-2} and (25 patients

- 8 males and 17 females, mean age = 69 +/- 11 years; 12 AK, 7 BD and 6 sBCC) at 18.5 Jcm^{-2} as well as at the end of light irradiation. The $SmbO_2$ was calculated by spectroscopic quantification of the two chromophores oxyhaemoglobin (HbO_2) and deoxyhaemoglobin (Hb), using previously validated 'in house' optical reflectance spectroscopy (ORS) instrumentation (School of Physics, University of Exeter, UK) [96]. Light from a stabilised quartz tungsten halogen white light source was delivered to the skin via a fibre optic probe. Backscattered light was collected by six concentric fibres set 250 μm from the source enabling depths of 200 μm to be monitored which approximated to the depth of the lesions being investigated [97]. Backscattered spectra ranging from 470-1120 nm were recorded in 0.05 seconds through a grating spectrometer and charge-coupled device camera and processed with custom written Windows-based software. The concentrations of HbO_2 and Hb were derived from the modified Beer-Lambert law using a four component multi-linear regression algorithm on a narrow spectral range (500-600 nm) where a linear relationship between scattering of blood and wavelength was assumed. To obtain spectra from the blood volume alone, an initial reference spectrum from the surrounding interstitium of the lesion was acquired by applying sufficient pressure on the probe to occlude the microvessels [96, 98]. The mean blood oxygen saturation was derived from the measured concentrations of HbO_2 and Hb and defined as oxygen saturation (%) = [HbO_2] x 100 / ([HbO_2] + [Hb]). This oxygen saturation was the mean blood oxygen saturation across the arterioles capillaries and venules in the cutaneous microcirculation under investigation. For each time point the oxygen saturation within the tissue was monitored for 60 seconds. Consistent probe placement within the lesion limited the effect of the heterogeneous microvasculature. Reproducibility studies of probe placement on normal skin produced a coefficient of variance (CV) of less than 7% (data not shown).

Furthermore, the skin microcirculation was studied with a well-established technique, laser Doppler fluximetry, which has previously been employed to monitor dermatological ALA-PDT [86, 99]. A Periscan PIM II perfusion imager (Perimed, Sweden) instrument was utilised to monitor perfusion within normal skin and the (pre)cancerous lesion treated with MAL-PDT. A single wavelength of low power (1 mW) laser light (670 nm) was directed onto the surface of the skin and the entire lesion scanned. Light backscattered from the tissue was collected by the photodetector, light scattered from moving objects (e.g. red blood cells) underwent frequency changes, or Doppler shift, whereas light backscattered from stationary objects remained unaltered. The magnitude and frequency distribution of the Doppler shift is a measure of the number and velocity of blood cells in the volume of tissue under investigation. The perfusion in the skin is quantified by the term flux (in arbitrary units) which is the product of the mean moving red blood cell velocity and the number of moving red blood cells. Following the scan, perfusion was monitored at a number of discrete points using the LDPIWin software (Perimed, Sweden) and the average perfusion of the lesion and normal skin was calculated, reducing the signal noise and the effects of spatial variations in the tissue. Patients (20 patients – 7 males and 13 females, average age = 69 years +/- 8.3 years; 9 AK, 4 BD and 7 sBCC) were monitored prior to light treatment, during light irradiation (at the half way stage) and following the completion of treatment for a maximum of 90 seconds. To ensure the continuity of the system a calibration box was scanned before and after every patient and no significant variation was observed ($p = 0.53$; data not shown). Skin temperature was monitored with a digital thermometer (Fluke Ltd, UK) during the acquisition of both the oxygen saturation and perfusion measurements.

The normality of the fluorescence data set was analysed with the Kolmogorov-Smirnov test. Normally distributed data were either analysed with the unpaired t-test or ANOVA analysis for between group comparisons or the paired t-test or repeated measures ANOVA for intra patient data. Least squares regression analysis and Spearman Rank analysis was utilised to determine the relationship between changes in oxygen saturation and PpIX concentration during treatment.

RESULTS

Prior to image acquisition the synthetic PpIX standard was monitored and over the course of these investigations no significant difference in the grayscale intensity was recorded (p = 0.95, data not shown).

PpIX Fluorescence Accumulation and Dissipation during Dermatological PDT

The images acquired from the licensed indications (25 AK, 25 BD and 25 sBCC) indicated that the majority underwent detectable fluorescence changes during the first and second MAL-PDT treatments (Figure 1). Subsequent analysis (Figure 2) demonstrated a significant increase in fluorescence intensity within all three distinct lesion types at the end of the three hour MAL application period ($p < 0.001$ and $p < 0.01$ respectively), followed by a significant decrease ($p < 0.001$ and $p < 0.01$ respectively) post irradiation during both the first and second treatments. The area of normal skin monitored concurrently produced no significant changes in fluorescence during the treatment procedure ($p = 0.84$ (1st treatment) and $p = 0.55$ (2nd treatment), data not shown). For both the first and second treatments no significant differences were observed between the distinct lesion types in terms of the fluorescence accumulation (ANOVA; 1st treatment $p = 0.95$; 2nd treatment $p = 0.71$) or dissipation (ANOVA; 1st treatment $p = 0.74$; 2nd treatment $p = 0.27$). The level of PpIX accumulation during both the first and second treatments after three hours MAL application was approximately equal ($p > 0.250$) to the dissipation observed during light irradiation on each occasion. However during the second treatment the total accumulation/dissipation of PpIX observed was statistically significantly lower than when compared to the initial treatment ($p < 0.01$ and $p < 0.05$ respectively for all three indications separately). Furthermore the area of fluorescence within the lesion was found to be significantly smaller ($p < 0.01$) on the second PDT treatment (data not shown). PpIX fluorescence distribution within lesions was also noted to vary greatly, with an approximately equal split between lesions demonstrating no variation (n=32, 43%) and lesions demonstrating significant ($p < 0.01$) variation (n=43, 57%).

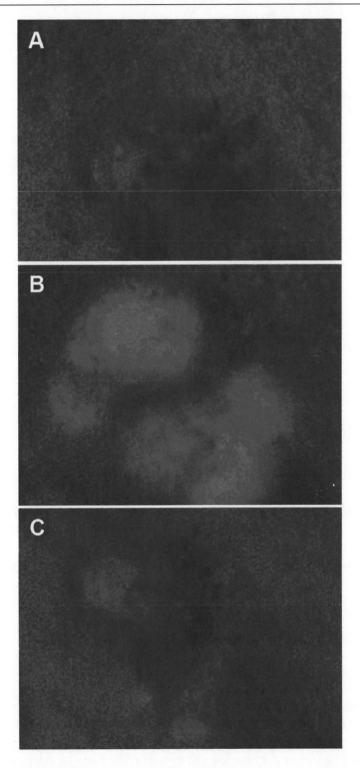

Figure 1. Colour images of PpIX fluorescence monitored during the PDT treatment process of a representative sBCC lesion A) before MAL application, B) after three hours MAL application and C) immediately following light irradiation.

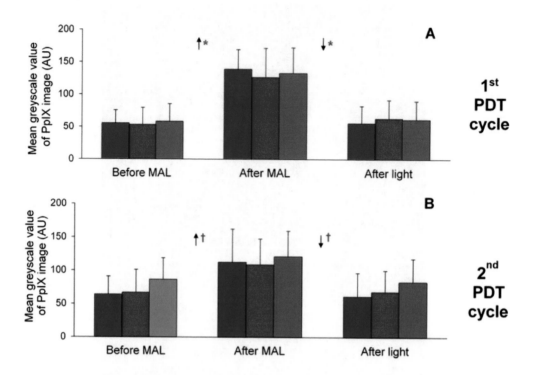

Figure 2. Mean PpIX fluorescence intensity observed at each time point monitored during the PDT treatment process within licensed lesions (25 AK - blue bars; 25 BD – red bars; 25 sBCC – green bars) undergoing their A) first and B) second MAL-PDT treatment. * $p < 0.001$ and $^{†} p < 0.01$ ANOVA +/- standard deviation.

The three licensed lesion types were each observed to undergo two distinct changes in fluorescence (Figure 2) during the first and second PDT treatments, whilst areas of surrounding normal skin remained unaltered. Firstly following the three hour MAL application a statistically significant increase in fluorescence was observed during both the first and second PDT treatments. This increase in fluorescence was attributed to the conversion of MAL via the haem biosynthesis pathway to the photosensitiser PpIX [100]. The second change in fluorescence was observed immediately following light irradiation where statistically significant decreases in fluorescence were detected during both the first and second treatments. The decrease in fluorescence during light treatment was attributed to the photobleaching of PpIX as a result of the production of singlet oxygen [4]. The fluorescence changes monitored correlated well with our current understanding of the accumulation and dissipation of PpIX during standard dermatological MAL-PDT [4, 59]. The level of accumulation and dissipation of fluorescence in individual lesion types during MAL-PDT was approximately equal with no significant difference observed between these two measurements. This indicated that the light dose employed was photobleaching all the accumulated PpIX within the lesions during the course of the treatment process. Furthermore all three licensed lesion types were observed to respond in a similar manner and it is widely reported that the standard licensed MAL-PDT treatment protocol has been observed to be similarly efficacious in each of these applications [3, 27, 35, 101-102]. It is important to note however, that inter patient variation was large and whilst the data presented here represents all of the lesions monitored, a small number of lesions did not follow the general trend of significant accumulation and dissipation of fluorescence. Within the data set there were several examples of lesions which either showed limited accumulation and subsequent dissipation of PpIX or demonstrated significant accumulation but limited dissipation of the photosensitiser. The former issue was most likely due to inadequate lesion preparation or insufficient cream application, whereas the latter could be due to the light placement, the relationship between PpIX concentrations and photobleaching or alternatively whether air cooling was employed as a method of pain relief. Significant changes in fluorescence were also recorded during the second PDT treatment, indicating that this process was worthwhile. However, the accumulation and dissipation of the photosensitiser was significantly lower than observed for the first treatment, indicating that the first treatment effectively destroyed the majority of cancerous and pre-cancerous tissue, whilst the second treatment removed the remaining diseased cells. This was further represented by the decrease observed in the size of the fluorescent area following the application of MAL for the second treatment cycle (data not shown).

PpIX Fluorescence and Clinical Outcome

The mean PpIX photobleaching of licensed dermatological lesions (37 AK, 29 BD and 34 sBCC) undergoing MAL-PDT was observed to be significantly different between lesions that were observed to be completely clear versus those that were only partially cleared by the treatment regime when examined clinically at three months (Figure 3). Changes in fluorescence intensity of 50% and 60% were significantly more likely within the complete responder group when compared with the partial responders group ($p < 0.01$ and $p < 0.001$ respectively).

Previous studies have shown a positive correlation between PpIX photobleaching and the induced cellular damage, indicating that greater PpIX photobleaching results in more efficacious PDT [50-51,103-104]. Our clinical findings support and extend this evidence base, demonstrating that the percentage change in fluorescence during MAL-PDT light irradiation of licensed dermatological lesions was indeed associated with improved clinical outcome, which was observed three months after treatment (Figure 3). Comparisons were only made between complete and partial responders in this study due to the lack of non-responders (only one patient showed no response to PDT treatment using our standard PDT treatment protocol). The clearance rates (complete clearance 72% and partial clearance 27%) obtained were also consistent with the published literature, which indicates that this standard MAL-PDT treatment regime is able to produce effective clearance in these approved dermatological indications [45, 89]. It therefore appears that with further investigation, the potential exists to follow PpIX photobleaching during clinical MAL-PDT and utilise this information as a predictive tool in determining potential clinical outcome at the time of treatment. These data currently suggest that a threshold percentage change of 60% could be applied to determine whether an additional PDT treatment cycle may be beneficial to ensure complete clearance of the lesion in the majority of patients.

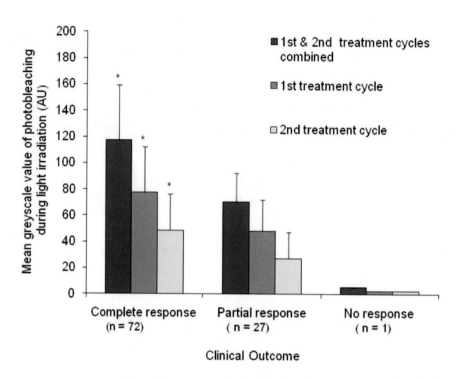

Figure 3. Mean PpIX photobleaching of lesions (37 AK, 29 BD and 34 sBCC) observed to undergo complete, partial and no response at 3 months following MAL-PDT. * indicates significance at $p <$ 0.005 Mann Whitney U test between the complete and partial responders +/- standard deviation.

Effect of Air Cooling Pain Relief

The effect of utilising the air cooling device as pain relief during irradiation was also investigated within licensed dermatological lesions (AK, BD and sBCC) undergoing standard MAL-PDT. A significant reduction ($p < 0.001$) in the PpIX photobleaching that occurred over the course of the light irradiation period was recorded within patients who had utilised the air cooling device versus those who had not used the device (Figure 4A). Furthermore, when considering clinical outcome of these lesions at three months, complete responders were more likely to be patients who hadn't used air cooling for pain relief with 82% of these patients achieving a complete response in comparison with only a 68% complete response in the air cooling group (Figure 4B). When these observed values were compared with 'predicted' response rates (80% complete clearance) based on the literature [3], the clearance rates in the air cooling pain relief group were significantly lower ($p < 0.01$) than that expected, whilst the results of the non-air cooling group were similar ($p = 0.62$).

These fluorescence results indicate that not all the PpIX present following MAL application was utilised during light irradiation for PDT when the air cooling device was employed at this time point in the treatment process. This was in contrast to the standard (non-air cooling) group who dissipated all the PpIX they accumulated during light irradiation, suggesting that maximal ROS production and therefore treatment efficacy occurred within this group. This hypothesis is supported by the significant difference in clinical clearance recorded between the two groups of patients at three months follow-up and therefore suggests that utilisation of air cooling during light irradiation should be avoided where possible as it lowers the potential efficacy of the treatment. The most likely explanation for these observed differences is that the air cooling device produces substantial localised cooling of the treatment area, inducing vasoconstriction, which in turn reduces oxygenation limiting the production of PDT-induced ROS and thus reducing treatment efficacy. However this is yet to be studied in detail and the investigation reported here was retrospective, non-randomised and simply observational in nature. The results do suggest that patients should be encouraged to try treatment without using an air cooling device if possible or to delay its utilisation. We now utilise a simple water spray for pain management where necessary, prior to offering the air cooling pain relief option to our patients.

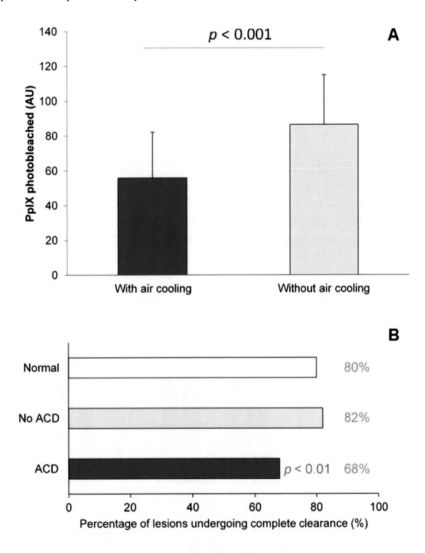

Figure 4. Effect of air cooling pain relief on lesions (AK, BD and sBCC) undergoing MAL-PDT A) percentage change in PpIX fluorescence during irradiation (+/- standard deviation) and B) observed complete response rates at three months compared with 'predicted' response rates based on the literature [3].

Effect of Acral Lesion Location

Lesions treated with MAL-PDT located at non-acral sites (n=104) were observed to undergo statistically greater changes in fluorescence ($p < 0.05$) after the three hour MAL application (Figure 5A) and following the light irradiation of the lesion (Figure 5B; $p < 0.001$) than lesions located at acral sites (n=96). When the histologically distinct lesions were considered individually, the change in fluorescence following the application of MAL was noted to be statistically reduced ($p < 0.01$) in acral AK lesions when compared to non-acral AK lesions (Figure 5A). In contrast the accumulation of fluorescence following MAL application in BD and sBCC were similar for acral and non-acral sites ($p = 0.63$ and $p = 0.70$ respectively; data not shown). Acral AK lesions were also observed to undergo a significantly reduced ($p < 0.05$) percentage change in fluorescence during light irradiation than observed with the non-acral AK lesions (Figure 5B). Although the non-acral BD appeared to undergo reduced photobleaching during light irradiation this difference did not reach significance over acral lesions ($p = 0.08$) and no significant difference was observed between acral and non acral sBCC ($p = 0.54$; data not shown). Two-way ANOVA analysis indicated no significant difference between lesion type in terms of the percentage change in fluorescence either after MAL application or during light irradiation ($p = 0.94$ and $p = 0.14$ respectively). Significance only arose from comparison of the different anatomical locations treated. A significantly lower percentage of acral lesions were also observed to undergo complete clinical clearance (Figure 5C) when compared with non-acral lesions (68% versus 85%; $p < 0.010$). This was also true for AK lesions alone (Figure 5C), with 85% of non-acral AK lesions been completely clear after three months and only 61% of acral AK undergoing complete clearance ($p < 0.05$). No significant difference was observed between the clearance rates in non-acral and acral BD (81% versus 69%) and sBCC lesions (87% versus 82%) (data not shown).

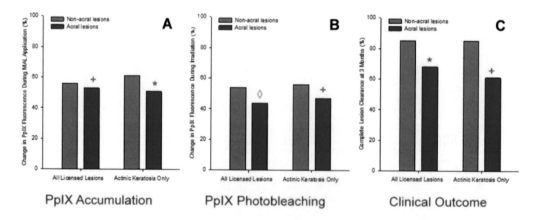

PpIX Accumulation   PpIX Photobleaching   Clinical Outcome

Figure 5. Bar charts indicating A) the percentage change in PpIX fluorescence after 3 hours MAL application, B) the percentage change in PpIX fluorescence during light irradiation and C) the clinical outcome observed at three months within all acral and non-acral licensed lesions (AK, BD and sBCC) and AK acral and non-acral lesions alone undergoing MAL-PDT. +, * and ◊ indicate statistical significance at $p < 0.05$, $p < 0.01$ and $p < 0.001$ respectively, between acral and non-acral sites.

These clinical outcome results confirm those of previous studies, which have recorded MAL-PDT being less effective in the treatment of AK when the lesions were located on the extremities/acral locations [105-110]. Furthermore, significantly less PpIX was observed in this investigation to be available following MAL application for activation during irradiation, potentially accounting for the significantly reduced effect of MAL-PDT in acral lesions. When the lesion types were considered individually only AK differed significantly in terms of the fluorescence changes witnessed. The direct comparison of PpIX accumulation and photobleaching of lesions located at acral and non-acral sites suggested that PpIX accumulation was observed to be significantly greater ($p < 0.001$) than PpIX photobleaching when all 96 acral lesions were considered and when the 51 acral BD lesions were considered. This indicated that not all the PpIX produced in these lesions was utilised during the treatment, therefore potentially reducing treatment efficacy. Monitoring fluorescence during clinical MAL-PDT has therefore provided an insight into the limited efficacy of the treatment of acral skin lesions. Firstly the significant reduction ($p < 0.05$) in the level of PpIX attained following the application of the topical prodrug in acral skin was probably due to limited prodrug penetration through the stratum corneum into the diseased cells below. This reduction in PpIX accumulation may be a result of a thicker stratum corneum in acral skin [111], which has previously been demonstrated to weakly negatively correlate with PpIX fluorescence [45] or alternatively the increased number of pilosebaceous units of the head may improve PpIX accumulation within non-acral skin regions [112]. Secondly, acral skin lesions were observed to undergo a statistically lower level ($p < 0.001$) of PpIX photobleaching during light irradiation. Due to the established relationship between PpIX photobleaching and the subsequent cellular damage/clinical outcome observed [50, 103-104], this reduction in PpIX photobleaching within acral lesions suggests lower levels of cellular damage/death and therefore an ultimately poorer clinical outcome as reported here.

PpIX Fluorescence During Light Delivery

The PpIX fluorescence results obtained when the light irradiation was briefly interrupted to take an additional measurement (Figure 6) determined that significant photobleaching ($p < 0.001$) occurred during the first half of the light delivery alone (0.0 - 18.5 Jcm^{-2}) as well as over the entire irradiation period (0.0 - 37.0 Jcm^{-2}); $p < 0.001$). However, the change in PpIX fluorescence (87% versus 60%) achieved during the second half of the light dose (18.5 - 37.0 Jcm^{-2}) was still found to be statistically significant ($p < 0.01$) indicating that this light delivery was still effectively inducing PDT effects.

The photobleaching of PpIX during MAL-PDT occurs as singlet oxygen reacts with PpIX resulting in the production of the chlorin, photoprotoporphyrin. Maximal PpIX photobleaching is desirable during clinical MAL-PDT because (as observed above) it is associated with an increased likelihood of complete clinical clearance being observed at three months after treatment. However, the ultimate goal of the treatment is to produce maximal damage to the tumour not destruction of the photosensitiser (as monitored via PpIX photobleaching), which is required to be present and active for as long as possible. So, as long as there is active drug (PpIX) left in the lesion, it is still feasible to cause more damage through further irradiation and so aiming to use all the PpIX in the treatment area until it is observed to be completed photobleached is a valid objective in this clinical scenario.

The image analysis undertaken here suggested that phased PpIX photobleaching occurred during MAL-PDT light delivery with a significantly greater decrease in PpIX fluorescence being observed during the first half of light treatment, when compared to the second half of light treatment. Whilst PpIX photobleaching was observed to be significantly greater in the initial phase of light irradiation, indicating maximal singlet oxygen production at this time, total photobleaching at the end of irradiation was observed to be significantly greater than that observed in the first half of irradiation alone ($p < 0.01$). This indicated that the delivery of the entire light dose was necessary to photobleach all the photosensitiser present in the treatment area and in some cases the data sets for individual patients indicated that the area could have benefitted from even more irradiation to ensure that the greatest PDT effect possible was produced (as would have been observed experimentally via all the accumulated PpIX being photobleached).

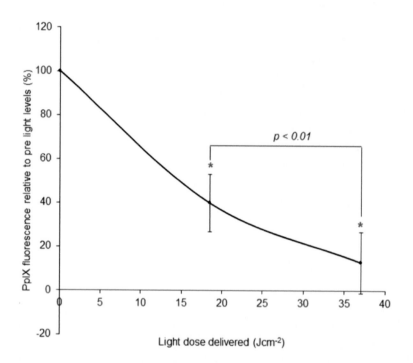

Figure 6. The percentage of PpIX fluorescence accumulated over the three hour drug light interval present at the beginning, middle and end of light irradiation for forty licensed lesions (AK, BD and sBCC) undergoing MAL-PDT +/- standard deviation. * indicates significance at $p < 0.001$.

These initial findings correspond with the literature [50, 59, 113-114], where *in vitro* and pre-clinical investigations have suggested a rapid initial phase of PpIX photobleaching within the first few minutes of treatment (1-10 Jcm^{-2}) followed by a second slower phase of PpIX decay. Unfortunately, continuous fluorescence monitoring of PpIX during light irradiation was not possible within this clinical study as these non-invasive optical measurements could not be acquired at the same time as PDT light irradiation was in process. Whilst continuous monitoring would have been preferred, the light source was paused for a maximum of 60 seconds to permit image acquisition, which should not have altered the treatment in a significant or adverse manner.

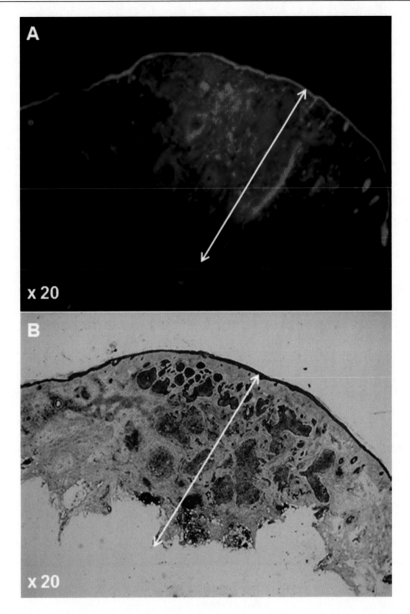

Figure 7. Distribution of PpIX fluorescence A) within a representative nBCC tumour 180 minutes following MAL application, presented with B) the corresponding H&E histological image. Arrows illustrate full extent of tumour depth.

Histological Assessment of Depth of PpIX Fluorescence

The distribution of MAL-induced PpIX within a representative nBCC, as measured by tumour fluorescence microscopy, is presented in Figure 7A. This tumour was excised three hours (the standard MAL-PDT drug light interval) after a single application of the prodrug cream. The corresponding H&E section is presented in Figure 7B and was used to identify the outline of the tumour, including its maximal depth as indicated by the arrow replicated on both corresponding images. Although the fluorescence concentration was not quantified, the sections collected at the different time points investigated demonstrated a gradual increase in depth of fluorescence over time, being the greatest observed after three hours cream application. The fluorescence was also noted to be fairly evenly distributed throughout the tumour after this time, suggesting good penetration of MAL over three hours, although this was not full thickness. None of the control tumours showed any significant fluorescence, confirming that without exogenous application of MAL, natural PpIX did not accumulate significantly within the cells of this nBCC tumour type. A high degree of tumour selectivity was also observed, with the surrounding normal skin showing only a thin layer of fluorescence in the epidermis alone. This selectivity between tumour and normal surrounding tissue is important during PDT treatment as it reduces the chance of phototoxic reaction in the surrounding normal skin at the time of light delivery, as it too also receives cream application and light irradiation. Table 1 shows the distribution of MAL as measured by depth of tumour fluorescence on microscopy in nBCCs at different time applications of MAL. Within this clinical pilot study there was no quantification of the fluorescence produced in the different lesions and it was difficult to compare fluorescence depth directly in view of the variation in site and thickness of the individual patient tumours. However, there appeared to be a definite trend towards relative increased depth of fluorescence as a percentage of tumour thickness, over time. It should be noted however, that at the standard MAL application time of three hours, the mean percentage of depth of PpIX fluorescence within the tumours was only 84% indicating that full thickness photosensitisation was not achieved.

Table 1. Relative histological thickness and depth of fluorescence within nBCC tumours following various times of MAL application

MAL Application Period (minutes)	Maximum histological (Breslow) thickness of each nBCC (n=3)			Group Mean
30	20	10	22	*17*
60	22	20	9	*17*
120	18	42	28	*29*
180	10	15	58	*28*
MAL Application Period (minutes)	Estimated depth of fluorescence within each nBCC (n=3)			Group Mean
30	7	2	2	*4*
60	10	5	4	*6*
120	15	22	18	*18*
180	10	10	50	*23*
MAL Application Period (minutes)	Relative depth (%) of fluorescence within each nBCC (n=3)			Group Mean
30	20	20	9	*16*
60	45	25	44	*38*
120	83	52	64	*66*
180	100	67	86	*84*

This histological investigation demonstrated that the distribution of MAL as determined by fluorescence microscopy was selectively taken up by the nBCC tumour with little or no fluorescence in the dermis. The fluorescence was seen at the greatest depths within tumours after three hours. This confirmed the findings of previous studies which showed that topical treatment with 160 mg/g MAL for 3 hours or 80 mg/g for 18 hours produced an adequate depth of porphyrin fluorescence throughout the thick tumours and was superior to other dose regimes and time applications studied [53]. This study also showed the relatively small or absent uptake of MAL in normal epidermis even after three hours, which confirms the relatively selective nature of MAL-PDT and the importance of removing any intact epidermis overlying the tumour prior to treatment. Preferential accumulation of PpIX in tumour cells appears to result not only from increased penetration of ALA or MAL through the abnormal epidermis but also to increased intracellular accumulation of PpIX in actively proliferating cells [115]. The fact that full thickness photosensitisation was not observed in all the tumours excised after three hours of MAL application, supports the current dermatological guidelines in respect to the treatment of nBCC with MAL-PDT [9] as well as the standard protocol to complete two MAL-PDT treatments a week apart for all but the most superficial precancerous lesions.

Effect of Iron Chelation on Histological and Clinical Outcome

These initial clinical pilot studies found the addition of the iron chelating agent CP94 to the ALA or MAL prodrug cream to be a simple pharmacological modification, which appeared to be safe, with no dose-limiting adverse events being noted in any of the patients treated. The histological response 6 weeks following the PpIX-PDT is presented in Table 2. In the CP94 control group there was no clinical response to the PDT treatment at 6 weeks. All other lesions showed some clinical response, with the clinical impression matching the histological response in all cases.

With ALA-PDT alone, 2 out of 6 histological specimens showed an actual increase in depth, or thickness, from the pre-treatment biopsy. Similarly four out of the six ALA + 5% CP94 treated nodular BCC group showed an increased thickness in the post treatment excision specimens. The reason for this could be twofold. Firstly any remaining BCC could have continued to grow in the 8-week period between biopsy and excision and secondly, the biopsy may not have been taken from the thickest part of the tumour even though it appeared to be so clinically. There was no significant improvement in response (i.e. reduction in tumour thickness) with the addition of 5% CP94 compared with the control groups (ALA alone or CP94 alone) ($p < 0.172$ and $p < 0.790$ respectively, unpaired student's t-test). With increasing concentrations of CP94 (10, 20 and 40%), the thickness of any tumour remaining in the excised specimens decreased in all cases. The addition of 40% CP94 showed a significant improvement in tumour response (i.e. reduction in tumour thickness after treatment) compared with both ALA and CP94 alone controls ($p < 0.001$ and $p < 0.001$ respectively, unpaired student's t-test). Some complete tumour responses were observed following PDT treatment (e.g. Figure 8), with 5 out of 6 showing complete or partial (greater than 50%) histological response in the ALA + 40% CP94 group. The BCC lesion in this group which showed no response was a thicker tumour with a thickness of 3 mm prior to treatment and it was noted that in general, in all groups, the tumours greater than 3 mm prior to treatment seemed to respond less well than tumours less than 3 mm thick pre-treatment. Table 2 demonstrates this increased trend towards complete clearance with increased concentrations of CP94. Overall there was a significant improvement in (histological) tumour response with the addition of the CP94 iron chelator (p < 0.001 ANOVA).

Table 2. Mean change in histological depth of nBCC lesions six weeks after receiving a single treatment cycle of ALA-PDT or MAL-PDT plus increasing amounts of the iron chelating agent, CP94

ALA-PDT + CP94		MAL-PDT + CP94	
Treatment Group	Mean Change in Histological Depth	Treatment Group	Mean Change in Histological Depth
40% CP94 alone	+0.33 mm	---	---
ALA + 0% CP94	-0.30 mm	MAL + 0% CP94	+2.13 mm
ALA + 5% CP94	+0.33 mm	---	---
ALA + 10% CP94	-0.78 mm	---	---
ALA + 20% CP94	-0.97 mm	MAL + 20% CP94	-0.43 mm
---	---	MAL + 30% CP94	-1.37 mm
ALA + 40% CP94	-1.41 mm	MAL + 40% CP94	-1.43 mm

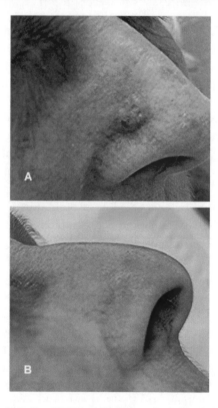

Figure 8. nBCC photographed A) before PDT and B) six weeks following PDT conducted with a single cycle of the licensed ALA-PDT protocol augmented with an iron chelating agent by simply adding 20% CP94 to the prodrug cream.

The ALA-PDT pilot study above was extended in an additional 12 patients, replacing the ALA with MAL and again increasing the concentration of CP94 (0% - 40%). No adverse effects above that normally experienced with MAL-PDT were reported from any of the participants and liver function tests also remained normal following treatment. All of the tumours from the participants treated with MAL alone had increased in depth 6 weeks following treatment and all of the patients treated with MAL + CP94 (20%, 30% and 40%) experienced reductions in tumour depth 6 weeks following treatment. Only one tumour was completely clinically resolved at 6 weeks and this tumour was in the MAL + 40% CP94 treated group (Table 2).

These studies have therefore produced encouraging results with regard to complete clearance of nBCC using the novel iron chelator, CP94 with no prior lesion preparation and only one cycle of enhanced PDT treatment. A single standard PpIX-induced PDT treatment would not normally be expected to clear these lesions. Standard routine therapy with MAL, involves two treatments seven days apart plus careful debulking of lesions before treatment. The treatment modification presented here is therefore of great interest. In general the average tumour thickness among the groups receiving the combined treatment was fairly similar, however individually there was variation. This however, is an inherent problem in a study where patients were allocated to the various treatment groups in strict order rather than stratified by tumour thickness.

These findings are in contrast to studies using other iron chelating agents particularly DFO, where the addition of DFO to the higher ALA dose being employed in clinical treatment did not significantly enhance PpIX levels, when examined in matched lesions in the same patient [116]. CP94 however is of lower molecular weight and higher lipophilicity than DFO. It is also neutrally charged in both iron free and iron complexed forms enabling it to move freely in and out of cells by simple diffusion [117]. CP94 consequently enters the intracellular iron pools more readily and it is this factor which is most likely to account for the increased effect of CP94 over DFO. Experimental studies support the efficacy of CP94 in the enhancement of ALA-PDT in normal and malignant colon tissue in animal models [118-119] as well as cultured cells [120] and CP94 has been found to be superior to DFO in a direct *in vitro* comparison [121]. The ability of CP94 to increase PpIX levels, particularly in deeper cells where the concentration of ALA or MAL would be low and PpIX production could have occurred at sub-lethal levels (as observed at three hours in the histological excision study described above), may explain the increased effect observed in the deeper nodular tumours investigated. PpIX fluorescence was not assessed in this clinical safety study but should form the basis of future work when optimising the treatment parameters prior to conducting a randomised controlled trial of this promising intervention.

Effect of Wavelength on PDT Effect *In Vivo*

The mean area of necrosis (mm^2) produced by systemic ALA-PDT (50 mg/kg ALA i.v.) in the normal rat colon with each laser/wavelength delivering a light dose of 100 J (100 mW) is presented in Figure 9. There was little difference between the area of necrosis produced if the copper vapour laser was used to deliver the energy dose at either 635 nm or 630 nm. When the laser diode set at 628 nm, was employed however, a significantly smaller area of necrosis was produced (635 nm = 32 mm^2 and 628 nm = 11 mm^2) ($p < 0.02$). This indicated that the area of necrosis produced by ALA-PDT (using these parameters in this model) was affected by the slight difference in wavelength of the excitation light, making a significant difference to the outcome of the treatment. It is known that 635 nm is a better excitation wavelength of ALA induced PpIX *in vivo* than 630 nm [122] and as the wavelength is shifted either further towards the blue or into the red, less energy will be absorbed by the drug. Comparisons have already been made between a copper vapour laser and diode laser at a wavelength suitable for mTHPc excitation (652 nm) [123]. At this wavelength, however, using this photosensitiser, no difference between the lasers (as determined by the outcome of the treatment) was observed. It is therefore unlikely that the use of a different type of laser can account for the difference observed here, whereas the small shift in wavelength away from the maximum of the narrow PpIX absorption peak in the red region could.

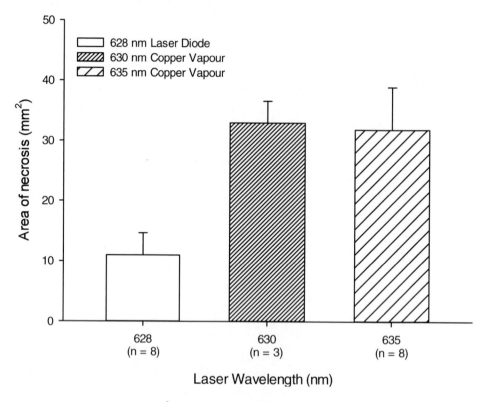

Figure 9. Mean area of necrosis (mm^2) produced in the normal rat colon as a function of laser and wavelength. 50 mg/kg ALA i.v. was administered 75 minutes prior to 100 J of light (100 mW). Error bars as determined by the standard error of the mean. 630 nm copper vapour data included from Messmann et al. (1995) [93].

Perfusion and Oxygen Saturation During Dermatological PDT

Perfusion within twenty dermatological lesions (9 AK, 4 BD and 7 sBCC) was monitored before and after as well as in the middle of the irradiation period of the standard MAL-PDT protocol (Figure 10). During the first half of light irradiation perfusion within the AK and sBCC lesions increased significantly ($p < 0.01$) and then remained at a similar level until the end of the light delivery ($p = 0.16$). The change in perfusion during the first half of light treatment was significantly greater ($p < 0.01$) than the changes during the second half of the irradiation. These trends were not observed in the small number of BD lesions included in this part of the investigation.

Significantly increased perfusion following light irradiation has previously been noted following the light irradiation stage of ALA-PDT treatment of BCC (where a light dose of 60 Jcm^{-2} was delivered at 100 $mWcm^{-2}$) [86]. Our findings have suggested that perfusion does not solely increase or decrease during MAL-PDT, rather perfusion initially increases before beginning to decrease and this corresponds with previous research suggesting that the original concept of unidirectional perfusion changes during PDT was misconceived [74].

When oxygen saturation was monitored in ten patients (3 AK, 3 BD and 4 sBCC) after only one minute of light delivery had occurred (4.75 Jcm^{-2}), a significant decrease ($p < 0.005$) had already occurred (Figure 11A). The overall level of oxygen depletion continued to increase until the full light dose (37.00 Jcm^{-2}) had been delivered. When the change in oxygen saturation that occurred within the first minute of irradiation was subsequently plotted against the change in PpIX fluorescence (which was also found to be significant; $p < 0.001$) over the same time period (Figure 11B), a strong linear relationship between these two parameters was revealed ($r^2 = 0.786$, $p < 0.001$).

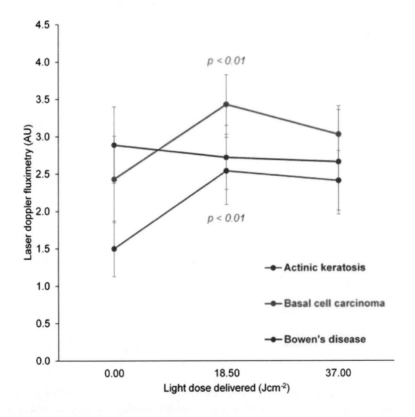

Figure 10. Mean perfusion as a function of the light dose delivered to licensed lesions (9 AK, 7 sBCC and 4 BD) undergoing MAL-PDT +/- standard deviation. The irradiation was interrupted briefly half-way through the light delivery.

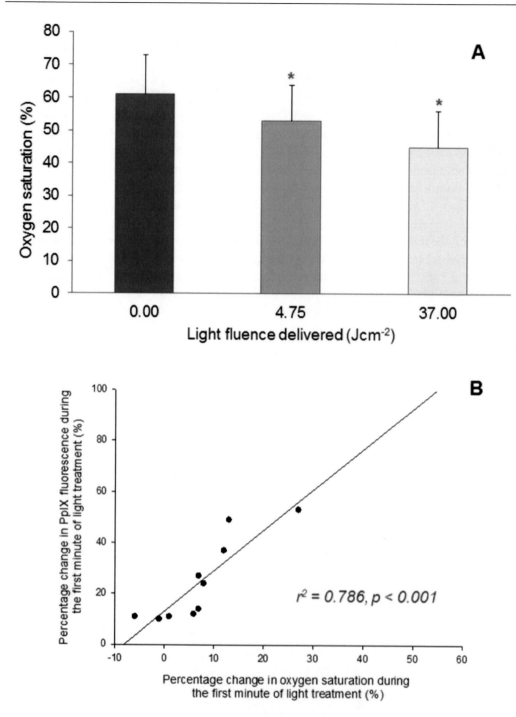

Figure 11. Licensed dermatological lesions undergoing MAL-PDT (n = 10) were monitored before light application, after one minute of light delivery and immediately following the irradiation period. A) Mean oxygen saturation as a function of the light dose delivered (+/- standard deviation; * indicates statistical significance at $p < 0.005$ from the pre-irradiation measurement) and B) linear regression (and coefficient) of the change in oxygen saturation and change in PpIX fluorescence that occurred during the first minute of irradiation.

These data provide clinical evidence that the effects are similar to those previously observed in animals. Rapid reductions in the pO_2 are observed immediately after the initiation of light treatment during PDT [79, 82, 85, 124]. Figure 11A indicates that the pO_2 is significantly depleted within the initial 4.75 Jcm^{-2} of light delivery and then remains at a similar level for the remainder of treatment. This suggests that it is the very early stages of irradiation where the maximal photochemical reactions take place. The reduction in oxygen saturation during MAL-PDT is proposed to occur primarily as a result of oxygen consumption during the photochemical reactions within cells and to a lesser extent, damage to the localised microvasculature may also be involved [78]. Mean blood oxygen saturation can only provide a measure of the oxygen content of the blood in the lesion during irradiation and is not a direct measure of tissue oxygenation. However, when considered in conjunction with the perfusion data also presented here, which demonstrated the vasodilatory effect of PDT irradiation it is reasonable to attribute this fall in oxygen saturation to an increase in oxygen consumption during light irradiation.

When considered concurrently, the oxygen saturation data, perfusion data and PpIX fluorescence changes suggest that on the initiation of light irradiation, singlet oxygen/other ROS are rapidly produced via photochemical reactions. Hence the pool of available oxygen and ground state PpIX are reduced, via photochemical consumption and singlet oxygen destruction respectively. The rapid oxygen consumption would produce significant reductions in the partial pressure of oxygen and therefore potentially the development of a hypoxic environment. This may initiate hypoxia induced vasodilation leading initially to increased perfusion as observed to replenish the depleted oxygen supply. These data also demonstrate that the oxygen saturation remains low for the remainder of treatment, therefore suggesting that the increased perfusion either does not significantly replenish the partial pressure of oxygen in the tissue or it continues to be consumed by photochemical reactions as the light delivery is continued. It can be concluded however, that oxygen consumption is reduced in the latter stages of irradiation as no significant alterations in this parameter were observed at the monitoring points investigated during the second half of treatment (data not shown). This probably occurs as a result of the significant reduction in PpIX availability (due to its photochemical destruction/photobleaching). As a result the perfusion in the tissue being treated may potentially decrease from this point onwards.

CONCLUSION

These investigations have demonstrated the capacity of a non-invasive imaging system (Dyaderm) to detect fluorescence changes during standard clinical dermatological MAL-PDT for licensed indications (AK, BD and sBCC). The fluorescence changes arise as a result of the accumulation and dissipation of porphyrins and previous studies have indicated that the photosensitiser PpIX is the dominant porphyrin to accumulate within cells after MAL application [47-48]. In addition a synthetic PpIX standard was utilised during the comprehensive validation of our image analysis system, which has indicated that the mean greyscale values calculated related to the PpIX concentration employed [56].

Statistically significant changes in PpIX fluorescence were observed to occur during both the first and second MAL-PDT treatments and all three licensed indications (AK, BD and sBCC) responded in a similar manner, supporting the one treatment regimen fits all protocol currently adopted for dermatological MAL-PDT. It was also demonstrated that whilst the second treatment undergoes statistically smaller changes in fluorescence intensity than during the first treatment, these changes were noted to be significant indicating that application of a second treatment was efficacious and therefore worthwhile. Taking additional fluorescence images half way through the light delivery also indicated that the majority of PpIX photobleaching during MAL-PDT occurred in the first half of the light dose, however the entire light dose routinely utilised for dermatological MAL-PDT (37 Jcm^{-2}) was required for maximal effect.

Consideration of clinical outcome determined at three months follow-up, also indicated that it may be possible in the future to utilise the PpIX photobleaching observed during the light irradiation period to give an indication of likely treatment outcome whilst the PDT treatment process is still in progress, with larger changes in PpIX photobleaching being associated with subsequent complete lesion clearance. A significant reduction in PpIX photobleaching was observed in the patients who utilised an air cooling device as a form of pain relief during MAL-PDT. Furthermore this observation was linked to a significantly reduced complete response rate at three months follow-up, indicating that this device reduced PDT efficacy. These findings suggest that utilisation of air cooling pain relief should be avoided/delayed where possible, in preference to other pain management strategies that do not adversely affect treatment outcome. As with previous investigations, a significantly reduced clinical clearance rate was also observed in acral lesions. Monitoring PpIX fluorescence throughout the MAL-PDT treatment process, suggested that significantly reduced PpIX accumulation occurred within acrally located lesions during the MAL application period and this subsequently limited PDT efficacy (as indicated by significantly reduced photobleaching) on irradiation. Future work should aim to resolve this issue (limited PpIX accumulation) to improve MAL-PDT effectiveness in acrally located lesions. *In vivo* investigation of the effect of excitation wavelength on the effectiveness of ALA-PDT, indicated that a small shift in wavelength (from 635 nm to 628 nm) significantly reduced the necrosis produced in this model, reinforcing the importance of matching the light source employed to the absorption spectrum of PpIX for maximal PDT outcome.

Histological examination of excised nBCC skin cancers after MAL application indicated that PpIX fluorescence preferentially accumulated within the tumour cells, rather than the normal surrounding tissue and was at its greatest observed depth after three hours cream application, although full thickness photosensitisation was not achieved following a single application of the prodrug cream in these relative thick dermatological skin cancers. The addition of the hydroxypyridinone iron chelating agent, CP94 to routine dermatological PpIX-induced PDT was found to be a simple and safe pharmacological modification. There was a trend of increasing efficacy with increasing CP94 dose, which may indicate that with further work this technique of enhancement may increase the proportion of BCC that can be treated by this modality in the future.

Furthermore, a rapid decline in oxygen saturation was observed to occur during dermatological MAL-PDT following the initiation of irradiation and this finding was found to be linearly related to the PpIX photobleaching that also occurred during this same time period. An increase in perfusion was also initially recorded within lesions during light irradiation, which then plateaued or declined as the irradiation continued. It is hypothesised that this increase in perfusion occurred in an attempt to replenish tissue oxygen depletion produced by the PDT process proceeding but was eventually outstripped. As PDT is an oxygen dependent process these findings indicate that oxygen availability may be limiting overall treatment effectiveness.

The findings of these investigations taken as a whole indicate that the mechanism of action of dermatological PDT is complex and depends on adequate PpIX accumulation throughout the full thickness of the lesion, delivery of the total light dose at the right wavelength and time as well as sufficient oxygen availability throughout irradiation. Excellent technique, lesion preparation and cream application is therefore essential for the success of PDT treatments as well as appropriate lesion selection in the first place. Furthermore, as PpIX photobleaching during irradiation can be utilised as a surrogate marker of PDT effectiveness, any intervention that reduces this observation or any application where this occurs in a less than optimal manner should be avoided wherever possible or requires enhancement for maximal PDT efficacy to occur respectively. Opportunities therefore still exist to further improve topical PpIX-induced PDT outcomes and widen the application of this modality to dermatological conditions not presently adequately covered by the highly effective standardised protocols currently being employed for licensed clinical indications.

ACKNOWLEDGEMENTS

We would like to thank all of our colleagues, collaborators and patients for their assistance with this research as well as the Duchy Health Charity Ltd and Killing Cancer for their generous financial support.

REFERENCES

[1]   Henderson, BW; Dougherty, T. How does photodynamic therapy work? *Photochem Photobiol,* 1992;55:145-57.

[2]   Luna, MC; Ferrario, A; Wong, S; Fisher, AM; Gomer, CJ. Photodynamic therapy-mediated oxidative stress as a molecular switch for the temporal expression of genes ligated to the human heat shock promoter. *Cancer Res,* 2000;60:1637-44.

[3]   Braathen, LR; Szeimies, RM; Basset-Seguin, N; Bissonnette, R; Foley, P; Pariser, D; Roelandts, R; Wennberg, AM; Morton, CA. Guidelines on the use of photodynamic therapy for nonmelanoma skin cancer: An international consensus. International Society for Photodynamic Therapy in Dermatology, 2005. *J Am Acad Dermatol,* 2007;56:125-43.

[4]   Peng, Q; Berg, K; Moan, J; Kongshaug, M; Nesland, JM. 5-Aminolevulinic acid-based photodynamic therapy: principles and experimental research. *Photochem Photobiol,* 1997;65:235-51.

[5]   Nowis, D; Makowski, M; Stoklosa, T; Legat, M; Issat, T; Golab, J. Direct tumor damage mechanisms of photodynamic therapy. *Acta Biochim Pol,* 2005;52:339-52.

[6]   Ackroyd, R; Kelty, C; Brown, N; Reed, M. The history of photodetection and photodynamic therapy. *Photochem Photobiol,* 2001;74:656-69.

[7]   Allison, RR; Downie, GH; Cuenca, R; Hu, XH; Childs, CJ; Sibata, CH. Photosensitizers in clinical PDT. *Photodiagnosis Photodynamic Therapy,* 2004;1:27-42.

[8]   Brown, SB; Brown, EA; Walker, I. The present and future role of photodynamic therapy in cancer treatment. *Lancet Oncol,* 2004;5:497-508.

[9]   Morton, CA; Szeimies, RM; Sidoroff, A; Braathen, LR. European guidelines for topical photodynamic therapy part 1: treatment delivery and current indications - actinic keratoses, Bowen's disease, basal cell carcinoma. *J Eur Acad Dermatol Venereol,* 2013;27:536-44.

[10]   Malik, Z; Lugaci, H. Destruction of erythroleukaemic cells by photoactivation of endogenous porphyrins. *Br J Cancer,* 1987;56:589-95.

[11]   Kennedy, JC; Pottier, RH; Pross, DC. Photodynamic therapy with endogenous protoporphyrin IX: basic principles and present clinical experience. *J Photochem Photobiol B,* 1990;6:143-8.

[12]   Dailey, HA. Enzymes of heme biosynthesis. *JBIC,* 1997;2:411-7.

[13]   Ericson, MB; Wennberg, A; Larkö, O. Review of photodynamic therapy in actinic keratosis and basal cell carcinoma. *Ther Clin Risk Manag,* 2008;4:1-9.

[14]   Moan, J; Sommer, S. Oxygen dependence of the photosensitizing effect of hematoporphyrin derivative in NHIK 3025 cells. *Cancer Res,* 1985;45:1608-10.

[15]   Castanoa, AP; Demidova, TN; Hamblin, MR. Mechanisms in photodynamic therapy: part one - photosensitizers, photochemistry and cellular localization. *Photodiagnosis Photodyn Ther,* 2004;1:279-83.

[16]   Plaetzer, K; Kiesslich, T; Oberdanner, CB; Krammer, B. Apoptosis Following Photodynamic Tumor Therapy: Induction, Mechanisms and Detection. *Current Pharma Design,* 2005;11:1151-5.

[17]   Flora, SJS. Structural, chemical and biological aspects of antioxidants for strategies against metal and metalloid exposure. *Oxid Med Cell,* 2009;2:191-206.

[18]   Ryter, SW; Alam, J; Choi, AM. Heme oxygenase-1/carbon monoxide: from basic science to therapeutic applications. *Physiol Rev,* 2006;86:583-650.

[19]   Sutton, HC; Winterbourn, CC. On the participation of higher oxidation states of iron and copper in Fenton reactions. *Free Rad Biol Med,* 1989;6:53-60.

[20]   Pourzand, C; Watkin, RD; Brown, JE; Tyrrell, RM. Ultraviolet A radiation induces immediate release of iron in human primary skin fibroblasts: The role of ferritin. *Proc Natl Acad Sci* USA,1999;96:6751-6.

[21]   Mroz, P; Yaroslavsky, A; Kharkwal, GB; Hamblin, MR. Cell Death Pathways in Photodynamic Therapy of Cancer. *Cancers,* 2011;3:2516-39.

[22]   Kessel, D; Vicente, MG; Reiners, JJ. Initiation of apoptosis and autophagy by photodynamic therapy. *Autophagy,* 2006;2:289-90.

[23]   Kessel, D; Vicente, MG; Reiners, JJ. Initiation of apoptosis and autophagy by photodynamic therapy. *Lasers Surg Med,* 2006;38:482-8.

[24]   Luo, Y; Chang, CK; Kessel, D. Rapid initiation of apoptosis by photodynamic therapy. *Photochem Photobiol,* 1996;63:528-34.

[25]   Wallach, D; Varfolomeev, EE; Malinin, NL; Goltsev, YV; Kovalenko, AV; Boldin, MP. Tumor necrosis factor receptor and Fas signaling mechanisms. *Annu Rev Immunol,* 1999;17:331-67.

[26] Zhuang, S; Demirs, JT; Kochevar, IE. Protein kinase C inhibits singlet oxygen-induced apoptosis by decreasing caspase-8 activation. *Oncogene,* 2001;20:6764-76.

[27] Morton, CA; McKenna, KE; Rhodes, LE. Guidelines for topical photodynamic therapy: update. *Br J Dermatol,* 2008;159:1245-66.

[28] Svanberg, K; Andersson, T; Killander, D; Wang, I; Stenram, U; Andersson-Engels, S; Berg, R; Johansson, J; Svanberg, S. Photodynamic therapy of non-melanoma malignant tumours of the skin using topical delta-amino levulinic acid sensitization and laser irradiation. *Br J Dermatol,* 1994;130:743-51.

[29] Dirschka, T; Radny, P; Dominicus, R; Mensing, H; Brüning, H; Jenne, L; Karl, L; Sebastian, M; Oster-Schmidt, C; Klövekorn, W; Reinhold, U; Tanner, M; Gröne, D; Deichmann, M; Simon, M; Hübinger, F; Hofbauer, G; Krähn-Senftleben, G; Borrosch, F; Reich, K; Berking, C; Wolf, P; Lehmann, P; Moers-Carpi, M; Hönigsmann, H; Wernicke-Panten, K; Hahn, S; Pabst, G; Voss, D; Foguet, M; Schmitz, B; Lübbert, H; Szeimies, RM. Photodynamic therapy with BF-200 ALA for the treatment of actinic keratosis: results of a multicentre, randomized, observer-blind phase III study in comparison with a registered methyl-5-aminolaevulinate cream and placebo. *Br J Dermat,* 2012;166:137-46.

[30] Tyrrell, J; Morton, C; Campbell, S; Curnow, A. Comparison of PpIX accumulation and destruction during methyl-aminolevulinate photodynamic therapy (MAL-PDT) of skin tumours located at acral and non-acral sites. *Br J Dermat,* 2011;164:1362-8.

[31] Bogaards, A; Sterenborg, HJ; Trachtenberg, J; Wilson, BC; Lilge L. In vivo quantification of fluorescent molecular markers in real-time by ratio imaging for diagnostic screening and image-guided surgery. *Lasers in Surgery and Medicine,* 2007;39:605-13.

[32] Neville, JA; Welch, E; Leffell, DJ. Management of nonmelanoma skin cancer in 2007. *Nat Clin Pract Oncol,* 2007;4:462-9.

[33] Green, A. Changing patterns in incidence of non-melanoma skin cancer. *Epithelial Cell Biol,* 1992;1:47-51.

[34] Annemans, L; Caekelbergh, K; Roelandts, R; Boonen, H; Leys, C; Nikkels, AF; van Den Haute, V; van Quickenborne, L; Verhaeghe, E; Leroy, B. Real-life practice study of the clinical outcome and cost-effectiveness of photodynamic therapy using methyl aminolevulinate (MAL-PDT) in the management of actinic keratosis and basal cell carcinoma. *Eur J Dermatol,* 2008;18:539-46.

[35] Basset-Seguin, N; Ibbotson, SH; Emtestam, L; Tarstedt, M; Morton, C; Maroti, M; Calzavara-Pinton, P; Varma, S; Roelandts, R; Wolf, P. Topical methyl aminolaevulinate photodynamic therapy versus cryotherapy for superficial basal cell carcinoma: a 5 year randomized trial. *Eur J Dermatol,* 2008;18:547-53.

[36] Kaufmann, R; Spelman, L; Weightman, W; Reifenberger, J; Szeimies, RM; Verhaeghe, E; Kerrouche, N; Sorba, V; Villemagne, H; Rhodes, LE. Multicentre intraindividual randomized trial of topical methyl aminolaevulinate-photodynamic therapy vs. cryotherapy for multiple actinic keratoses on the extremities. *Br J Dermatol,* 2008;158:994-9.

[37] Morton, CA; Horn, M; Leman, J; Tack, B; Bedane, C; Tijoe, M; Ibbotson, S; Khemis, A; Wolf, P. Comparison of topical methyl aminolevulinate photodynamic therapy with cryotherapy or Fluorouracil for treatment of squamous cell carcinoma in situ: Results of a multicenter randomized trial. *Arch Dermatol,* 2006; 142:729-35.

[38] Morton, CA. Methyl aminolevulinate (Metvix) photodynamic therapy - practical pearls. *J Dermatolog Treat*, 2003;14:23-6.

[39] Foley, P. Clinical efficacy of methyl aminolevulinate (Metvix) photodynamic therapy. *J Dermatolog Treat*, 2003;14:15-22.

[40] Szeimies, R; Ibbotson, S; Murrell, D; Rubel, D; Frambach, Y; de Berker, D; Dummer, R; Kerrouche, N; Villemagne, H; Excilight Study Group.. A clinical study comparing methyl aminolevulinate photodynamic therapy and surgery in small superficial basal cell carcinoma (8-20 mm), with a 12-month follow-up. *J Eur Acad Dermatol Venereol*, 2008;22:1302-11.

[41] Scott, MA; Hooper, C; Sahota, A; Springett, R; McIlroy, BW; Bown, SG; Macrobert, AJ.. Fluorescence Photodiagnosis and Photobleaching Studies of Cancerous Lesions using Ratio Imaging and Spectroscopic Techniques. *Lasers Med Sci*, 2000;15:63-72.

[42] Wennberg, AM; Gudmundson, F; Stenquist, B; Ternesten, A; Molne, L; Rosen, A; Larko O.. In vivo detection of basal cell carcinoma using imaging spectroscopy. *Acta Derm Venereol*, 1999;79:54-61.

[43] Ackermann, G; Abels, C; Karrer, S; Baumler, W; Landthaler, M; Szeimies, RM. Fluorescence-assisted biopsy of basal cell carcinomas. *Hautarzt*, 2000;51:920-4.

[44] Siewecke, C; Szeimies, RM. PDT and fluorescence diagnosis in dermatology. *Hospital Pharmacy Europe*, 2004;May/June:49-52.

[45] Smits, T; Kleinpenning, MM; Blokx, WA; van de Kerkhof, PC; van Erp, PE; Gerritsen, MJ. Fluorescence diagnosis in keratinocytic intraepidermal neoplasias. *Journal of the American Academy of Dermatology*, 2007;57:824-31.

[46] Bogaards, A; Aalders, MC; Zeyl, CC; de Blok, S; Dannecker, C; Hillemanns, P; Stepp, H; Sterenborg, HJ.. Localization and staging of cervical intraepithelial neoplasia using double ratio fluorescence imaging, *J Biomed Opt;* 2002;7:215-20.

[47] Hua, Z; Gibson, SL; Foster, TH; Hilf, R. Effectiveness of delta-aminolevulinic acid-induced protoporphyrin as a photosensitizer for photodynamic therapy in vivo. *Cancer Research*, 1995;55:1723-31.

[48] Loh, CS; Vernon, D; MacRobert, AJ; Bedwell, J; Bown, SG; Brown, SB. Endogenous porphyrin distribution induced by 5-aminolaevulinic acid in the tissue layers of the gastrointestinal tract. *Journal of Photochemistry and Photobiology*, 1993;20:47-54.

[49] Andersson-Engels, S; Klinteberg, C; Svanberg, K; Svanberg, S. In vivo fluorescence imaging for tissue diagnostics. *Physics in Medicine and Biology*, 1997;42:815-24.

[50] Boere, IA; Robinson, DJ; de Bruijn, HS; van den Boogert, J; Tilanus, HW; Sterenborg, HJ; de Bruin, RW. Monitoring in situ dosimetry and protoporphyrin IX fluorescence photobleaching in the normal rat esophagus during 5-aminolevulinic acid photodynamic therapy. *Photochem Photobiol*, 2003;78:271-7.

[51] Ericson, MB; Sandberg, C; Stenquist, B; Gudmundson, F; Karlsson, M; Ros, AM; Rosén, A; Larkö, O; Wennberg, AM; Rosdahl I.. Photodynamic therapy of actinic keratosis at varying fluence rates: assessment of photobleaching, pain and primary clinical outcome. *Br J Derm*, 2004;151:1204-12.

[52] Loschenov, VB; Konov, VI; Prokhorov, AM. Photodynamic Therapy and Fluorescence Diagnostics. *Laser Physics*, 2000;10:1188-1207.

[53] Peng, Q; Soler, AM; Warloe, T; Nesland, JM; Giercksky, KE. Selective distribution of porphyrins in skin thick basal cell carcinoma after topical application of methyl 5-aminolevulinate. *Journal of Photochemistry and Photobiology*, 2001;62:140-5.

[54] Fauteck, JD; Ackermann, G; Birkel, M; Breuer, M; Moor, AC; Ebeling, A; Ortland, C. Fluorescence characteristics and pharmacokinetic properties of a novel self-adhesive 5-ALA patch for photodynamic therapy of actinic keratoses. *Arch Dermatol Res,* 2008;300:53-60.

[55] Jaap de, L; van der Beek, N; Neugebauer, WD; Bjerring, P; Neumann, HA. Fluorescence detection and diagnosis of non-melanoma skin cancer at an early stage. *Lasers in Surgery and Medicine,* 2009;41:96-103.

[56] Tyrrell, J; Campbell, S; Curnow, A. The validation of a non-invasive fluorescence imaging system to monitor clinical dermatological photodynamic therapy. *Photodiagnosis Photodyn Ther,* 2010;7:86-97.

[57] Cottrell, WJ; Paquette, AD; Keymel, KR; Foster, TH; Oseroff, AR. Irradiance-dependent photobleaching and pain in delta-aminolevulinic acid-photodynamic therapy of superficial basal cell carcinomas. *Clin Cancer Res,* 2008;14:4475-83.

[58] Wennberg, AM. Pain, pain relief and other practical issues in photodynamic therapy. *Australasian Journal of Dermatology,* 2005;46:S3-S4.

[59] Kruijt, B; de Bruijn, HS; van der Ploeg-van den Heuvel, A; de Bruin, RW; Sterenborg, HJ; Amelink, A; Robinson, DJ. Monitoring ALA-induced PpIX photodynamic therapy in the rat esophagus using fluorescence and reflectance spectroscopy. *Photochem Photobiol,* 2008;84:1515-27.

[60] Lindeburg, KE; Brogaard, HM; Jemec, GB. Pain and photodynamic therapy. *Dermatology (Basel, Switzerland),* 2007;215:206-8.

[61] Morton, CA. Photodynamic therapy for nonmelanoma skin cancer and more? *Arch Dermatol.* 2004;140:116-20.

[62] Grapengiesser, S; Ericson, M; Gudmundsson, F; Larko, O; Rosen, A; Wennberg, AM. Pain caused by photodynamic therapy of skin cancer. *Clinical and Experimental Dermatology.* 2002;27:493-7.

[63] Morton, CA; MacKie, RM. Photodynamic Therapy for Basal Cell Carcinoma: Effect of Tumour Thickness and Duration of Photosensitizer Application on Response. *Arch Dermatol.* 1998;134:248-9.

[64] Morton, CA; Whitehurst, C; McColl, JH; Moore, JV; MacKie, RM. Photodynamic therapy for large or multiple patches of Bowen disease and basal cell carcinoma. *Arch Dermatol.* 2001;137:319-24.

[65] Wiegell, SR; Skiveren, J; Philipsen, PA; Wulf, HC. Pain during photodynamic therapy is associated with protoporphyrin IX fluorescence and fluence rate. *Br J Dermatol.* 2008;158:727-33.

[66] Holmes, MV; Dawe, RS; Ferguson, J; Ibbotson, SH. A randomized, double-blind, placebo-controlled study of the efficacy of tetracaine gel (Ametop) for pain relief during topical photodynamic therapy. *Br J Dermatol,* 2004;150;337-40.

[67] Paoli, J; Halldin, C; Ericson, MB; Wennberg, AM. Nerve blocks provide effective pain relief during topical photodynamic therapy for extensive facial actinic keratoses. *Clin Exp Dermatol,* 2008;33:559-64.

[68] Halldin, CB; Paoli, J; Sandberg, C; Gonzalez, H; Wennberg, AM. Nerve blocks enable adequate pain relief during topical photodynamic therapy of field cancerization on the forehead and scalp. *Br J Dermatol,* 2009;160:795-800.

[69]   Pagliaro, J; Elliott, T; Bulsara, M; King, C; Vinciullo, C. Cold air analgesia in photodynamic therapy of basal cell carcinomas and Bowen's disease: an effective addition to treatment: a pilot study. *Dermatol Surg, 2004*;30:63-6.

[70]   Serra-Guillen, C; Hueso, L; Nagore, E; Vila, M; Llombart, B; Requena Caballero, C; Botella-Estrada, R; Sanmartinm, O; Alfaro-Rubio, A; Guillen, C.. Comparative study between cold air analgesia and supraorbital and supratrochlear nerve block for the management of pain during photodynamic therapy for actinic keratoses of the frontotemporal zone. *Br J Dermatol, 2009*;161:353-6.

[71]   Calzavara-Pinton, PG; Venturini, M; Sala, R. Photodynamic therapy: update 2006. Part 1: Photochemistry and Photobiology. *J Eur Acad Dermatol Venereol,* 2007;21:293-302.

[72]   Fuchs, J; Thiele, J. The role of oxygen in cutaneous photodynamic therapy. *Free Radic Biol Med,* 1998;24:835-47.

[73]   Henderson, BW; Fingar, VH. Relationship of tumor hypoxia and response to photodynamic treatment in an experimental mouse tumor. *Cancer Res,* 1987;47: 3110-4.

[74]   Busch, TM. Local physiological changes during photodynamic therapy. *Lasers Surg Med,* 2006;38:494-9.

[75]   Chen, Q; Huang, Z; Chen, H; Shapiro, H; Beckers, J; Hetzel, FW.. Improvement of tumor response by manipulation of tumor oxygenation during photodynamic therapy. *Photochem Photobiol,* 2002;76:197-203.

[76]   Tromberg, BJ; Orenstein, A; Kimel, S; Barker, SJ; Hyatt, J; Nelson, JS; Berns, MW.. In vivo tumor oxygen tension measurements for the evaluation of the efficiency of photodynamic therapy. *Photochem Photobiol,* 1990;52:375-85.

[77]   Mitchell, JB; McPherson, S; DeGraff, W; Gamson, J; Zabell, A; Russo A.. Oxygen dependence of hematoporphyrin derivative-induced photoinactivation of Chinese hamster cells. *Cancer Res,* 1985;45:2008-11.

[78]   Busch, TM; Hahn, SM; Evans, SM; Koch, CJ.. Depletion of tumor oxygenation during photodynamic therapy: detection by the hypoxia marker EF3 [2-(2-nitroimidazol-1[H]-yl)-N-(3,3,3-trifluoropropyl)acetamide]. *Cancer Res,* 2000;60:2636-42.

[79]   Curnow, A; Haller, JC; Bown, SG. Oxygen monitoring during 5-aminolaevulinic acid induced photodynamic therapy in normal rat colon. Comparison of continuous and fractionated light regimes. *J Photochem Photobiol B,* 2000;58:149-55.

[80]   Pogue, BW; O'Hara, JA; Goodwin, IA. Wilmot, CJ; Fournier, GP; Akay, AR; Swartz, H.. Tumor PO(2) changes during photodynamic therapy depend upon photosensitizer type and time after injection. *Comp Biochem Physiol A Mol Integr Physiol, 2002*;132:177-84.

[81]   Henderson, BW; Gollnick, SO; Snyder, JW; Busch, TM; Kousis, PC; Cheney, RT; Morgan, J.. Choice of oxygen-conserving treatment regimen determines the inflammatory response and outcome of photodynamic therapy of tumors. *Cancer Res,* 2004;64:2120-6.

[82]   Sitnik, TM; Hampton, JA; Henderson, BW. Reduction of tumour oxygenation during and after photodynamic therapy in vivo: effects of fluence rate. *Br J Cancer,* 1998;77:1386-94.

[83] Busch, TM; Wileyto, EP; Emanuele, MJ; Del Piero, F; Marconato, L; Glatstein, E; Koch, CJ.. Photodynamic therapy creates fluence rate-dependent gradients in the intratumoral spatial distribution of oxygen. *Cancer Res,* 2002;62:7273-9.

[84] Robinson, DJ; de Bruijn, HS; van der Veen, N; Stringer, MR; Brown, SB; Star, WM.. Protoporphyrin IX fluorescence photobleaching during ALA-mediated photodynamic therapy of UVB-induced tumors in hairless mouse skin. *Photochem Photobiol,* 1999;69:61-70.

[85] Thompson, MS; Johansson, A; Johansson, T; Andersson-Engels, S; Svanberg, S; Bendsoe, N; Svanberg, K.. Clinical system for interstitial photodynamic therapy with combined on-line dosimetry measurements. *Appl Opt,* 2005;44:4023-31.

[86] Enejder, AM; af Klinteberg, C; Wang, I; Andersson-Engels, S; Bendsoe, N; Svanberg, S; Svanberg, K.. Blood perfusion studies on basal cell carcinomas in conjunction with photodynamic therapy and cryotherapy employing laser-Doppler perfusion imaging. *Acta Derm Venereol,* 2000;80:19-23.

[87] Schacht, V; Szeimies, RM; Abels, C. Photodynamic therapy with 5-aminolevulinic acid induces distinct microcirculatory effects following systemic or topical application. *Photochem Photobiol Sci,* 2006;5:452-8.

[88] Herman, MA; Fromm, D; Kessel, D. Tumor blood-flow changes following protoporphyrin IX-based photodynamic therapy in mice and humans. *J Photochem Photobiol B,* 1999;52:99-104.

[89] Morton, CA; Brown, SB; Collins, S; Ibbotson, S; Jenkinson, H; Kurwa, H; Langmack, K; McKenna, K; Moseley, H; Pearse, AD; Stringer, M; Taylor, DK; Wong, G; Rhodes, LE. Guidelines for topical photodynamic therapy: report of a workshop of the British Photodermatology Group. *Br J Dermatol,* 2002;146:552-67.

[90] National Institute of Health and Care Excellence (NICE), Photodynamic therapy for non-melanoma skin tumours (including premalignant and primary non-metastatic skin lesions). *Interventional Procedures Guidance* [IPG155]. 2006.

[91] Morton, CA; Mackie, RM; Whitehurst, C; Moore,JV; McColl, JH.. Photodynamic therapy for basal cell carcinoma: effect of tumour thickness and duration of photosensitiser application on response. *Arch Dermatol,* 1998;134:248-9.

[92] Barr, H; MacRobert, AJ; Tralau, CJ; Boulos, PB; Bown, SG. The significance of the nature of the photosensitisers for photodynamic therapy: quantitative and biological studies in the colon. *Br J Cancer,* 1990;62:730-5.

[93] Messmann, H; Mlkvy, P; Buonaccorsi, G; Davies, CL; MacRobert, AJ; Bown, SG. Enhancement of photodynamic therapy with 5-aminolaevulinic acid-induced porphyrin photosensitisation in normal rat colon by threshold and light fractionation studies. *Br J Cancer,* 1995;72:589-94.

[94] Barr, H; Tralau, CJ; MacRobert, AJ; Krasner, N; Boulos, PB; Clark, CJ; Bown, SG. Photodynamic therapy in the normal rat colon with phthalocyanine sensitisation. *Br J Cancer,* 1987;56:111-8.

[95] Tyrrell, J; Campbell, S; Curnow, A. Protoporphyrin IX photobleaching during the light irradiation phase of standard dermatological methyl-aminolevulinate photodynamic therapy. *Photodiagnosis and Photodynamic Therapy,* 2010;7:232-8.

[96] Thorn, CE. *The Regulation of Cutaneous Microvascular Haemodynamics as determined by Optical Reflectance Spectroscopy;* the Role of Vasomotion In: Peninsula

Postgraduate Health Institute, Vol. PhD. Exeter: Universities of Exeter and Plymouth. 2008; 281.

[97]   Meglinsky, IV; Matcher, SJ. Modelling the sampling volume for skin blood oxygenation measurements. *Med Biol Eng Comput,* 2001;39:44-50.

[98]   Merschbrock, U; Hoffmann, J; Caspary, L; Huber, J; Schmickaly, U; Lübbers, DW.. Fast wavelength scanning reflectance spectrophotometer for noninvasive determination of hemoglobin oxygenation in human skin. *Int J Microcirc Clin Exp,* 1994;14:274-81.

[99]   Palsson, S; Gustafsson, L; Bendsoe, N; Soto Thompson, M; Andersson-Engels, S; Svanberg, K.. Kinetics of the superficial perfusion and temperature in connection with photodynamic therapy of basal cell carcinomas using esterified and non-esterified 5-aminolaevulinic acid. *Br J Dermatol,* 2003;148:1179-88.

[100] Peng, Q; Warloe, T; Berg, K; Moan, J; Kongshaug, M; Giercksky, KE; Nesland, JM. 5-Aminolevulinic acid-based photodynamic therapy. Clinical research and future challenges. *Cancer,* 1997;79:2282-308.

[101] Morton, C; Horn, M; Leman, J; Tack, B; Bedane, C; Tjioe, M; Ibbotson, S; Khemis, A; Wolf, P. Comparison of topical methyl aminolevulinate photodynamic therapy with cryotherapy or Fluorouracil for treatment of squamous cell carcinoma in situ: Results of a multicenter randomized trial. *Arch Dermatol,* 2006; 142:729-35.

[102] Calzavara-Pinton, PG; Venturini, M; Sala, R. Photodynamic therapy: update 2006. Part 2: Clinical results. *J Eur Acad Dermatol Venereol,* 2007;21:439-51.

[103] Ascencio, M; Collinet, P; Farine, MO; Mordon, S. Protoporphyrin IX fluorescence photobleaching is a useful tool to predict the response of rat ovarian cancer following hexaminolevulinate photodynamic therapy. *Lasers Surg Med,* 2008;40:332-41.

[104] Robinson, DJ; de Bruijn, HS; van der Veen, N; Stringer, MR; Brown, SB; Star, WM. Fluorescence photobleaching of ALA-induced protoporphyrin IX during photodynamic therapy of normal hairless mouse skin: the effect of light dose and irradiance and the resulting biological effect. *Photochem Photobiol,* 1998;67:140-9.

[105] Fink-Puches, R; Hofer, A; Smolle, J; Kerl, H; Wolf, P.. Primary clinical response and long-term follow-up of solar keratoses treated with topically applied 5-aminolevulinic acid and irradiation by different wave bands of light. *J Photochem Photobiol B,* 1997;41:145-51.

[106] Itoh, Y; Ninomiya, Y; Henta, T; Tajima, S; Ishibashi, A.. Topical delta-aminolevulinic acid-based photodynamic therapy for Japanese actinic keratoses. *J Dermatol,* 2000;27:513-8.

[107] Jeffes, EW; McCullough, JL; Weinstein, GD; Fergin, PE; Nelson, JS; Shull, TF; Simpson, KR; Bukaty, LM; Hoffman, WL; Fong, NL.. Photodynamic therapy of actinic keratosis with topical 5-aminolevulinic acid. A pilot dose-ranging study. *Arch Dermatol,* 1997;133:727-32.

[108] Szeimies, RM; Karrer, S; Sauerwald, A; Landthaler, M.. Photodynamic therapy with topical application of 5-aminolevulinic acid in the treatment of actinic keratoses: an initial clinical study. *Dermatology,* 1996;192:246-51.

[109] Kurwa, HA; Yong-Gee, SA; Seed, PT; Markey, AC; Barlow, RJ.. A randomized paired comparison of photodynamic therapy and topical 5-fluorouracil in the treatment of actinic keratoses. *J Am Acad Dermatol,* 1999;41:414-8.

[110] Piaserico, S; Belloni Fortina, A; Rigotti, P; Rossi, B; Baldan, N; Alaibac, M; Marchini, F.. Topical photodynamic therapy of actinic keratosis in renal transplant recipients. *Transplant Proc,* 2007;39:1847-50.

[111] Sandby-Moller, J; Poulsen, T; Wulf, HC. Epidermal thickness at different body sites: relationship to age, gender, pigmentation, blood content, skin type and smoking habits. *Acta Derm Venereol,* 2003;83:410-3.

[112] Jun, MS; Choi, HS; Han, I; Kim, M; Kim, JC.. In vitro and ex vivo protoporphyrin IX expression induced by 5-aminolevulinic acid in human pilosebaceous unit. *J Dermatol Sci,* 2005;40:68-70.

[113] Dysart, JS; Patterson, MS. Photobleaching kinetics, photoproduct formation, and dose estimation during ALA induced PpIX PDT of MLL cells under well oxygenated and hypoxic conditions. *Photochem Photobiol Sci,* 2006;5:73-81.

[114] Sheng, C; Hoopes, PJ; Hasan, T; Pogue, BW. Photobleaching-based dosimetry predicts deposited dose in ALA-PpIX PDT of rodent esophagus. *Photochem Photobiol,* 2007;83:738-48.

[115] Rittenhouse-Diakun, K; Van Leengoed, H; Morgan, J. The role of transferrin receptor (CD71) in photodynamic therapy of activated and malignant lymphocytes using the heme precursor delta-aminolevulinic acid (ALA). *Photochem Photobiol,* 1995;61:523-86.

[116] Choudry, K; Brooke, RCC; Farrer, W; Rhodes, LE. The effect of an iron chelating agent on protoporphyrin IX levels and phototoxicity in topical 5-aminolaevulinic acid photodynamic therapy. *Br J Dermatol,* 2003;149:124-30.

[117] Hoyes, KP; Porter, JB. Subcellular distribution of desferrioxamine and hydroxypyridin-4-one chelators in K562 cells affects chelation of intracellular iron pools. *Br J Haematol,* 1993;85:393-400.

[118] Curnow, A; McIlroy, BW; Postle-Hacon, MJ; Porter, JB; MacRobert, AJ; Bown, SG.. Enhancement of 5-aminolaevulinic acid induced photodynamic therapy using iron chelating agents. *Br J Cancer,* 1998;78:1278-82.

[119] Curnow, A; MacRobert, A; Bown, S. Comparing and combining light fractionation and iron chelation to enhance experimental photodynamic therapy with aminolevulinic acid. *Lasers in Surg and Med,* 2006;38:325-31.

[120] Bech, O; Phillips, D; Moan, J; MacRobert, AJ. A hydroxypyridinone (CP94) enhances protoporphyrin IX formation in 5-aminolaevulinic acid treated cells. *J Photochem Photobiol B: Biol,* 1997;41:136-44.

[121] Pye, A; Curnow, A. Direct comparison of delta-aminolevulinic acid and methyl-aminolevulinate-derived protoporphyrin IX accumulations potentiated by desferrioxamine or the novel hydroxypyridinone iron chelator CP94 in cultured human cells. *Photochem Photobiol,* 2007;83:766–73.

[122] Szeimies, RM; Abels, C; Fritsh, C; Karrer, S; Steinbach, P; Baumler, W; Goerz, G; Goetz, AE; Landthaler, M. Wavelength dependency of photodynamic effects after sensitisation with 5-aminolaevulinic acid in vitro and in vivo. *The Journal of Investigative Dermatology,* 1995;105:672-7.

[123] De Jode, ML; McGilligan, JA; Dilkes, MG; Cameron, I; Grahn, MF; Williams, NS. An in vivo comparison of the photodynamic action of a new diode laser and a copper vapour dye laser at 652 nm. *Lasers in Medical Science, 1996*;11:117-21.

[124] Henderson, BW; Busch, TM; Snyder, JW. Fluence rate as a modulator of PDT mechanisms. *Lasers Surg Med,* 2006;38:489-93.

In: Photodynamic Therapy
Editor: Adrian G. Hugo

ISBN: 978-1-63463-857-9
© 2015 Nova Science Publishers, Inc.

Chapter 4

NANOTECHNOLOGY-BASED CANCER PHOTODYNAMIC THERAPY

Elisa Panzarini* and Luciana Dini

Department of Biological and Environmental Science and Technology (Di.S.Te.B.A.),
University of Salento, Lecce, Italy

ABSTRACT

The increasing incidence of cancer and the search for the development of more effective therapies with minimal side effects have prompted studies to find alternative new treatments. Among new therapies, PhotoDynamic Therapy (PDT) appears a promising modality in cancer treatment with the lowest rates of side effects over traditional modalities as surgery, ionizing radiation and chemotherapy. PDT is currently used in the clinic for the treatment of several types of tumors, i.e. lung, gastrointestinal tract, head and neck, bladder, prostate, non melanoma skin cancers, and actinic keratosis but also for non oncology applications in ophthalmology, dermatology, cardiology, virus inactivation and blood purification.

PDT exploits the interaction between light, tissue molecular oxygen and PhotoSensitizer (PS). These three components are mandatory for the photodynamic reaction that produces Reactive Oxygen Species (ROS) which by interacting with neighboring lipids and proteins, cause acute injury to tumor microvascular, blood vessel blockage, cell death and immune responses.

This has brought about an active pursuit of new PDT agents that can be optimized for the unique set of photophysical characteristics that are required for a successful clinical agent. Many of the PS under investigation are already commercially available, but most of them show prolonged skin phototoxicity, extended retention in the host organism, low extinction coefficient and absorption peak at short wavelengths, low photostability, limited range of solvent conditions and loss of photodynamic activity in aqueous media. In particular, the majority of PS in the clinical use or under preclinical study are hydrophobic and strongly aggregate in aqueous media, thus resulting in a reduction of the photosensitizing efficacy.

* Corresponding author: Dr. Elisa Panzarini, Department of Biological and Environmental Sciences and Technologies (Di.S.Te.B.A.), University of Salento, Prov.le Lecce-Monteroni, 73100 Lecce, Italy, e-mail: elisa.panzarini@unisalento.it; phone: +390832298614; fax: +390832298937.

The recent application of NanoMaterials (NMs) in biomedicine offers excellent prospects for circumventing these PSs drawbacks. For examples, the aggregation tendency may be minimized by using a nanostructured photosensitive molecular structure. The selective release and accumulation of PSs at the targeted tissue can be enhanced by using nanocarriers. Among the many NMs already exploited in oncomedicine, like polymeric NanoParticles (NPs), dendrimers, liposomes, polymersomes, polymeric micelles, nanospheres, fullerenes, Quantum Dots (QDs), SuperParamagnetic Iron Oxide NanoParticles (SPIONs) and metallic and non-metallic NPs, researchers are searching for the most suitable NM for PDT use. Liposomes, polymeric NPs, gold NPs, QDs and UpConvertingNanoParticles (UCNPs) are particularly promising to circumvent photobleaching and low tissue penetration of PSs.

In this chapter we will overview the most important and recent developments of NMs for cancer PDT.

Keywords: Photodynamic therapy; NanoMaterials (NMs); drug delivery; nanocarriers; PhotoSensitizers (PSs); cancer therapy

1. INTRODUCTION

Surgery, radiation therapy, chemotherapy and, more recently, immunotherapy are the current clinical strategies to counteract cancer. Unfortunately each of these strategies presents disadvantages, leading to different side effects. For example, surgical removal of tumor is ineffective in the presence of metastasis or when tumor is allocated near sensitive areas; radiotherapy can frequently damage also normal cells, lead to formation of scar tissues or induce immunosuppression; chemotherapy rises undesirable systemic toxic side effects [1] and cancer cells can acquire resistance to chemotherapeutics [2].

Therefore, the goal of the current cancer research is overcoming these limitations. To this end, two different approaches are under investigation: i) the development of alternative treatments resulting safer and/or more beneficial than surgery, chemotherapy or radiotherapy and ii) the improvement of conventional cancer treatments exploiting nanomedicine approaches.

A promising new strategy is PhotoDynamic Therapy (PDT), that is gaining acceptance as a technique for cancer treatment in recent years. It has emerged in management of several types of cancer, i.e., early lung cancer, Barrett's esophagus, bladder cancer, head and neck cancer and skin cancer [3]. Currently, PDT is also clinical used in many non-cancerous diseases, such as macular degeneration, actinic keratosis, psorias, rheumatoid arthritis, dental infections, herpes simplex, Candida albicans, ecc. [4-7].

PDT is based on the destructive power of singlet oxygen ($^1O_2$) and other cytotoxic Reactive Oxygen Species (ROS) produced when non- or weakly-toxic photosensitizer drugs (PSs) are activated by light with appropriate wavelength in the presence of O_2. PDT comprises three phases: excitation of PS, generation of cytotoxic molecules and cells response [3].

A light with an appropriate wavelength, chosen from visible to near-infrared in relation to the maximum absorption wavelength of the PS, activates the PS, that moves from its singlet ground state (S_0) to the short-lived first excited singlet-state (S_1). The S_1 PS can come back to the S_0 state by emitting fluorescence or phosphorescence or it can undergo to intersystem crossing with spin inversion. The S_1 PS converts to the long-lived excited triplet state (T_1) that transfers its energy to biomeolecules to generate ROS through photo-oxidative reactions. Three types of photo-oxidative reactions are known. In the Type I reaction, the PS interacts with ground-state molecular oxygen to produce superoxide anion ($O_2^{\cdot-}$) radicals, hydrogen peroxides (H_2O_2) and hydroxyl radicals ($\cdot OH$); in the so called Type II reaction, the direct transfer of energy from the triplet state PS to the ground state molecular oxygen forms highly-reactive $^1O_2$ [8]; in the Type III reaction, also known as the modified type I (MTO), the long-lived triplet PS directly reacts with biological substrates in the absence of oxygen [9]. The Type II reaction predominates over the others during photosensitization process. In addition, since Type II reaction presents the higher reactive properties, the $^1O_2$ causes irreversible effects, that include microvascular acute injury, blood vessel blockage in the tumor area, cancer cell death and immune responses [10]. Microvascular collapse, fast observed following PDT, can lead to severe and persistent post-PDT tumor hypoxia. The effects induced by PDT on tumor microvascular network are due to vessel constriction, macromolecular vessel leakage, leukocyte adhesion and thrombus formation. The phenomena are linked to platelet activation and aggregation and to thromboxane release upon the inhibition of production/release of nitric oxide by the endothelial cells. PDT induces the death of cancer cells by the concomitantly occurrence of apoptosis, necrosis, and autophagy; however, apoptosis is the preferred path to cell death as also supported by our recent evidences [11-13]. In addition, PDT promotes anti cancer immune response through anti-tumor activity of PDT-induced inflammatory cells that massively release powerful inflammatory mediators regulating a massive neutrophils, mast cells and monocytes/macrophages homing in the tumor site and leading to a long-term anti-tumor immune response [14].

The success of PDT strictly depends on the efficient $^1O_2$ production, that in turn is determined by the selective PS accumulation in malignant cells and by the selective light irradiation. The generation of $^1O_2$ depends on the chemical properties of PS, light intensity and wavelength, and O_2 concentration. Because of the very limited lifetime (less than 3.5 µs) and diffusion length of $^1O_2$ (from 0.001 to 0.02 µm) [15], the localization of the PS is very influential to the induction and to the extent of damage. In general, the damage is confined to the cellular site of PS concentration, that, in turn, strictly depends on PS chemistry and pharmacokinetic, and on the cancer microenvironment, characterized by low pH value [16], overexpression of low density lipoprotein receptor [17], poorly developed lymphatic drainage [18], and tumor-associated macrophages [19]. On the other hand, light is a very limiting factor in PDT. In fact, it is well known that its tissue penetration is a very complex phenomenon due to the fact that the light is either scattered or absorbed in relation to tissue type and light wavelength [20]. In particular, shorter wavelength (less than 650 nm) have lower tissue penetration and high absorption causing skin photosensitivity; conversely, wavelength longer than 850 nm are not sufficient to trigger $^1O_2$ generation. Therefore, the maximum efficiency in PDT occurs within the so called "phototherapeutic window" whose approximate range is 650-850 nm [21].

In searching for overcoming these drawbacks and for better strengthening the therapeutic application of PDT, nanotechnology, nowadays widely used in medicine, represents a very powerful tool [22]. Nanotechnology is also an emerging active research area in the PDT field. In this respect, the incorporation of PSs in nanocarriers can improve tumor targeting and intracellular delivery of the PS payload in particular for those PS that cannot properly accumulate inside the tumor cells. Indeed, most of PSs are hydrophobic and aggregate under physiological conditions, significantly reducing the ROS production [23]. On the other hand, accumulation at malignant sites of water-soluble PSs is not high enough for clinical use. The recent interest in NanoMaterials (NMs) as drug carriers is due to the fact that they (i) can transport hydrophobic drugs in blood, (ii) have large surface area modifiable to acquire additional chemical/biochemical properties and selective targeting, (iii) are efficiently taken up by cells, (iv) can allow a controlled release of drugs, (v) can be synthesized through numerous strategies [24].

It is worth noting that PSs nanocarriers can also have role in the phototoxicity process representing an additional active intermediary in photodynamic reactions (NM can *per se* photogenerate ROS and thus they can be considered a PS) and participating in PS excitation[25-29].

A valuable advantage of the use of nanocarriers relays in that the release of PS for photodynamic reaction is not required; in fact, since ROS represent the therapeutic agent, it is only essential their diffusion out of nanocarriers.

In the following sections, we report the state of the art in the nanomedical approaches for advanced cancer PDT.

2. ENGINEERED NANOSTRUCTURAL MATERIALS FOR APPLICATION IN CANCER PDT

In PDT, engineered NMs can be exploited mainly as nanocarriers for delivery or active targeting of PSs or, as in some instances reported, representing themselves a PS, being able to absorb light and switch to an excited state leading to photochemical generation of ROS. In fact, NMs possess an extinction coefficient of appreciable size in an appropriate region of electromagnetic spectrum.

2.1. NMs as PS nanocarriers. The potential of nanocarriers as transporting vehicles for imaging and therapeutic payloads is extensively accepted [30, 31]. Owing to their ability to adapt to unique features of tumor sites, such as unique tumor microenvironment, in relation to material composition, size, shape, and surface properties, nanocarriers are currently used in cancer management [32].

Efficient and efficacious PSs delivery are the main challenge in PDT. Despite their effectiveness on tumor cells, PSs present several limitations and disadvantages in clinical applications, such as extended retention in the host organism, skin phototoxicity, low solubility in aqueous physiological environment, low accumulation and limited half-life within tissues [23]. One strategy that is promising in overcoming these limitations is the PS encapsulation in nanocarriers. In fact, nanoencapsulation allowing the incorporation of high PS amounts without activity loss or alteration, promote the selective PS accumulation in the diseased tissue, the delivery of therapeutic PS concentrations to the target tissue, the PS protection from degradation and clearance, the minimal drug leakage during transit to target, and the easy PS interaction with cells. Essential carrier prerequisites are biodegradability and minimally or no immunogenicity [24].

Nowadays, liposomes, polymeric and silica NPs are among the most studied PSs nanocarriers in the PDT [33].

2.1.1 Liposomes. Liposomes represent a significant percentage of the nanobiomedicine research today [34], playing an important role also in PDT [24, 35, 36].

Liposomes are nanosized artificially prepared spherical vesicles made of natural or synthetic derived phospholipids and cholesterol. The phospholipids form vesicles with single or multi concentric bilayers, with an aqueous phase inside and between the bilayers [37]. Thus, liposomes characterized by a hydrophilic and a hydrophobic region, allows the encapsulation and delivery of both hydrophilic and hydrophobic drugs. The presence of cholesterol controls membrane fluidity, increases stability and modulates membrane-protein interactions [38]. The variety of available phospholipids for liposome preparation and cholesterol influence liposomes size, charge, and surface properties dictating the drug delivery and release. Two modalities were described for the release from liposomes of the cargo; liposomes can fuse with cell membranes and thus release PS into the cytosol or can be internalized by phagocytes and their digestion inside endosomes or lysosomes allows the cytosolic PS release [38].

However, the interaction of conventional liposomes with ill tissue is influenced by short blood half-life (tens of minutes) that depends on the rate at which liposomes pass through the leaky tumoral vessels, on the poor lymphatic drainage, on the plasma proteins opsonization and on accumulation in liver, spleen, bone marrow and blood phagocytes. Therefore, liposomes can be modified to make them tumoritropic, "invisible" to lipoproteins opsonization and to phagocytes by using polyethylene glycol (PEG) that transform them in "sterically stabilized" or Stealth liposomes [39-41]. Physical and chemical factors, like heat, light, pH and target binding, can tightly allow liposomes to control PSs release. For example, a) thermosensitive liposomes, synthesized with temperature-sensitive lipids or coated with termosensitive polymers, disintegrate at 42°C favoring PS release [42]; b) addition of acid-sensitive molecules to the liposomal membrane allows PSs release between pH 5 and 6,3 [43]; c) photosensitive liposomes, composed of dimyristoylphosphatidylcholine (DMPC) or 1,2-destearoyl-sn-glycero-3-phosphocholine (DSPC), cholesterol and Zinc(II) phtalocyanine (ZnPc) release ZnPc, a second-generation sensitizer for PDT, upon light exposure [44]. A wide range of molecules such as glycoproteins, glycolipids, peptides, growth factors, and monoclonal antibodies, possessing high affinity for specific membrane markers on malignant cells can be attached on liposomal membrane to increase affinity for ill cells and allow a specific PSs target [45, 46]. The peptide, Ala-Pro-Arg-Pro-Gly (APRG), specific for angiogenic endothelial cells, can be conjugated to liposomes to suppress tumor growth through destruction of angiogenic vasculature [47]. Finally, the molecules can be attached directly or *via* spacer arm to phospholipid bilayer allowing also the binding of different purposes molecules, i.e., to increase the circulation half-life and/or hydrophilicity [48]. In this manner, the liposomes for PS delivery can be categorized as conventional, long circulating, actively targeted, triggered release and multifunctional platform.

In 2000, Visudyne was the first conventional liposomal PS introduced in the clinical practice for the treatment of age-related macular degeneration thus paving the way for the development of lipid carriers in PDT field. In particular, Visudyne is a lipid-formulated composition of benzoporphyrin derivative mono acid ring A (BPD-MA), or verteporfin, whose efficacy in suppressing tumor growth through tumor vasculature endothelial cells damage was demonstrated in 2004 by Oku's group [48]. Verteporfin possess several features of the ideal PS, as chemical stability, efficient singlet oxygen generation, fast clearance, etc. [23]. Visudyne allows blood delivery of hydrophobic BPD-MA, circumventing the tendency to self-aggregation in aqueous medium [49]. Indeed, the efficacy of liposomes to deliver different PSs in a variety of tumors [50], suggested by many *in vitro* and *in vivo* studies, is essentially based on the prevention of PSs aggregation.

Foslip is another conventional liposomal PS formulation currently in use. It is based on dipalmitoylphosphatidylcholine (DPPC) and Temoporfin [mTHPC-5,10,15,20-tetrakis(3-hydroxyphenyl)-chlorin] [51] that is one of the most potent second-generation PS approved by FDA in 2001 as Foscan [52]. In recent years, a liposomal formulation of mTHPC, called Fospeg, incorporating PEG to avoid reticuloendothelial system (RES)-trapping of Foslip has been largely investigated [53-55]. By comparing photodynamic activity of Foslip and Fospeg *vs* non-encapsulated mTHPC on different human tumor cell lines (lung, prostate, squamous cell carcinoma) it was demonstrated that cellular uptake of encapsulated mTHPC is higher than non-encapsulated one [53, 55]. In addition, encapsulation ensures higher photodynamic effects, cell death [56] and nucleic acid damage [57]. The high efficacy of encapsulated m-THPC in terms of reduction of the total time of treatment, tumor selectivity, tumor surrounding tissues damage and skin photosensitivity has also confirmed by many preclinical studies in animal models with xenografted tumor [41, 58, 59]. Fospeg seems to be more promising and advantageous than Foslip with respect to tumor uptake, blood plasma concentration[41] and neovascular vessels damage [60].

2.1.2 Polymeric NPs. Alternative to liposomes, biodegradable polymeric NPs are receiving great attention as systems to deliver both conventional antineoplastic drugs and PSs. The reasons can be found in their high drug loading, stability, controlled drug release, large variety of materials and manufacturing processes [61].

By varying chemical composition and architecture of polymers, polymeric NPs can accommodate PSs with different degrees of hydrophobicity, molecular weight and charge. Moreover, these nancarriers are also very versatile due to the possibility to modulate their surface properties, morphologies, and composition of polymer matrices for polymer degradation control and PSs release. Conversely, a major drawback of polymeric NPs is their recognition by the RES after intravenous administration and their accumulation in the spleen and liver. This fast removal decreases the time of polymeric NPs presence in the blood circulation. To overcome this limitation surface NPs can be modified by addition of polymers like PEG, polyglicolide (PGA), polylactide (PLA) and the copolymer poly(D,L-lactide-co-glycolide) (PLGA), composed of PLA and PGA in different concentration [62]. The investigation of biodegradable polymeric NPs for PDT began as early as 1990 and comprises hematoporphyrin [63] and tetrasulfonated zinc phtalocyanine (ZnPcS4) [64]. To overcome the poor carrier capacity and rapid drug release, second generation Pc derivatives were formulated in PEG NPs. These NPs caused tumor regression in 100% of EMT-6 tumor-bearing mice that demonstrate also a prolonged sensitivity towards PDT [65]. Because of their versatility, physical robustness, biocompatibility, high drug-loading efficiency, and controlled drug release almost all researches have utilized PLA and PLGA (50:50 and 75:25) NPs. PLGA-NPs have similar molecular weights but different copolymer molar ratios [66-68]. Although possessing the same characteristics in terms of polymer molecular weight, crystallinity, particle size and drug loading, the p-THPP loaded PLGA-NPs exhibited different *in vitro* photocytoxicity on EMT-6 mouse mammary tumor cells on the basis of copolymer molecular ratios, i.e., 50:50 PLGA>75:25 PLGA. In addition, PLGA- coated NPs are more phototoxic than PLA-coated one [67, 68].

The efficacy of PLGA NPs as carrier for verteporfin has been demonstrated. Since the size of the carrier is important for cellular and tissue uptake that directly affects the therapeutic activity of the delivered PSs, two types of verteporfin loaded PLGA NPs, 167 (small) and 370 nm (large) in diameter, were tested in EMT-6 mammary tumor cells in comparison with free verteporfin in aqueous medium. The results suggested that 1) encapsulated verteporfin has more photodynamic activity than free verteporfin and 2) small PLGA NPs are more effective to induce cell death respect large ones (69% and 29% reduction in cell viability respectively). This result has also been confirmed *in vivo* by using rhabdomyosarcoma-bearing DBA/2 mice where small PLGA NPs effectively control tumor growth for 20 days in mice [69]. PLGA NPs are interesting carrier also for two other types of PSs, ZnPc [70] and IndoCyanine Green (ICG) [71]. Hypericin-loaded NPs are also very effective in PDT of ovarian cancer as demonstrated by using NuTu-19 ovarian cancer cell model treated with a formulation of PLA NPs with size in the 200-300 nm range. The encapsulation enables the use of lower drug doses, minimizing possible side effects [72].

In addition to biodegradable polymeric carrier systems, non-biodegradable NPs can also be used as vehicle for PSs. Because of their inability to degrade and release drugs in controlled amounts, they were not considered suitable for drug delivery for long time. However, due to their facile synthesis and functionalization, and robustness of structure integrity, non-biodegradable NPs have recently receiving great interest. Indeed, since PS is not toxic *per se* but for its ability to produce ROS upon light excitation, to trigger the noxious effects on cancer cells it is not necessary the PS release but only the diffusion of cytotoxic species [73]. Thus, on the basis of porosity of silica-based spherical 30 nm sized NPs encapsulating 2-devinyl-2-(1-hexyloxyethyl) pyropheophorbide (HPPH) allow efficient generation and diffusion of singlet oxygen which easy enter into cultured UCl-107 and HeLa tumor cells and cause significant cell death [73]. The organically modified silica (ORMOSIL) HPPH-loaded NPs are even more stable [74]. Likewise, ORMOSIL Rose Bengal (RB)-loaded NPs, able to reduce cell proliferation in melanoma SK-MEL-28 cells [75], have relevant photostability, high photoproduction efficiency and ease diffusion of singlet oxygen through NPs pores. Polyacrylamide (PAA), a nontoxic, biologically inert and water-soluble substance for systemic administration, has also been used successfully in PDT to load PSs [76-78]. The effectiveness of free and *meta*-tetra(hydroxyphenyl)-chlorin (*m*-THPC)-loaded PAA NPs of 2- 3-nm in diameter in killing cultured rat C6 glioma cells was compared [79]. Cells were killed by either free or PAA-NPs-encapsulated *m*-THPC upon exposure to 650 nm light. However, since encapsulation reduces molecular aggregation in physiological solution, enhanced PS solubility, and singlet oxygen production and diffusion, and consequently cells were significantly damaged at low *m*-THPC concentration. The very low NPs size allows the removal from the body via renal clearance and decreases the risk of drug accumulation [79].

2.1.3 Gold NPs. Gold nanoparticles (AuNPs) possessing good biocompatibility, versatile surfaces, tunable sizes, and unique optical properties, represent a valuable tool to improve the targeting and efficacy for cancer treatments [80-82]. Phthalocyanine (Pc4)-NPs are ideally suited for PDT. In fact, their very low size (average diameter of 2-4 nm) ensures internalization by cells and delivery of Pc4 directly inside cells. The peculiar synthesis process allows that the Pc4, a hydrophobic PS, is bound in the monomeric form on the nanoparticle surface, absorbs radiation at 695 nm and efficiently produces the singlet oxygen causing apoptosis in HeLa cells [80].

PEGylation of AuNPs-Pc4 conjugates forms a cage around the NPs allowing and improving hydrophobic drug delivery, that in turn reduces the maximum drug accumulation time to the target tumor to only less than 2 hours, compared to 2 days for the free Pc4 [81]. In addition, the *in vivo* noncovalent delivery *via* AuNPs allows cancer drugs to penetrate deeper into the center of tumors. By using female athymic mice subcutaneously implanted with rat glioma (9L) cancer cells and successively injected with Pc4-AuNPs, the authors demonstrated *via* fluorescence imaging, elemental analysis, and histological staining that Pc4-AuNPs within hours (less than 6 hours) penetrates deeply into tumors where it is rapidly released and fastly (after 7 days)excreted from the body by renal clearance and hepatobiliary system without inducing systemic toxic effects [82].

Besides the role as simple carrier for PSs, NMs, formulated with specific moieties possessing affinity for receptors overexpressed on the tumor cells and their vasculature but not on normal cells, can also be useful tools to improve PSs tumor selectivity [83]. The advantage of selective delivery is that PSs will accumulate only in tumor tissue ensuring increment of overall efficacy of PDT and decrement of collateral damage to surrounding normal cells.

Indeed, tumor vasculature represents the main target in the eradication of vascularized tumor by PDT; angiogenesis-targeted PDT ensures destruction of reforming vasculature and suppresses tumor recurrence after single PDT [84]. Different types of nanocarriers, such as NPs, liposomes, and nanogels, different types of cellular targets, such as integrin $\alpha v \beta 3$, VEGFR, CD44 receptor, and cell surface glycoprotein, and different types of PSs, such as Pyropheophorbide A, 5-ALA, Photofrin, ZnPc, Chlorin e6, and BPD-MA, involved in active targeting of PSs are reported in [85].

2.2 NMs as active participants in photodynamic reaction. An alternative exploitation of NMs in the PDT realm is their use as PSs or as agents able to improve photodynamic reaction by enhancing singlet oxygen production.

2.2.1. NMs as photosensitizers. An alternative approach to existing PSs is the use of semiconductor NMs, like zinc oxide (ZnO) NPs, titanium dioxide (TiO$_2$) NPs and QDs, composed of alloys of pairs of group II-IV (e.g., ZnO, ZnS, CdSe) or group III-V (e.g., GaAs, InN, InP, AlAs, TiO$_2$) elements. Both ZnO and TiO$_2$ can produce ROS (mainly hydroxyl radical, superoxide anion, and singlet oxygen) [86, 87] upon UV irradiation and visible light, in particular blue light [88].

TiO$_2$-NPs that are non toxic *per se* in experimental *in vivo* and *in vitro* models [89], possess photocatalyst properties and thus can trigger cell death *via* oxidization of cell membrane proteins and lipids. Their efficacy against several tumor cell lines has been widely demonstrated [90-93]). Unfortunately, the major drawback for clinical use of TiO$_2$-NPs is their aggregation in aqueous solution that suppresses their photocatalytic effect. Yamaguchi and coworkers [94] have coated TiO$_2$-NPs with PEG and demonstrated *in vitro* on C6 rat glioma cells, that the efficiency in inducing cell death by 50 nm TiO$_2$-NPs/PEG is greater than insoluble one. More than 90% of cells were killed and the cytotoxicity depends on TiO$_2$-NPs/PEG concentration and the energy dose of UV irradiation. In addition, by using C6 glioma spheroids model that simulates the cellular microenvironment within a tumor mass, TiO$_2$-NPs/PEG suppress efficiently tumor growth under UV irradiation by eliciting apoptosis [94]. The ability of TiO$_2$-NPs/PEG *vs* uncoated TiO$_2$-NPs to counteract tumors has been demonstrated also *in vivo*, by using female BALB/c-nude mice first inoculated with U87 glioma cells then injected with TiO$_2$-NPs and irradiated with UVA. Glioma undergoes to pronounced areas of necrosis, elevated indices of apoptosis and delayed tumor growth, leading to increased survival of mice [95].

Similar to TiO_2-NPs, ZnO nanorods were used to assess their photodynamic effects on human hepatocarcinoma SMMC-7221 cells [96]. The viability of SMMC-7221 cells treated with ZnO nanorods and UV irradiation remarkably decreased in a dose-dependent manner while ROS formation damaged cell membrane (mainly by lipid peroxidation), nuclei acids and proteins causing apoptotic cell death. An improved anti-tumor activity was gained by a double treatment modality, PDT *via* UV irradiation of ZnO nanorods and chemotherapy *via* safe delivery of daunorubicin (DNR) achieved by combining ZnO nanorods with DNR i.e. DNR-ZnO nanocomposites. The comparison of the therapeutic effects of TiO_2- and ZnO-NPs did not show differences in photodynamically-induced anticancer activity in SMMC-7721 [97]. However, the need of ZnO-NPs high concentration and their low efficiency, still represents significant drawbacks in clinical use. In order to improve the photodynamically-induced anticancer profiles of ZnO-NPs, Ismail and coworkers [98] doped the NPs with metal, such as Fe^{3+}, Ag^+, Pb^{2+}, and Co^{2+}, or coated them with silicate and evaluated the effects on human liver adenocarcinoma cells HepG2 under UV irradiation. ZnO-NPs doped with metal ions display an anti-proliferative effect on HepG2 cells due to high generation of ROS, on the other hand silica-coated ZnO-NPs did not show any anti-proliferative activity under UV irradiation.

Similarly to semiconductor NPs, QDs, possessing high quantum yields, high photostability, and narrow and tunable by size fluorescent emission, can transfer energy to surrounding O_2 and generate UV irradiation-mediated ROSand thus QDs can be considered as potential PSs [26]. QDs are typically composed of cadmium selenide (CdSe), cadmium sulfide, indium arsenide and indium phosphide. Few studies showed that photoactivation of CdSe or CdTe-core QDs generated ROS that in turn caused cell death [99-101]. Recently, to selectively deliver CdTe(S)-QDs to cells Morosini et al., [102] conjugate QDs with folic acid, knows as an optimal targeting ligand for selective delivery to cancer tissues, using different spacers (PEG or Jeffamine D-400). The toxic photodynamic effects against human head and neck carcinoma KB cells overexpressing folic acid receptor (FR-α) and human colon cancer HT-29 cells lacking FR-α of folic acid-conjugated QDs were confirmed on KB cells irradiated with 515 or 658 nm light [102]. 60 nm sized graphene QDs (GQDs) irradiated with 470 nm blue light cause in U251 human glioma cells photodynamically-induced cell death through apoptotic and autophagic processes. The reduction of cell viability depends on the photoexposure duration and GQDs concentration [103]. The effectiveness of GQDs in PDT (white light, 400-800 nm, irradiation) was also assayed by Ge et al., [104] in *in vitro* experiments (induction of cell death in HeLa cells) and *in vivo* model (destruction of tumor mass in female BALB/nu mice with subcutaneous breast cancer xenografts).

2.2.2. NMs as enhancers of singlet oxygen production by PSs. As intriguing as the capacity of NMs to act as PSs is the ability of some NMs to also enhance the singlet oxygen production by classic PSs in case of possible light-mediated energy transfer between molecules.

The first demonstration of the NMs use to facilitate excitation of a PS is dated to 2003, when *Samia* et al., [105] used 5 nm CdSe QDs linked to Pc4. The combination of QDs and Pc4 enabled the use of an excitation wavelength at which PS alone does not absorb but allowed the indirect excitation of Pc4 at 488 nm through a Fluorescence Resonance Energy Transfer (FRET) mechanism. Likewise, carbon QDs-protoporphyrin IX conjugate extends the tissue penetration capability of protoporphyrin IX both *in vitro*, by using HeLa cells, and *in vivo*, in tumors induced in C3H/HeN mice using a syngenic radiation-induced fibrosarcoma mouse tumor model. The excitation wavelength used at 800 nm is in the phototherapeutic window and can penetrate tissue four times deeper than the 630 nm generally used for clinical PDT, thus offering the potential to access more deeply located tumors [106]. Same findings were reported by using QDs conjugated with sulphonated aluminum phtalocyanines (AlPcSs). QDs indirectly excite AlPcSs upon 532 nm irradiation, which is the absorption region of QDs but not of AlPcSs, producing singlet oxygen *via* FRET with efficiency around 80%. In this form, AlPcS-QDs can kill human nasopharyngeal carcinoma KB cells [107].

Au-based NMs can be used to enhance singlet oxygen production from PSs by exploiting surface plasmon resonance phenomenon that is based on the interaction of the conduction electrons of metal nanostructures with incoming light [108]. Zhao et al.,[109] in 2010 and successively Khlebstov et al.,[110] in 2011 demonstrated the efficient generation of singlet oxygen and death induction in human breast adenocarcinoma cell line (MDA-MB-231) and HeLa cells by nanocomposites comprising a gold nanorod core [109] or gold-silver nanocage [110] and a mesoporous silica shell doped with hematoporfirin and Yb-2,4-dimethoxyhematoporphyrin respectively. It is worth noting that, these nanocomposites in a single platform are potential theranostic agents, used for bioimaging through IR-luminescence and for therapy *via* singlet-oxygen generation.

395 nm irradiation of 5-ALA/AuNPs conjugates enhances PDT efficacy *vs* 5-ALA alone in human fibrosarcoma [111] and chronic myelogenous leukemia K562 cells [112]. Recently, Hadizadeh et al., [113] demonstrated that in the epidermoid carcinoma A431 cells, there is a synergistic effect on the inhibition of cell growth between 5-ALA-PDT and AuNPs. The cells firstly incubated with AuNPs for 18h and then added with 5-ALA for additional 4h before 630 nm irradiation, showed 90-95% cell death *vs* 45-50% measured with 5-ALA-PDT alone.

Gold nanorods conjugated with rose Bengal (RB), a well known anionic PS with a singlet oxygen quantum yield of nearly 76% under 532 nm green light irradiation, can combine 532 nm irradiation PDT and photothermal therapy (PTT) under 810 nm near-infrared (NIR) irradiation leading human oral squamous carcinoma Cal-27 cells to die; moreover, gold nanorods also enhanced RB uptake by cancer cells [114]. In particular, RB-gold nanorods in Cal-27 cancer cells: i) induce more photodynamically-mediated cytotoxicity than pure RB in a dose-dependent manner; ii) cause mainly ROS-mediated apoptotic cell death; iii) trigger PTT effects under NIR light irradiation. In addition, in hamster cheek pouch model, one of the most widely accepted oral cancer models for its similarity with tumorigenesis and progression of human oral cancer, the combined PDT-PTT treatment with RB-gold nanorods leads to 95.5% tumor inhibition at the 10th day and allows the repetition of the treatment without tissue toxicity [114].

3. FUTURE PERSPECTIVES IN NANOTECHNOLOGY-BASED PDT

A new type of PSs potentially usable in PDT is based on photon upconverting NPs (UCNPs).

In upconversion (UC) process, the sequential absorption of two or more photons leads to the emission of light at shorter wavelength than the excitation wavelength allowing efficient excitation even at low excitation densities [115]. Photon upconverting materials convert lower-energy light to higher-energy light through excitation with multiple photons. In particular, UCNPs are modified nanometer-sized composites which generate higher energy light from lower energy radiation, generally NIR or IR, by using transition metal, lanthanide, or actinide ions doped into a solid-state host [116].

The first test about the efficacy of UCNPs in PDT use $NaYF_4:Yb^{3+},Er^{3+}$ silica-coated NPs doped with merocyanine-540 PS and excited at 974 nm. They efficiently kill breast cancer MCF-7 cells but are ineffective *in vivo* due to the fact that the NPs cannot be activated at depth in animal tissue [28]. Only in 2011, Wang et al.,[117] are able to shown the effectiveness of UC- NPs also *in vivo* by using UCNPs containing ce6 intratumoral injected into 4T1 subcutaneous tumors, growing on backs of Balb/c mice, followed by 980 nm laser irradiation. Tumors in mice disappeared in 2 weeks after PDT and any tumor regrowth and over 60 days survival of mice are observed [117].

Recently, it has been demonstrated the possibility to load $NaYF_4:Yb^{3+},Er^{3+}$ UCNPs with doxorubicin (Dox) allowing a synergistic chemo-PTD [118]. Dox-loaded UCNPs irradiated with 980 nm laser in MDA-MB-231 cells induce ROS production through the conversion of NIR light to UV light that activates photodynamic reactions and efficiently deliver DOX in cancer cells allowing a significant growth inhibition of MDA-MB-231 cells based on synergistic effect of PDT and chemotherapy [118]. The same findings are reported by using U87-MG human glioblastoma cancer cells and MCF-7 cells [119].

CONCLUSION

The rapid growth of nanotechnology deeply potentiates the field of cancer management in terms of diagnosis and therapy. Nanotechnology applications play a key role also in PDT. PDT has emerged as one of the important therapeutic options in management of cancer over current cancer treatments, due to its advantages, consisting of selective and irreversible destruction of diseased tissue without damaging adjacent healthy ones. However, there are still several technical difficulties (listed below) in the application of PDT in cancer to gain general clinical acceptance.

1. Currently approved PDT PSs absorb below 700 nm where light penetration is low, thus limiting PDT application at superficial lesions and, in parallel, they are not light source that can easy reach body cavities;
2. Most existing PSs are hydrophobic and aggregate under physiological conditions, thus making ineffective their parenteral administration;
3. The accumulation selectivity to diseased tissues is often not high enough for clinical use.

NMs allow to circumvent these drawbacks by encapsulating PSs. In addition, the accumulation can be very selective by modifying the surface of NMs with monoclonal antibodies or specific tumor-seeking molecules.

Moreover, instead of mere carriage, the NMs can actively participate in photodynamic reaction either by acting as PSs themselves *via* singlet oxygen production under irradiation or as transducers of NIR radiation by emitting wavelength exciting attached PSs. Further, the most recent papers demonstrate the possibility to carry out a double treatment modality, i.e., PDT and chemotherapy, by exploiting photon upconversion process NPs-mediated.

Thus, it is easy to forecast that the continue to grow of nanotechnology and its application to cancer PDT will potentiate this treatment that will become ever more convincing.

REFERENCES

[1]   Darzynkiewicz Z, Traganos F, Wlodkowic D. Impaired DNA damage response-an Achilles' heel sensitizing cancer to chemotherapy and radiotherapy. *Eur. J. Pharmacol.* 2009;625:143-50. doi: 10.1016/j.ejphar.2009.05.032.

[2]   Luqmani YA. Mechanisms of Drug Resistance in Cancer Chemotherapy. *Med. Princ. Pract.* 2005;1:35-48. doi:10.1159/00008618.

[3]   Triesscheijn M, Baas P, Schellens JH, Stewart FA. Photodynamic therapy in oncology. *Oncologist.* 2006;11:1034-44. doi: 10.1634/theoncologist.11-9-1034.

[4]   Kharkwal GB, Sharma SK, Huang YY, Dai T, Hamblin MR. Photodynamic therapy for infections: clinical applications. *Lasers Surg. Med.* 2011;43:755-67. doi: 10.1002/lsm.21080.

[5]   Gursoy H, Ozcakir-Tomruk C, Tanalp J, Yilmaz S. Photodynamic therapy in dentistry: a literature review. *Clin. Oral Investig.* 2013;17:1113-25. doi: 10.1007/s00784-012-0845-7.

[6]   Wan MT, Lin JY. Current evidence and applications of photodynamic therapy in dermatology. *Clin. Cosmet Investig. Dermatol.* 2014;7:145-63. doi: 10.2147 /CCID.S35334.

[7]   Lyon JP, Moreira LM, de Moraes PC, dos Santos FV, de Resende MA. Photodynamic therapy for pathogenic fungi. *Mycoses.* 2011. doi: 10.1111/j.1439-0507.2010.01966.x.

[8]   Plaetzer K, Krammer B, Berlanda J, Berr F, Kiesslich T. Photophysics and photochemistry of photodynamic therapy: fundamental aspects. *Lasers Med. Sci.* 2009;24:259-68. doi: 10.1007/s10103-008-0539-1.

[9]   Gal D. Effect of photosensitizers in chemical and biological processes: the MTO mechanism in photodynamic therapy. *Biochem. Biophys. Res. Commun.* 1992;186:1032-6. doi:10.1016/0006-291X(92)90850-K.

[10] Skupin-Mrugalska P, Sobotta L, Kucinska M, Murias M, Mielcarek J, Duzgunes N. Cellular changes, molecular pathways and the immune system following photodynamic treatment. *Curr. Med. Chem.* 2014;21:4059-73. doi:10.2174/0929867321666140 826120300.

[11] Panzarini E, Tenuzzo B, Dini L. Photodynamic therapy*Ann. N Y Acad. Sci.* 2009;171:617-26. doi: 10.1111/j.1749-6632.2009.04908.x.

[12] Dini L, Inguscio V, Tenuzzo B, Panzarini E. Rose bengal acetate photodynamic therapy*Cancer Biol. Ther.* 2010;10:1048-55. doi: 10.4161/cbt.10.10.13371.

[13] Panzarini E, Inguscio V, Dini L. Timing the multiple cell death*Cell Death Dis.* 2011. doi: 10.1038/cddis.2011.51.

[14] Garg AD, Nowis D, Golab J, Agostinis P. Photodynamic therapy*Apoptosis.* 2010;15:1050-71. doi: 10.1007/s10495-010-0479-7.

[15] Hatz S, Lambert JD, Ogilby PR. Measuring the lifetime of singlet oxygen in a single cell: addressing the issue of cell viability. *Photochem. Photobiol. Sci.* 2007;6:1106-16. doi:10.1039/B707313E.

[16] Pottier R, Kennedy JC. The possible role of ionic species in selective biodistribution of photochemotherapeutic agents toward neoplastic tissue. *J. Photochem. Photobiol.B.* 1990;8:1-16.

[17] Allison BA, Pritchard PH, Levy JG. Evidence for low-density lipoprotein receptor-mediated uptake of benzoporphyrin derivative. *Br. J. Cancer.* 1994;69:833-9.

[18] Roberts WG, Hasan T. Role of neovasculature and vascular permeability on the tumor retention of photodynamic agents. *Cancer Res.* 1992;52:924-30.

[19] Hamblin MR, Newman EL. On the mechanism of the tumour-localising effect in photodynamic therapy. *J. Photochem. Photobiol.* B. 1994;23:3-8.

[20] Wilson BC, Jeeves WP, Lowe DM. In vivo and post mortem measurements of the attenuation spectra of light in mammalian tissues. *Photochem. Photobiol..* 1985;42:153-62. doi:10.1111/j.1751-1097.1985.tb01554.x.

[21] Szaciłowski K, Macyk W, Drzewiecka-Matuszek A, Brindell M, Stochel G. Bioinorganic photochemistry: frontiers and mechanisms. *Chem. Rev.* 2005;105:2647-94. doi:10.1021/cr030707e

[22] Peer D, Karp JM, Hong S, Farokhzad OC, Margalit R, Langer R. Nanocarriers as an emerging platform for cancer therapy. *Nat. Nanotechnol.* 2007;2:751-60. doi: 10.1038/nnano.2007.387.

[23] Allison RR, Sibata CH. Oncologic photodynamic therapy photosensitizers: a clinical review. *Photodiagnosis Photodyn Ther.* 2010;7:61-75. doi: 10.1016/j.pdpdt. 2010.02.001.

[24] Konan YN, Gurny R, Allémann E. State of the art in the delivery of photosensitizers for photodynamic therapy. *J. Photochem. Photobiol B.* 2002;66:89-106. doi:10.1016 /S1011-1344(01)00267-6.

[25] Samia AC, Chen X, Burda C. Semiconductor quantum dots for photodynamic therapy. *J. Am. Chem. Soc.* 2003;125:15736-7. doi:10.1021/ja0386905

[26] Bakalova R, Ohba H, Zhelev Z, Ishikawa M, Baba Y. Quantum dots as photosensitizers? *Nat. Biotechnol.* 2004;22:1360-1. doi:10.1038/nbt1104-1360.

[27] Chen W, Zhang J. Using nanoparticles to enable simultaneous radiation and photodynamic therapies for cancer treatment. *J. Nanosci. Nanotechnol.* 2006;6:1159-66.

[28] Zhang P, Steelant W, Kumar M, Scholfield M. Versatile photosensitizers for photodynamic therapy at infrared excitation. *J. Am. Chem. Soc.* 2007;129:4526-7. doi:10.1021/ja0700707.

[29] Menon JU, Jadeja P, Tambe P, Vu K, Yuan B, Nguyen KT. Nanomaterials for photo-based diagnostic and therapeutic applications. *Theranostics.* 2013;3:152-66. doi:10.7150/thno.5327.

[30] Sharma P, Brown S, Walter G, Santra S, Moudgil B. Nanoparticles for bioimaging. *AdvColloid Interface Sci.* 2006;123-126:471-85. doi:10.1016/j.cis.2006.05.026.

[31] Ferrari M. Cancer nanotechnology: opportunities and challenges. *Nat. Rev. Cancer.* 2005;5:161-71. doi:10.1038/nrc1566.

[32] Danhier F, Feron O, Préat V. To exploit the tumor microenvironment: Passive and active tumor targeting of nanocarriers for anti-cancer drug delivery. *J. Control Release.* 2010;148:135-46. doi:10.1016/j.jconrel.2010.08.027.

[33] Lim CK, Heo J, Shin S, Jeong K, Seo YH, Jang WD, et al., Nanophotosensitizers toward advanced photodynamic therapy of Cancer. *Cancer Lett.* 2013;334:176-87. doi:10.1016/j.canlet.2012.09.012.

[34] Kim KY. Nanotechnology platforms and physiological challenges for cancer therapeutics. *Nanomedicine.* 2007;3:103-10. doi:org/10.1016/j.nano.2006.12.002

[35] Huang YY, Sharma SK, Dai T, Chung H, Yaroslavsky A, Garcia-Diaz M, et al., Can nanotechnology potentiate photodynamic therapy. *Nanotechnol. Rev.* 2012;1:111-146. doi:10.1515/ntrev-2011-0005.

[36] Veres D, Bőcskei-Antal B, Voszka I, Módos K, Csík G, Kaposi AD, et al., Comparison of binding ability and location of two mesoporphyrin derivatives in liposomes explored with conventional and site-selective fluorescence spectroscopy. *J. Phys. Chem. B.* 2012;116:9644-52. doi:10.1021/jp304712n.

[37] Vemuri S, Rhodes CT. Preparation and characterization of liposomes as therapeutic delivery systems: a review. *Pharm Acta Helv.* 1995;70:95-111.

[38] Samad A, Sultana Y, Aqil M. Liposomal drug delivery systems: an update review. *CurrDrug Deliv.* 2007;4:297-305. doi:10.2174/156720107782151269.

[39] Lasic DD, Martin FJ, Gabizon A, Huang SK, Papahadjopoulos D. Sterically stabilized liposomes: a hypothesis on the molecular origin of the extended circulation times. *Biochim. Biophys. Acta* 1991;1070:187-92. doi:10.1016/0005-2736(91)90162-2.

[40] Francis GE, Delgado C, Fisher D, Malik F, Agrawal AK. Polyethylene Glycol Modification: Relevance of Improved Methodology to Tumour Targeting. *J. DrugTargeting.* 1996;3:321-40. doi:10.3109/10611869608996824.

[41] Bovis MJ, Woodhams JH, Loizidou M, Scheglmann D, Bown SG, Macrobert AJ. Improved in vivo delivery of m-THPC via pegylated liposomes for use in photodynamic therapy. *J. Control Release.* 2012;157:196-205. doi: 10.1016 /j.jconrel.2011.09.085.

[42] Bikram M, West JL. Thermo-responsive systems for controlled drug delivery. *ExpertOpin. Drug Deliv.* 2008;5:1077-91. doi:10.1517/17425247.5.10.1077.

[43] Powell ME, Hill SA, Saunders MI, Hoskin PJ, Chaplin DJ. Human tumor blood flow is enhanced by nicotinamide and carbogen breathing. *Cancer Res.* 1997;57:5261-4.

[44] Aygun A, Torrey K, Kumar A, Stephenson LD. Investigation of factors affecting controlled release from photosensitive DMPC and DSPC liposomes. *Appl. Biochem.Biotechnol.* 2012;167:743-57. doi: 10.1007/s12010-012-9724-6.

[45] Bakowsky H, Richter T, Kneuer C, Hoekstra D, Rothe U, Bendas G, et al., Adhesion characteristics and stability assessment of lectin-modified liposomes for site-specific drug delivery. *Biochim. Biophys. Acta.* 2008;1778:242-49. doi:10.1016/j.bbamem. 2007.09.033

[46] Mastrobattista E, Koning GA, Storm G. Immunoliposomes for the targeted delivery of antitumor drugs. *Adv. Drug Deliv. Rev.* 1999;40:103-27. doi:10.1016/S0169-409X(99)00043-5.

[47] Ichikawa K, Hikita T, Maeda N, Yonezawa S, Takeuchi Y, Asai T, et al., Antiangiogenic photodynamic therapy (PDT) by using long-circulating liposomes

modified with peptide specific to angiogenic vessels. *Biochim. Biophys. Acta.* 2005;1669:69-74. doi:10.1016/j.bbamem.2005.02.003.

[48] Ichikawa K, Takeuchi Y, Yonezawa S, Hikita T, Kurohane K, Namba Y, et al., Antiangiogenic photodynamic therapy (PDT) using Visudyne causes effective suppression of tumor growth. *Cancer Lett.* 2004;205:39-48. doi:10.1016/j.canlet.2003.10.001.

[49] Aveline BM, Hasan T, Redmond RW. The effects of aggregation, protein binding and cellular incorporation on the photophysical properties of benzoporphyrin derivative monoacid ring A (BPDMA). *J. Photochem. Photobiol. B.* 1995;30:161-9.

[50] Master A, Livingston M, Sen Gupta A. Photodynamic nanomedicine in the treatment of solid tumors: perspectives and challenges. *J. Control Release.* 2013;168:88-102. doi:10.1016/j.jconrel.2013.02.020.

[51] Kachatkou D, Sasnouski S, Zorin V, Zorina T, D'Hallewin MA, Guillemin F, Bezdetnaya L. Unusual photoinduced response of mTHPC liposomal formulation (Foslip). *Photochem. Photobiol.* 2009;85:719-24. doi: 10.1111/j.1751-1097.2008.00466.x.

[52] Senge MO, Brandt JC. Temoporfin (Foscan, 5,10,15,20-tetra(mhydroxyphenyl) chlorin) – a second-generation photosensitizer. *Photochem. Photobiol.* 2011;87:1240-69. doi: 10.1111/j.1751-1097.2011.00986.x.

[53] Compagnin C, Moret F, Celotti L, Miotto G, Woodhams JH, MacRobert AJ, et al., Meta-tetra(hydroxyphenyl)chlorin-loaded liposomes sterically stabilised with poly(ethylene glycol) of different length and density: characterisation, in vitro cellular uptake and phototoxicity. *Photochem. Photobiol. Sci.* 2011;10:1751-9. doi: 10.1039/c1pp05163f.

[54] Reshetov V, Kachatkou D, Shmigol T, Zorin V, D'Hallewin MA, Guillemin F, et al., Redistribution of meta-tetra(hydroxyphenyl)chlorin (m-THPC) from conventional and PEGylated liposomes to biological substrates. *Photochem. Photobiol. Sci.* 2011;10:911-9. doi: 10.1039/c0pp00303d.

[55] Petri A, Yova D, Alexandratou E, Kyriazi M, Rallis M. Comparative characterization of the cellular uptake and photodynamic efficiency of Foscan® and Fospeg in a human prostate cancer cell line. *Photodiagnosis Photodyn Ther.* 2012;9:344-54. doi: 10.1016/j.pdpdt.2012.03.008.

[56] Gyenge EB, Hiestand S, Graefe S, Walt H, Maake C. Cellular and molecular effects of the liposomal mTHPC derivative Foslipos in prostate carcinoma cells in vitro. *Photodiagnosis Photodyn Ther.* 2011;8:86-96. doi: 10.1016/j.pdpdt.2011.02.001.

[57] Kiesslich T, Berlanda J, Plaetzer K, Krammer B, Berr F. Comparative characterization of the efficiency and cellular pharmacokinetics of Foscan- and Foslip-based photodynamic treatment in human biliary tract cancer cell lines. *Photochem. Photobiol. Sci.* 2007;6:619-27. doi:10.1039/B617659C.

[58] de Visscher SA, Kaščáková S, de Bruijn HS, van den Heuvel Av, Amelink A, Sterenborg HJ, et al., Fluorescence localization and kinetics of mTHPC and liposomal formulations of mTHPC in the window-chamber tumor model. *Lasers Surg. Med.* 2011;43:528-36. doi: 10.1002/lsm.21082.

[59] Lassalle HP, Dumas D, Gräfe S, D'Hallewin MA, Guillemin F, Bezdetnaya L. Correlation between in vivo pharmacokinetics, intratumoral distribution and

photodynamic efficiency of liposomal mTHPC. *J. Control Release.* 2009;134:118-24. doi: 10.1016/j.jconrel.2008.11.016.

[60] Pegaz B, Debefve E, Ballini JP, Wagnières G, Spaniol S, Albrecht V, et al., Photothrombic activity of m-THPC-loaded liposomal formulations: pre-clinical assessment on chick chorioallantoic membrane model. *Eur. J. Pharm. Sci.* 2006;28:134-40. doi:10.1016/j.ejps.2006.01.008.

[61] van Nostrum CF. Polymeric micelles to deliver photosensitizers for photodynamic therapy. *Adv. Drug Deliv. Rev.* 2004;56:9-16. doi:10.1016/j.addr.2003.07.013.

[62] McCarthy JR, Kelly KA, Sun EY, Weissleder R. Targeted delivery of multifunctional magnetic nanoparticles. *Nanomedicine.* 2007;2:153-67. doi:10.2217/17435889.2.2.153.

[63] Brasseur N, Brault D, Couvreur P. Adsorption of hematoporphyrin onto polyalkylcyanoacrylate nanoparticles: carrier capacity and drug release. *Int. J. Pharm.* 1991;70:129-35. doi:10.1016/0378-5173(91)90172-K.

[64] Labib A, Lenaerts V, Chouinard F, Leroux JC, Ouellet R, van Lier JE. Biodegradable nanospheres containing phthalocyanines and naphthalocyanines for targeted photodynamic tumor therapy. *Pharm Res.* 1991;8:1027-31.

[65] Allemann E, Brasseur N, Benrezzak O, Rousseau J, Kudrevich SV, Boyle RW, et al., PEG-coated poly(lactic acid) nanoparticles for the delivery of hexadecafluoro zinc phthalocyanine to EMT-6 mouse mammary tumours. *J. Pharm. Pharmacol.* 1995;47:382-7.

[66] Panyam J, Labhasetwar V. Biodegradable nanoparticles for drug and gene delivery to cells and tissue. *Adv. Drug Deliv. Rev.* 2003;55:329-47. doi:10.1016/S0169-409X(02)00228-4.

[67] Konan YN, Berton M, Gurny R, Allemann E. Enhanced photodynamic activity of meso-tetra(4-hydroxyphenyl)porphyrin by incorporation into sub-200 nm nanoparticles. *Eur. J. Pharm. Sci.* 2003;18:241-9. doi:10.1016/S0928-0987(03)00017-4.

[68] Konan YN, Cerny R, Favet J, Berton M, Gurny R, Allemann E. Preparation and characterization of sterile sub-200 nmmeso-tetra(4-hydroxylphenyl)porphyrin-loaded nanoparticles for photodynamic therapy. *Eur. J. Pharm. Biopharm.* 2003;55:115-24. doi:10.1016/S0939-6411(02)00128-5.

[69] Konan-Kouakou YN, Boch R, Gurny R, Allemann E. In vitro and in vivo activities of verteporfi n-loaded nanoparticles. *J. Control Release.* 2005;103:83-91. doi:10.1016/j.jconrel.2004.11.023.

[70] Ricci-Junior E, Marchetti JM. Zinc(II) phthalocyanine loaded PLGA nanoparticles for photodynamic therapy use. *Int. J. Pharm.* 2006;310:187-95. doi:10.1016/j.ijpharm.2005.10.048.

[71] Saxena V, Sadoqi M, Shao J. Polymeric nanoparticulate delivery system for Indocyanine green: biodistribution in healthy mice. *Int. J. Pharm.* 2006;308:200-4. doi:10.1016/j.ijpharm.2005.11.003.

[72] Zeisser-Labouebe M, Lange N, Gurny R, Delie F. Hypericin-loaded nanoparticles for the photodynamic treatment of ovarian cancer. *Int. J. Pharm.* 2006;326:174-81. doi:10.1016/j.ijpharm.2006.07.012.

[73] Roy I, Ohulchanskyy TY, Pudavar HE, Bergey EJ, Oseroff AR, Morgan J, et al., Ceramic-based nanoparticles entrapping water-insoluble photosensitizing anticancer drugs: a novel drug-carrier system for photodynamic therapy. *J. Am. Chem. Soc.* 2003;125:7860-5. doi:10.1021/ja0343095.

[74] Ohulchanskyy TY, Roy I, Goswami LN, Chen Y, Bergey EJ, Pandey RK, et al., Organically modified silica nanoparticles with covalently incorporated photosensitizer for photodynamic therapy of cancer. *Nano Lett.* 2007;7:2835-42. doi:10.1021/nl0714637.

[75] Gianotti E, Martins Estevão B, Cucinotta F, Hioka N, Rizzi M, et al., An efficient rose bengal based nanoplatform for photodynamic therapy. *Chemistry.* 2014;20:10921-5. doi:10.1002/chem.201404296.

[76] Tang W, Xu H, Kopelman R, Philbert MA. Photodynamic characterization and in vitro application of methylene blue-containing nanoparticle platforms. *Photochem. Photobiol.* 2005;81:242-9. doi:10.1111/j.1751-1097.2005.tb00181.x.

[77] Tang W, Xu H, Park EJ, Philbert MA, Kopelman R. Encapsulation of methylene blue in polyacrylamide nanoparticle platforms protects its photodynamic effectiveness. *Biochem. Biophys. Res. Commun.* 2008;369:579-83. doi: 10.1016/j.bbrc.2008.02.066.

[78] Reddy GR, Bhojani MS, McConville P, Moody J, Moffat BA, Hall DE, et al., Vascular targeted nanoparticles for imaging and treatment of brain tumors. *Clin Cancer Res.* 2006;12:6677-86. doi: 10.1158/1078-0432.CCR-06-0946.

[79] Gao D, Xu H, Philbert MA, Kopelman R. Ultrafine hydrogel nanoparticles: synthetic approach and therapeutic application in living cells. *Angew Chem. Int. Ed. Engl.* 2007;46:2224-7. doi:10.1002/anie.200603927.

[80] Wieder ME, Hone DC, Cook MJ, Handsley MM, Gavrilovic J, Russell DA. Intracellular photodynamic therapy with photosensitizer-nanoparticle conjugates: cancer therapy using a ' Trojan horse '. *Photochem. Photobiol. Sci.* 2006;5:727-34. doi:10.1039/B602830F.

[81] Cheng YC, Samia A, Meyers JD, Panagopoulos I, Fei B, Burda C. Highly efficient drug delivery with gold nanoparticle vectors for in vivo photodynamic therapy of cancer. *J. Am. Chem. Soc.* 2008;130:10643-7. doi:10.1021/ja801631c.

[82] Cheng Y, Meyers JD, Broome AM, Kenney ME, Basilion JP, Burda C. Deep penetration of a PDT drug into tumors by noncovalent drug-gold nanoparticle conjugates. *J. Am. Chem. Soc.* 2011;133:2583-91. doi: 10.1021/ja108846h.

[83] Sharman WM, van Lier JE, Allen CM. Targeted photodynamic therapy via receptor mediated delivery systems. *Adv. Drug Deliv. Rev.* 2004;56:53-76. doi:10.1016/j.addr.2003.08.015.

[84] Weiss A, den Bergh Hv, Griffioen AW, Nowak-Sliwinska P. Angiogenesis inhibition for the improvement of photodynamic therapy: the revival of a promising idea. *Biochim. Biophys. Acta.* 2012;1826:53-70. doi: 10.1016/j.bbcan.2012.03.003.

[85] Lim CK, Heo J, Shin S, Jeong K, Seo YH, Jang WD, et al., Nanophotosensitizers toward advanced photodynamic therapy of Cancer. *Cancer Lett.* 2013;334:176-87. doi:10.1016/j.canlet.2012.09.012.

[86] Konaka R, Kasahara E, Dunlap WC, Yamamoto Y, Chien KC, Inoue M. Irradiation of titanium dioxide generates both singlet oxygen and superoxide anion. *Free Radic. Biol. Med.* 1999;27:294-300. doi:10.1016/S0891-5849(99)00050-7.

[87] Xu J, Sun Y, Huang J, Chen C, Liu G, Jiang Y, et al., Photokilling cancer cells using highly cell-specific antibody-TiO(2) bioconjugates and electroporation. *Bioelectrochemistry.* 2007;71:217-22. doi:10.1016/j.bioelechem.2007.06.001.

[88] Rehman S, Ullah R, Butt AM, Gohar ND. Strategies of making TiO_2 and ZnO visible light active. *J. Hazard Mater.* 2009;170:560-9. doi:10.1016/j.jhazmat.2009.05.064.

[89] Fabian E, Landsiedel R, Ma-Hock L, Wiench K, Wohlleben W, van Ravenzwaay B. Tissue distribution and toxicity of intravenously administered titanium dioxide nanoparticles in rats. *Arch. Toxicol.* 2008;82:151-7. doi: 10.1007/s00204-007-0253-y

[90] Cai R, Hashimoto K, Itoh K, Kubota Y, Fujishima A. Photo-killing of malignant cells with ultrafine TiO2 powder. *Bull Chem. Soc. Jpn.* 1991;64:1268-73.

[91] Cai R, Kubota Y, Shuin T, Sakai H, Hashimoto K, Fujishima A. Induction of cytotoxicity by photoexcited TiO$_2$ particles. *Cancer Res.* 1992;52:2346-8.

[92] Kubota Y, Shuin T, Kawasaki C, Hosaka M, Kitamura H, Cai R, et al., Photokilling of T-24 human bladder cancer cells with titanium dioxide. *Br. J. Cancer.* 1994;70:1107-11.

[93] Zhang AP, Sun YP. Photocatalytic killing effect of TiO$_2$ nanoparticles on Ls-174-t human colon carcinoma cells. *World J. Gastroenterol.* 2004;10:3191-3.

[94] Yamaguchi S, Kobayashi H, Narita T, Kanehira K, Sonezaki S, Kubota Y, et al., Novel photodynamic therapy using water-dispersed TiO$_2$ -polyethylene glycol compound: evaluation of antitumor effect on glioma cells and spheroids in vitro. *Photochem. Photobiol..* 2010;86:964-71. doi:10.1111/j.1751-1097.2010.00742.x.

[95] Wang C, Cao S, Tie X, Qiu B, Wu A, Zheng Z. Induction of cytotoxicity by photoexcitation of TiO2 can prolong survival in glioma-bearing mice. *Mol. Biol. Rep.* 2011;38:523-30. doi:10.1007/s11033-010-0136-9.

[96] Zhang H, Chen B, Jiang H, Wang C, Wang H, Wang X. A strategy for ZnO nanorod mediated multi-mode cancer treatment. *Biomaterials.* 2011;32:1906-14. doi:10.1016/j.biomaterials.2010.11.027.

[97] Zhang H, Shan Y, Dong L. A comparison of TiO2 and ZnO nanoparticles as photosensitizers in photodynamic therapy for cancer. *J. Biomed. Nanotechnol.* 2014;10:1450-7. doi:org/10.1166/jbn.2014.1961

[98] Ismail AF, Ali MM, Ismail LF. Photodynamic therapy mediated antiproliferative activity of some metal-doped ZnO nanoparticles in human liver adenocarcinoma HepG2 cells under UV irradiation. *J.Photochem. Photobiol. B.* 2014;138:99-108. doi: 10.1016/j.jphotobiol.2014.04.006.

[99] Anas A, Akita H, Harashima H, Itoh T, Ishikawa M, Biju V. Photosensitized breakage and damage of DNA by CdSe-ZnS quantum dots. *J. Phys. Chem. B.* 2008;112:10005-11. doi: 10.1021/jp8018606.

[100] Cho SJ, Maysinger D, Jain M, Röder B, Hackbarth S, Winnik FM. Long-term exposure to CdTe quantum dots causes functional impairments in live cells. *Langmuir.* 2007;23:1974-80. doi:10.1021/la060093j.

[101] Liang J, He Z, Zhang S, Huang S, Ai X, Yang H et al., Study on DNA damage induced by CdSe quantum dots using nucleic acid molecular "light switches" as probe. *Talanta.* 2007:71:1675-8. doi:10.1016/j.talanta.2006.07.048.

[102] Morosini V, Bastogne T, Frochot C, Schneider R, François A, Guillemin F, et al., Quantum dot-folic acid conjugates as potential photosensitizers in photodynamic therapy of cancer. *Photochem. Photobiol. Sci.* 2011;10:842-51. doi: 10.1039/c0pp00380h.

[103] Markovic ZM, Ristic BZ, Arsikin KM, Klisic DG, Harhaji-Trajkovic LM, Todorovic-Markovic BM, et al., Graphene quantum dots as autophagy-inducing photodynamic agents. *Biomaterials.* 2012;33:7084-92. doi: 10.1016/j.biomaterials.2012.06.060.

[104] Ge J, Lan M, Zhou B, Liu W, Guo L, Wang H, et al., A graphene quantum dot photodynamic therapy agent with high singlet oxygen generation. *Nat. Commun.* 2014. doi: 10.1038/ncomms5596.

[105] Samia AC, Chen X, Burda C. Semiconductor quantum dots for photodynamic therapy. *J. Am. Chem. Soc.* 2003;125:15736-7. doi:10.1021/ja0386905.

[106] Fowley C, Nomikou N, McHale AP, McCaughan B, Callan JF. Extending the tissue penetration capability of conventional photosensitisers: a carbon quantum dot-protoporphyrin IX conjugate for use in two-photon excited photodynamic therapy. *Chem. Commun.* 2013;49:8934-6. doi:10.1039/c3cc45181j.

[107] Li L, Zhao JF, Won N, Jin H, Kim S, Chen JY. Quantum dot-aluminum phthalocyanine conjugates perform photodynamic reactions to kill cancer cells via fluorescence resonance energy transfer. *Nanoscale Res. Lett.* 2012;7:386. doi: 10.1186/1556-276X-7-386.

[108] Csaki A, Schneider T, Wirth J, Jahr N, Steinbruck A, Stranik O, et al., Molecular plasmonics: light meets molecules at the nanoscale. *Philos Transact A. Math Phys. Eng. Sci.* 2011;369:3483-96. doi:10.1098/rsta.2011.0145.

[109] Zhao T, Wu H, Yao SQ, Xu QH, Xu GQ. Nanocomposites containing gold nanorods and porphyrin-doped mesoporous silica with dual capability of two-photon imaging and photosensitization. *Langmuir.* 2010;26:14937-42. doi: 10.1021/la102556u.

[110] Khlebtsov B, Panfilova E, Khanadeev V, Bibikova O, Terentyuk G, Ivanov A, et al., Nanocomposites containing silica-coated gold-silver nanocages and Yb-2,4-dimethoxyhematoporphyrin: multifunctional capability of IR-luminescence detection, photosensitization, and photothermolysis. *ACS Nano.* 2011;5:7077-89. doi: 10.1021/nn2017974.

[111] Oo MK, Yang X, Du H, Wang H. 5-aminolevulinic acid-conjugated gold nanoparticles for photodynamic therapy of cancer. *Nanomedicine.* 2008;3:777-86. doi: 10.2217/17435889.3.6.777.

[112] Xu H, Liu C, Mei J, Yao C, Wang S, Wang J, et al., Effects of light irradiation upon photodynamic therapy based on 5-aminolevulinic acid-gold nanoparticle conjugates in K562 cells via singlet oxygen generation. *Int. J. Nanomedicine.* 2012;7:5029-38. doi: 10.2147/IJN.S33261.

[113] Hadizadeh M, Fateh M. Synergistic Cytotoxic Effect of Gold Nanoparticles and 5-Aminolevulinic Acid-Mediated Photodynamic Therapy against Skin Cancer Cells. *IranJ. Med. Sci.* 2014;39:452-8.

[114] Wang B, Wang JH, Liu Q, Huang H, Chen M, Li K, et al., Rose-bengal-conjugated gold nanorods for in vivo photodynamic and photothermal oral cancer therapies. *Biomaterials.* 2014;35:1954-66. doi: 10.1016/j.biomaterials.2013.11.066.

[115] Haase M, Schafer H. Upconverting nanoparticles. *Angew Chem. Int. Ed. Engl.* 2011;50:5808-29. doi:10.1002/anie.201005159.

[116] Boyer JC, Vetrone F, Cuccia LA, Capobianco JA. Synthesis of colloidal upconverting NaYF4 nanocrystals doped with Er3+, Yb3+ and Tm3+, Yb3+ via thermal decomposition of lanthanide trifluoroacetate precursors. *J. Am. Chem. Soc.* 2006;128:7444-5. doi:10.1021/ja061848b

[117] Wang C, Tao H, Cheng L, Liu Z. Near-infrared light induced in vivo photodynamic therapy of cancer based on upconversion nanoparticles. *Biomaterials.* 2011;32:6145-54. doi: 10.1016/j.biomaterials.2011.05.007.

[118] Yin M, Ju E, Chen Z, Li Z, Ren J, Qu X. Upconverting Nanoparticles with a Mesoporous TiO2 Shell for Near-Infrared-Triggered Drug Delivery and Synergistic Targeted Cancer Therapy. *Chemistry.* 2014;20:14012-7. doi: 10.1002/chem.201403733.
[119] Yuan Y, Min Y, Hu Q, Xing B, Liu B. NIR photoregulated chemo- and photodynamic cancer therapy based on conjugated polyelectrolyte-drug conjugate encapsulated upconversion nanoparticles. *Nanoscale.* 2014;6:11259-72. doi: 10.1039/c4nr03302g.

In: Photodynamic Therapy
Editor: Adrian G. Hugo

ISBN: 978-1-63463-857-9
© 2015 Nova Science Publishers, Inc.

Chapter 5

PHOTODYNAMIC THERAPY IN ANIMAL HEALTH

Michelle Peneluppi Silva* and Antonio Olavo Cardoso Jorge
Department of Biosciences and Oral Diagnosis,
Institute of Science and Technology, UNESP – Univ Estadual Paulista, São José dos
Campos, SP, Brazil

ABSTRACT

Photodynamic therapy (PDT) is a treatment option indicated for various therapeutic protocols, such as local infections, bacteria, fungi and cancer. In veterinary medicine, studies are also being carried out to make the PDT a safe and effective treatment option for animals. In the literature, there are reports of studies about this therapeutic modality demonstrating encouraging clinical results using different classes of photosensitizers and types of light sources. PDT is based on chemical activation of a substance through visible light, generating oxygen radicals and causing destruction of the target tissue or cell without developing resistance. Although studies in the literature reporting the use of PDT with their advantages and disadvantages, it is still considered as a new and promising treatment for neoplastic and non-neoplastic diseases, and its potential, either as single treatment or in combination with conventional therapy, has much yet to be explored. This chapter attempts to provide the reader, succinctly, the advance of photodynamic therapy in veterinary medicine until today, seeking a cure for potentially fatal diseases or even better quality of life for the veterinary patient. Many of these discoveries become a chance to be applied in humans due to similarities in the etiopathogeny of some diseases.

INTRODUCTION

Although the concept of photodynamic therapy is old, its application in medicine has expanded over the past 30 years (Daniell, Hill, 1991; Ackroyd et al., 2001; Lucroy, 2005). Whereas in human medicine photodynamic therapy is safe, satisfactory and recognized treatment option in several indications, it is still little known and, unfortunately, no

---

* M.P. Silva (corresponding author): michellepeneluppi@gmail.com.

established treatment option for pets. Many photosensitizers and light sources have been used and clinical results published (Buchholz, Walt, 2013).

By combining the use of photosensitizing substance and light for antimicrobial treatment, photodynamic therapy is called Antimicrobial Photodynamic Therapy (Wainwright, Crossley, 2004). It also has other names such as Photodynamic inactivation or photoactivated disinfection (Bonsor et al., 2006; Nagata et al., 2012.). For the cancer treatment, PDT is also known as photochemotherapy or chemotherapy by light activated (Dougherty, 1993; Lucroy, 2002).

The PDT used as primary or adjunctive therapy in malignant or benign tumors or in non-neoplastic diseases is of great interest for cancer patients, both in veterinary and human medicine. The treatment is non-invasive and can reduce or eliminate morbidity and potentially dangerous side effects of surgery, chemotherapy or radiation (Campbell et al., 2002).

Thus, PDT is a therapeutic modality in development in the treatment of neoplastic and non-neoplastic diseases in human and veterinary medicine (Reeds et al., 2004; Morton et al., 2006; Osaki et al., 2006; Calista, Coccia, 2008; Puizina-Ivic et al., 2008; Rossi et al., 2008; Wang et al., 2008; Tierney et al., 2009; Osaki et al., 2009; Barnes et al., 2010).

WHY APPLY PHOTODYNAMIC THERAPY IN VETERINARY MEDICINE?

In the past, PDT was rarely applied in veterinary medicine for cancer treatment (Buchholz, Walt, 2013). Nowadays, it represents new alternative treatment for solid and superficials tumors with 1.5 to 2 cm deep (Liu et al., 2011).

In the treatment of exotic animals, PDT is potentially useful due to the minimal adverse effects compared to radiotherapy or chemotherapy, and how it is applied in small dimensions, provides better vascular access. Generally, it is performed in a single session, providing fewer problems with general anesthesia and repeated vascular access (Lucroy, 2005).

The selectivity of PDT in cancer treatment differs brusquely of all harmful effects caused by chemotherapy to the organism and the potential damage to normal tissues developed by the use of radiation therapy. The development of multidrug resistance and tumor hypoxia, which confer resistance to chemotherapy and radiation, respectively, may limit the effectiveness of conventional treatment modalities (Lucroy, 2005).

The extent of squamous cell carcinoma in equine affecting eyelid and orbital tissue, often results in eye distortion, impaired function of the eyelids, loss of vision and, in some cases, the healthy animal euthanasia (Giuliano et al., 2008), since many of these animals are show horse and horseback riding.

However, before submitting an animal for PDT, some laboratory and imaging tests are strictly necessary, as complete hemogram, biochemistry profile, thorax radiography, ultrasonography and aspiration cytology in regional lymph nodes. If identified metastasis, PDT is not the ideal treatment choice. In cases of kidney or liver disease, increases the anesthetic risk and difficulty of metabolism and elimination of the photosensitizer (Lucroy, 2005).

Thus, we explain that the major advantages of PDT among many others are: specificity in detection tumor cells, easily application, low potential for drug resistance, low toxicity, be minimally invasive, well tolerated and not damage the structure and function of tissues and organisms healthy (Liu et al., 2011). There are no reports of resistance to PDT in tumors in vivo and the mechanisms by which they can activate the immune system to prevent or delay recurrence of the tumor or metastasis (Lucroy et al., 2000).

Photodynamic therapy is not limited to oncology, this therapeutic modality has also been used successfully in the treatment of infections caused by microorganisms such as bacteria (Hamblin, Hasan, 2004; Wong et al., 2005), fungi and virus (Mohr et al., 1995; Friedberg et al., 2001; Smijs, Schuitmaker, 2003; Wainwright, 2004).

MECHANISM OF PHOTODYNAMIC THERAPY ACTION

Photodynamic therapy is successfully performed through the perfect combination of light source, substance called photosensitizer and presence of oxygen to generate reactive oxygen species (ROS) and selectively destroy the affected area (Liu et al., 2011). In the absence of any of these three elements, the phototoxic effects will not occur correctly (Konopka, Goslinski, 2007; Hamblin, Hasan, 2004).

The photosensitizer accumulates mainly in the affected area and activated in the presence of light (Moore, Ogilvie, 2001), passing to the excited state. One of the ways in which excited molecules return to the ground state is through transferring energy directly to oxygen, forming highly reactive singlet oxygen responsible for the death of target cells; characterizing the type II reaction (Daniell, Hill, 1991). Vascular and cell damage contribute to kill the target (Henderson, Dougherty, 1992; Dougherty, 2002; Triesscheijn et al., 2006). Alternatively, excited molecules may transfer energy to intermediate molecules that react with oxygen to produce free radicals, called Type I reaction (Lucroy et al., 2000).

The PDT only occurs by combining and activation appropriate of photosensitizer, light source and oxygen molecules. The photosensitizer has no biological effect until activated by light, and the light does not present enough intensity to cause tissue damage. Reactive oxygen species generated during PDT have very short half-life, limiting damage to adjacent areas (Henderson, Dougherty, 1992).

In PDT, cell death occurs mainly through the activation of oxygen free radicals, resulting in disruption of cell membrane, breaks lipoprotein and damage in nucleic acid (Campbell et al., 2002).

MECHANISM OF ACTION IN CANCER CELLS

The mechanism of PDT action depends on the capture photosensitizer by cancer cells or other areas of therapeutic interest as neovascular regions, followed by selective irradiation with appropriate wavelength visible light absorbed by the photosensitizer, activating systematically or locally. In the presence of oxygen, irradiation leads to the production of reactive oxygen species (ROS) locally generated, including singlet oxygen, hydroxyl radical or superoxide anion which inducing cytotoxicity (Dougherty et al., 1998; Lucroy et al., 1999; MacDonald, Dougherty, 2001; Lucroy, 2005), apoptosis, vascular stasis, subsequent ischemic necrosis and inflammation (Lucroy, 2005).

When the photosensitizer agent is exposed to light with certain wavelength, energy is transferred in the form of electrons to the components of the cell (type I reaction) or molecular oxygen (type II reaction) inducing cell damage and destruction of neoplastic cells (Vrouenraets et al., 2003; Giuliano et al., 2007). Thus, the photosensitizer accumulates into the neoplastic cells after oral, intravenous or topical administration (Buchholz et al., 2007).

MECHANISM OF ACTION IN MICROORGANISMS

As an alternative to traditional antimicrobial treatment, antimicrobial photodynamic therapy has been increasingly used during the last decades to destroy microorganisms. This technique can be used in microbiological control environment, surfaces and localized infections by numerous pathogens (Hamblin, Hasan, 2004; Jori et al., 2011).

Several microbial cells are susceptible to photo-oxidation effect caused by singlet oxygen, including inactivation of enzymes and other proteins, lipid peroxidation, resulting in lise of the cell membrane, lysosomes, mitochondria (Pereira-Gonzales, Maisch, 2012) and DNA (Romanova et al., 2003; Soukos, Goodson, 2011).

Microbial selectivity observed in PDT may occur due to differences in the pharmacokinetics of mammalian cells and microorganisms and not by specific recognition events (Soukos et al., 1996; O'Riordan et al., 2005). Unlike conventional antimicrobial therapy, PDT offers minimal opportunity for development of resistance by microorganisms, because their cytotoxic effects are caused by ROS as done mostly by activated phagocytic immune cells (Hamblin, Hasan, 2004; Konopka, Goslinski, 2007). In addition, pathogens exposed to PDT, which demonstrated insufficient microbicidal effect, remains with inhibited virulence factors and reduced antibiotic resistance (Kato et al., 2013).

PHOTOSENSITIZER

Numerous studies have been conducted over the years to develop new and better photochemical sensitizers (Faustino et al., 2000; Kanai et al., 2000; Rosenkranz et al., 2000; Vrouenraets et al., 2000; Whiteacre et al., 2000; Campbell et al., 2002). The ideal photosensitizer is one that can be produced in pure form, not metabolized by the organism, absorbs light of wavelength easily transmitted through tissue, produces efficiently singlet oxygen or other active intermediate oxidants and rapidly removed after treatment (Allison et al., 1993; Ronn et al., 1997; Campbell et al., 2002; Lucroy, 2002). A major concern in developing the ideal photosensitizer is prolonged skin photosensitivity (Dougherty et al., 1998).

In animals, photosensitizers may be administered systemically (orally or intravenously) or topically. In systemic application, the patient may have generalized sensitivity to light and, therefore, can no longer be exposed to it. Many photosensitizers, particularly first generation, have the disadvantage of long generalized photosensitivity (several weeks). With topical application, this does not occur, but on the other hand, the photosensitizer has a limited depth of the diffusion in tissues (Svaasand et al., 1996; Buchholz,Walt, 2013).

The distribution of the photosensitizer is a key factor in the effectiveness of treatment with PDT (Rousset et al., 2000; Chowdhary et al., 2003). To begin the therapy, the patient receives pre or pro-formed photosensitizer. The pre-formed photosensitizers are generally administered intravenously, may accumulate in neoplastic tissues due to its chemical properties, such as affinity for collagen synthesis and binding to lipoprotein receptors, both common in tumors (Allison et al., 1994; Dougherty et al., 1998).

Important to emphasize that, after an interval of 24 to 72 hours, in the treatment of tumors, the photosensitizer is excreted by most normal tissues, but remains inside the cancer cells, creating a favorable drug-concentration relationship for PDT. Some photosensitizers, such as hematoporphyrin derivatives, can remain on the skin for up to 8 weeks after administration, causing complications as prolonged skin photosensitivity (Wolfsen, Ng, 2002; Lucroy, 2005).

Pro-photosensitizers, such as 5-aminolevulinic acid, is administered topically, orally or intravenously in the unactivated form (Lucroy et al., 1999; Lucroy et al., 2003; Ridgway, Lucroy, 2003). ALA is metabolized within 2 to 6 hours in an active photosensitizer protoporphyrin IX by malignant epithelial cells. Protoporphyrin IX can be detected at lower concentrations in normal epithelium after several hours and not detectable in mesenchymal tissues, making PDT with ALA highly specific for carcinomas treatment (Lucroy, 2005).

With the new generation of photoactive agents under development to reduce the risk of undesirable side effects, the second generation photosensitizers include synthetic products of various groups such as porphyrins and porphycenes, chlorines, phthalocyanines, among others that have better pharmacological properties, including more efficient light absorbance and higher quantum yield of atomic oxygen (Giuliano et al., 2007).

SOME PHOTOSENSITIZERS USED IN VETERINARY MEDICINE

Hematoporphyrin Monomethyl Ether

Hematoporphyrin monomethyl ether (HMME) belongs to the second-generation porphyrin derived photosensitizers formed by two monomers, 3 (1-methyloxyethyl) -8 (1-hydroxyethyl) deuteroporphyrin IX and 8 (1-methyloxyethyl) -3 (1-hydroxyethyl) deuteroporphyrin IX. Both have isomeric location. Experimental studies and clinical trials have demonstrated HMME has more selectivity for tumor tissue, greater photodynamic effect and low toxicity (Cheng et al., 2010). Under several experimental conditions, such as differences in dosing and exposure times, HMME remains, mainly, in the cytoplasm with low concentrations in the nucleus. In the cytosol, HMME distributes mostly in the mitochondria, endoplasmic reticulum, Golgi and lysosomes (Dai et al., 2009). Studies have been performed using HMME in PDT for treatment of canine breast cancer, but more knowledge is still necessary (Li et al., 2013).

Benzoporphyrin Derivative

Verteporfin, benzoporphyrin derivative, belongs to the porphyrin family, which contains aromatic heterocyclic cyclic molecules composed of four modified pyrrole units which are interconnected at their carbon atoms via methine bridges (Liu-Chittenden et al., 2012), belonging to the second generation photosensitizers, has been developed for the treatment of macular degeneration in humans (Brown, Mellish, 2001; Messmer, Abel, 2001; Marcus et al., 1994.; Panjehpour et al., 2002.; Houle, Strong, 2002; Lui et al., 2004) has also been used in the treatment of solid tumors (Marcus et al., 1994.; Panjehpour et al., 2002; Houle, Strong, 2002; Lui et al., 2004), presenting rapid accumulation inside neoplastic cells, about 3 hours, and elimination within a few days, when administered intravenously (Rousset et al., 2000; Houle, Strong, 2002; Chowdhary et al., 2003; Lui et al., 2004), thus reducing the risk of prolonged skin photosensitivity (Houle, Strong, 2002; Lui et al., 2004; Rowe et al., 2014). Furthermore, it shows maximum absorbance around 690 nm and this wavelength permits activation of the drug within the deeper portions of the target tissue in comparison with other photoactive agents (Giuliano et al., 2007).

Previous studies using verteporfin demonstrated the drug distribution in tumor tissues through the vascular location. The photosensitizer dissipates throughout the affected tissue in relatively homogeneous distribution in few hours after intravenous administration. Drug distribution also affects the mechanisms of tumor cell death (Durand, Aquino-Parsons, 2001; Chen et al., 2003; Pogue et al., 2005; Barnes et al., 2009) and tumor destruction is due mostly to vascular damage caused by irradiation applied shortly after drug administration, and direct death of cell parenchyma is the major mechanism of tumor cell death when the time interval between drug administration and light irradiation is 3 hours (Chen et al., 2005; Zhou et al., 2006; Barnes et al., 2009).

Palladium Bacteriopheophorbide

The synthesis of the photosensitizers family derived from photosynthetic pigments bacteriochlorophyll (Scherz et al., 1997; Scherz et al., 2003), effectively eradicate solid tumors, but through antivascular mechanism. Bacteriochlorophyll serine has been used successfully as PDT agent for treating melanoma and sarcoma (Kelleher et al., 1999; Zilberstein et al., 2001; Kelleher et al., 2003). Subsequently, the advanced drug Pd-bacteriopheophorbide, WST09®, was used in xenograft photodynamic treatment in various animal models and healthy dogs. Bacteriochlorophyll photosensitizers, including WST09®, exhibit characteristics photochemical and pharmacological advantages such as high extinction coefficient near infrared allowing treatment of large tumors with depth of 2 cm, rapid clearance from the circulation (<10 minutes) and skin and the treatment protocol for PDT is fast (10 minutes) in a single session that the photosensitizer and light are sequentially administered with no time lag in laboratory animals or during 20 minutes after drug infusion with overlapping lighting (17 minutes) in humans (Chen et al., 2002).

Pyropheophorbide-Alpha-Hexyl-Ether

The photosensitizer Pyropheophorbide-alpha-hexyl-ether (HPPH-23) has activation wavelength of 665 nm, based on studies with murine, is rapidly cleared from the normal skin, therefore, saving normal tissues of photosensitizing effect. Other advantages possibles as photosensitizer include purity, clearly defined chemical structure and high coefficient of elimination at the peak of absorption compared with porfimer sodium (Bellnier et al., 1993; Magne et al., 1997).

Hematoporphyrin Derivative

PDT with porfimer sodium, hematoporphyrin derivative, Photofrin®, has been applied to many neoplasias in dogs and cats (Klein, Roberts, 1993). The limitations of this photosensitizer as tumor therapeutic agent include limited tissue penetration due to the short wavelength of activation (630 nm) and prolonged skin photosensitization the patients to sunlight (Peaston et al., 1993; Allison, Sibata, 2010).

Methylene Blue

Phenothiazine derivatives photosensitizers, such as methylene blue, are widely used in studies involving PDT in microbial control. Combined with red light in appropriate parameters, the dose required for cytotoxicity in photodynamic microbial inactivation is, generally, less than required to cause damage to host cells such as keratinocytes, fibroblasts (Soukos et al., 1996), irrelevant toxicity in low concentrations (Lim et al., 2013). In innate immune cells can also initiate inflammatory responses that complement the resolution of infection (Soukos et al., 1996; Tanaka et al., 2012; Sellera et al., 2014a).

5-Aminolevulinic Acid

5-aminolevulinic acid (5-ALA) é is widely used in the treatment of tumors of human skin (Kennedy et al., 1990; Bexfield et al., 2008) and it is being much studied in veterinary medicine (Lucroy et al., 2003). 5-ALA can be administered topical, intravenous and parenteral (Marcus et al., 1996), preferentially absorbed by damaged keratin overlying the tumors, but has little penetration through the normal intact keratin (Kennedy et al., 1990; Bexfield et al., 2008). Although not photoactive by itself, when diffused into the cell, 5-ALA is converted to protoporphyrin IX, chemical product sensitive to light, by heme cycle. This activation results in cell death and vascular damage by the production of reactive oxygen species and immune activation against tumor cells (Garcia-Zuazaga et al., 2005; Bexfield et al., 2008).

Meta-Tetra(Hydroxyphenyl) Chlorin (mTHPC)

Meta-tetra(hydroxyphenyl) chlorin (mTHPC) belongs to the second generation of photosensitizers. It is a drug not metabolized and eliminated by the liver, single and stable molecular species with spectroscopic and thermodynamic properties documented. The biodistribution was reported in humans, dogs, rabbits and rats (Ronn et al., 1997). Compared to other photosensitizing agents, there are few reports of toxic effects (Ronn et al., 1997; Lofgren et al., 1994; Campbell et al., 2002). This has proved to be a promising photosensitizer for the treatment of squamous neoplasia in animal models (Lofgren et al., 1994; Andrejevic-Blant et al., 1997; Campbell et al., 2002) and human (Grosjean et al., 1996; Savary et al., 1998; Zellweger et al., 1999; Campbell et al., 2002).

Phthalocyanines

This dye family is potent photosensitizer (Allen et al., 2001; Allison, Sibata, 2010). Their structures are porphyrin based and generally include a central atom usually zinc, silicon or aluminum to increase singlet oxygen production. They have strong absorption bands in the 670 nm range, have fluorescent capabilities and can be activated clinically at 100 J/cm^2. As they are highly hydrophobic these photosensitizers are encapsulated by liposomes. These photosensitizer accumulate in mitochondria and apparently induces apoptosis. Depending on formulation, the drugs can clear the body in about 24 hours, minimizing photosensitivity. Treatment generally is initiated one hour after photosensitizer application. A topical formulation is also possible (Allison, Sibata, 2010).

Photodynamic treatments in cats and dogs suggest that some photosensitizers, such as aluminum phthalocyanine tetrasulfonate, are associated with idiosyncratic hepatic (Leach, Peaston, 1994), while other, ALA, cause dose-dependent hepatopathy (Lucroy et al., 2003). Phthalocyanine compounds are activated at wavelength of 675 nm and preliminary favorable results after treatment of squamous cell carcinoma in cats has been reported with PDT-based *chloraluminum sulfonated phthalocyanine* (Peaston et al., 1993).

The use of photosensitizer, such as substance already known or new drug with photosensitizing properties, requires much care and research. Besides being ideal choice for composing the triad of PDT (photosensitizer, light source and oxygen), capturing the light at the appropriate wavelength, it is necessary to know the pharmacokinetics, pharmacodynamics and metabolism of substance, absorbance spectrum, species animal to be treated, since some photosensitizers are well tolerated while others do not.

LIGHT SOURCE

Different types of light sources have been used, mainly Light Amplification by Stimulated Emission of Radiation, Laser, however, some studies have reported usage of Light Emitting Diode, LED. Laser is most frequently used as device distribution of light in PDT because it emits coherent and monochromatic light radiating with accurately the treatment region (Buchholz, Walt, 2013).

Recently, the uses of non-coherent light sources, with principal emphasis on LED, have been evaluated by using predetermined specific wavelength. These lights offer interesting cost-effective because they are portable and cheaper, facilitating application of PDT. The recent creation of these light sources together with topical photosensitizing agents caused the resurgence of exploration of PDT as an antimicrobial treatment (Wardlaw et al., 2012).

Other light sources such as halogen lamps have also become available for PDT. These, along with LED offer several advantages over laser, including lower cost of equipment, minimal risk of injuries in eye of responsible professional for the application and no need of special requirements in electrical installations. Limitations of non-coherent light sources include low power output and difficulty of channeling light through fiber optic networks (Giuliano et al., 2007; Brancaleon, Moseley, 2002).

The choice of photosensitizer determines the wavelength of light required for the treatment. The depth of light penetration depends on the wavelength of the light type light source and power output. Light in the spectral region of 600 to 700 nm penetrates 50 to 200% more than the light in the region 400 to 500 nm (Keijzer et al., 1989; Giuliano et al., 2007). Moreover, the penetration of light is also very dependent on the type of tissue involved. Tissues highly pigmented or high hemoglobin content such as muscle, may reduce the penetration depth of light (Bernstein et al., 1990; Giuliano et al., 2007).

ADVERSE EFFECT

The use of photodynamic therapy in veterinary patients requires some special care like appropriate contention of the patient during the procedure using general anesthesia and the protection of treated area against self-induced trauma through the use of bandages and /or elizabethan collars during the post treatment period. It is important to include the use of analgesics and anti-inflammatories (Lucroy et al., 1996; Buchholz, Walt, 2013).

Some side effects may be observed according to the type and concentration of the photosensitizer, the type and dose of light, target tissue (Hamblin, Hasan, 2004), via of administration and degree sensitivity of the patient. Side effects are mostly observed in patients submitted to cancer treatment, such as skin photosensitivity, nausea and vomiting. In the topical treatment, it can observe local sensitivity accompanied by pain, edema, erythema and itching (Zelickson, 2005; Sellera et al., 2014b). Most pet owners concerned about the post-treatment morbidity and quality of life for their pets (Lucroy et al., 1996).

THE ADVANCE OF PHOTODYNAMIC THERAPY IN VETERINARY MEDICINE

PDT is very indicated to the treatment of localized cancer, but not indicated in cases of metastasis (Lucroy, 2002). In addition to this treatment, photodynamic therapy has several other potential to be used in veterinary medicine, being effective in destruction of cutaneous bacteria and yeasts (Zeina et al., 2001; Lucroy, 2002), useful for the treatment of deep pyoderma and chronic otitis externa. Large areas of skin can be irradiated using optical fibers equipped with lenses of diffusion and external auditory canals can be irradiated with optical fibers that end in cylindrical diffusers. As the photosensitizer can be administered topically or parenterally, there are, several options in developing protocol useful antimicrobial PDT (Lucroy, 2002).

PDT has been shown emergent new therapy in veterinary ophthalmology for the treatment of periocular tumors (Giuliano et al., 2007). In cutaneous squamous cell carcinoma (Ruslander et al., 1997; Lucroy, 2007; Ferreira et al., 2009), became a treatment option, being first used in animals with spontaneous tumors with intravenous application of derivatives hematoporphyrin and laser irradiation (Thomas, Fox, 2002; Ferreira et al., 2009). These studies included animals with various types of tumors, the majority considered sensitive, indicating the clinical potential of this therapy in the treatment of cancer, identifying PDT as an important tool for oncologists and veterinary dermatologists (Lucroy et al., 1996; Lucroy, 2002; Ferreira et al., 2009).

Pythiosis, disease difficult to treat, has been described in humans, domestic and wild animals and aquatic birds (Santurio et al., 1998; Sallis et al., 2003; Santurio et al., 2003; Pupaibool et al., 2006; Rakich et al., 2005; Pérez et al., 2005; Pesavento et al., 2008; Videla et al., 2012; Pires et al., 2013), being the horse the most affected animal (Sallis et al., 2003) followed by the dog (Dykstra et al., 1999; Berryessa et al., 2008). There is little response to conventional or antimicrobial therapies available. Experimental therapies often seem promising in vitro, but when tested in vivo, the results are less promising with relapses that occur when treatment is discontinued (Dykstra et al., 1999; Berryessa et al., 2008; Mendoza et al., 2003; Mendoza, Newton, 2005; Pires et al., 2013). Study by Pires et al. (2013) evaluated the PDT as a novel and promising treatment, effective in this disease.

However, currently, many studies are still under development to establish correct application of PDT in various diseases affecting the different species of animals, evaluating the effectiveness of this new treatment modality in veterinary medicine.

PHOTODYNAMIC THERAPY IN DIFFERENT ANIMAL SPECIES

Cat

In cats, PDT with variety of photosensitizers and light sources has main indication cutaneous treatment, such as skin tumors, which often occur as squamous cell carcinoma, usually found in head areas, slightly pigmented. For early stages of this tumor, promising results have been published using new and selective drugs that reduce light sensitivity after systemic administration and increase the rate of response to treatment (Roberts et al., 1991; Buchholz et al., 2007; Buchholz, Walt, 2013).

Magne and colleagues (1997) evaluated the safety and efficacy of photodynamic therapy using a photosensitizer pyropheophorbide-alpha-hexyl-ether (HPPH-23) in the treatment of squamous cell carcinoma on skin face of cats. PDT was performed with pulsed argon laser 24 hours after administration the photosensitizer. After treatment, the tumors were evaluated in relation to rate of complete response and time of local control. There were no signs of clinical, haematological and biochemical toxicity after administration of the drug. However, it has been found morbidity in animal after treatment of large and invasive tumors of the nasal plane. Thus, the authors could conclude that PDT with photosensitizer HPPH-23 was safe and efficient in the treatment of early stage of squamous cell carcinoma of the nasal level and skin facial in cats. However, toxicity was detected after treatment of large tumors.

Bexfield and colleagues (2008) investigated the effect of PDT using photosensitizing agent 5-aminolevulinic acid (5-ALA), topically, and red light source of high intensity (635 nm) in superficial squamous cell carcinoma of the nasal plane in 55 cats. The animals were evaluated for adverse effects, response and control tumor: 96% responded to therapy, 85% showed a complete response and 11% partial. Animals with complete response to single treatment, the recurrence rate was 51% with an average time of 157 days (confidence interval of 95%, 109-205 days). The treatment was reapplied in 22 cats with median follow-up of 1146 days, with 45% of animals were alive and free of disease, 33% were euthanized due to tumor recurrence and 22% also euthanized for other reasons. According to the authors, were observed only transitory and level effects on local after treatment, such as erythema and edema. Thus, they concluded that PDT using 5-ALA and red light was safe, well tolerated and effective in treating superficial squamous cell carcinoma of the nasal plan cats and offers an alternative to conventional therapy. But although the initial response rate is high, this treatment did not cause lasting remission or cure in all cases.

In your studies, Ferreira et al. (2009) analyzed the action of PDT using hematoporphyrin derivative photosensitizer (Photogem®) and LED as the light source in 12 cats with squamous cell carcinoma cutaneous. The lesions were irradiated for 30 minutes after 24 hours of administration the photosensitizer. Clinical responses were classified as complete tumor remission with complete reepithelialization, partial remission (greater than 50% reduction) and without remission (less than 50% reduction). Tumors located in the pinna were treated with one (n = 3) or two (n = 4) application of PDT and had no response. The highly invasive tumors located in the nose and nasal plan also showed no response after two treatments (n = 2). PDT was combined with surgery in three cases. Two animals showed partial response and complete remission with single application of therapy 30 days after nasal surgery. Small and non-infiltrative lesions (n = 3) of the nasal plan had partial response with an application (n = 2) and complete after two applications (n = 1). According to the authors, this study showed that PDT using Photogem® and LED can provide local control of squamous cell carcinoma low grade in feline and concomitant treatment with PDT and surgery in more invasive cases may help prevent recurrence.

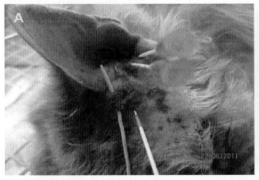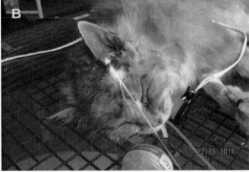

Figura 1. (a) Preparation of a cat for treatment with interstitial photodynamic therapy of a squamous cell carcinoma. (b) Control of fiber placement in the same patient seen in (a) usingthe aiming laser. Reproduced from Buchholz, Walt (2013). Photodiagnosis and Photodynamic Therapy, Reproduced with permission of Elsevier Limited.

Dog

PDT is applied for the treatment of various pathologies affecting dogs. Different types of photosensitizers which exhibit good tolerance for this specie have been used showing promising results.

One of PDT indications in dogs is urinary tract tumors. Another example is transmissible venereal tumor, which the use of PDT aims, beyond cure, minimize the effects of chemotherapy and radiotherapy and also reduces the number of sessions. Important studies on PDT application in mammary glands tumors of dogs were performed and results show great potential for use in humans due to similarities in the characteristics of developing these cancers (Pinho et al., 2012; Li et al., 2013).

Liu et al. (2011) studied apoptosis induced hematoporphyrin monomethyl ether (HMME), a promising and new photosensitizer related with porphyrin for photodynamic therapy, in CHMM cells, a cell line cancer on mammary gland of dogs. The CHMM cells were treated with HMME and He-Ne laser with a wavelength of 632.8 nm. Cell viability was determined using the trypan blue exclusion assay. Apoptosis was analyzed Hoechst 33258, AO/EB, Annexin V/PI staining and single-cell gel electrophoresis. The morphology of apoptosis was confirmed by Giemsa staining and transmission electron microscopy. Apoptosis rates increased after PDT-HMME treatment in a time-dependent manner. Analyzing the overall results, the authors demonstrated that apoptosis plays an important role in PDT induced HMME combined with irradiation by He-Ne laser in vitro in breast cancer cells in dogs, reducing the viability of these. The authors concluded that although one can not exclude the possibility that treatment with PDT-HMME can induce necrosis CHMM cells, the results of the experiment indicated that apoptosis is the main mechanism for cell death. This is confirmed by the reduction in cell viability of time-dependent manner, with cell death occurred 12 hours after PDT-HMME treatment. This pattern of death is consistent with the fact that induction of apoptosis requires transcription, translation and activation of signaling pathways for apoptosis. However, it should be noted that necrosis is not mutually exclusive of apoptosis, since they are intrinsically linked and necrotic characteristics were present in PDT-HMME induced apoptotic cells.

In your studies, Osaki and colleagues (2009) evaluated the efficacy of antivascular PDT using Benzoporphyrin derivative monoacid ring A (BPD-MA) for treatment of oral and nasal tumors in 14 dogs. At 15 min after initiating intravenous infusion of 0.5 mg/kg BPD-MA, tumors were irradiated with laser light at 690 nm emitted by a diode laser. The 1-year survival rate of 7 dogs with oral tumors was 71% and nasal tumors was 57%. Imaging of each tumor was performed by using angiographic computed tomography before and after each antivascular PDT. Contrast-enhanced tumors were observed before antivascular PDT, but these tumors were not enhanced with contrast medium following antivascular PDT. The autors concluded Antivascular PDT is suggested to be a promising treatment for dogs with oral and nasal tumors that cannot be effectively treated with current antitumor therapies. This therapy should be considered as a possible treatment in canine solid malignant tumors. Moreover, angiographic CT might play an extremely useful role in determining the therapeutic effect after antivascular PDT.

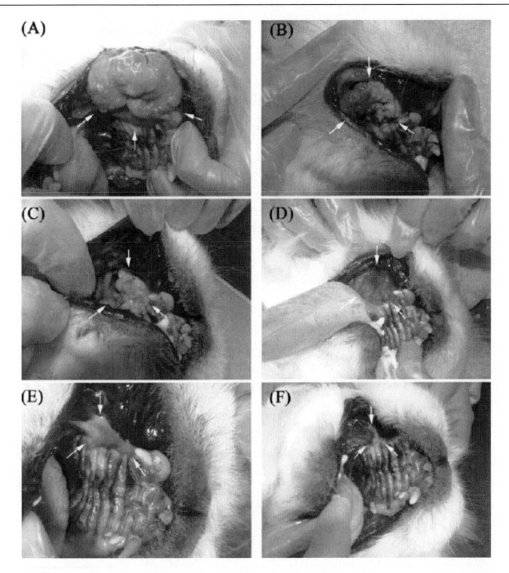

Figura 2. (A) before PDT (tumor locate maxilla), (B) 5 days after PDT (the tumor is atrophied), (C)12 days after PDT (necrotic tumor tissue sloughs away), (D) 12 days after PDT (after debridement), (E) 33 days after PDT (an ulcerative lesion) and (F) 96 days after PDT (the treated area is almost com-pletely covered with a normal oral mucosa). Arrows indicate the tumor and treated area. Reproduced from Osaki et al. (2009). The Journal of Veterinary Medical Science, Reproduced with permission of The Japanese Society of Veterinary Science.

Osaki and colleagues (2012) applied antivascular PDT benzoporphyrin derivative monoacid ring A and 690 nm laser in 5 years old with cross breed dog, eight months after the initial manifestation of chronic rhinosinusitis. Computed tomography (CT) showed opacities areas of soft tissue or fluid in the left nasal cavity and frontal sinus. The diagnosis of chronic sinusitis with polyps myxomatous was based on histology of biopsy samples, therefore, treatment with prednisolone was administered for one month. Although the clinical signs presented slightly improved, no changes on CT images were observed. After 11 days of antivascular PDT, CT revealed remarkable decrease in the opacity of soft tissue; whereas facial edema and sneezing were resolved. Three additional sessions PDT were performed at

114, 210 and 303 days after the first due to recurrence of clinical signs. According to the authors, the disease was well controlled for about 10 months by the antivascular PDT, however, the effectiveness of this treatment was insufficient, because was a disease with inflammation process, it could only be expected control, unlike tumor with potential for eradication. The authors observed good tolerance by the animal to the stipulated treatment and facial edema developed after a few days of each session did not require specific care. Thus, they concluded that antivascular PDT proved useful in the treatment of severe myxomatous polyps for which medical therapy is not effective. Therefore, this therapy can serve as an alternative for some cases medical treatment of nasal polyps.

Burch et al. (2009) in your studies verified the capacity of photodynamic therapy to treat large bone tumors due to the limitations of light penetration, determining whether may induce necrosis and, if possible, quantifying the volume of tissue treated. Seven dogs with spontaneous osteosarcoma of the distal radius were treated with PDT using verteporfin and irradiated with 690 nm diode laser for 5 minutes. Tumor regions were analyzed with magnetic resonance imaging (MRI) before and after 48 hours of treatment and volumes of hypointense regions compared. The treated limbs were amputated immediately after 48 hours images and sectioned corresponding to the axial MRI images. Histologically, tumor necrosis was identified and these areas correspond anatomically to the hypotensive tissue on MRI. The average volume of necrotic tissue observed after photodynamic therapy was 21305 mm^3 comparing to pre-treatment volume of 6108 mm^3. According to the authors, these data suggest that photodynamic therapy can penetrate in large bone tumors of dog and may complement the treatment of this pathology.

Li et al. (2013) analyzed the effect of PDT with Hematoporphyrin monomethyl ether (HMME) in the structure and dysfunction mitochondrial in cancer cells of mammary glands in dogs. Cancer cells were treated with HMME and He-Ne laser 632.8 nm. It was observed structural changes in the mitochondria with loss of potential in mitochondrial membrane. As a result, HMME-PDT increased mitochondrial reactive oxygen species, inhibited the enzymatic activities of mitochondrial, abolished mitochondrial ability in the uptake and release of calcium, and decreased mitochondrial ATPase activity. The combination of these factors led to accumulation of ROS in mitochondrial to high levels, which in turn contributed to HMME-PDT-induced damages of mitochondrial structure and mitochondrial dysfunction.

Sellera and colleagues (2013a) investigated the efficacy of PDT for the treatment of mixed breed adult canine oral papillomatosis. The patient presented with dysphagia, halitosis and oral multiple verrucous lesions. Major lesions in the oral mucosa, excluding tongue lesions, were injected with an aqueous methylene blue solution (300 uM) under general anesthesia. After 5 minutes, the lesions were irradiated with diode laser 660 nm perpendicular to the lesion during 3 minutes. The irradiated lesions were significantly smaller at the two weeks follow-up. The lesions on the tongue, which were not injected with methylene blue and irradiated, did not show visible changes. A complete reduction in the buccal and tongue lesions was observed 15 days after the second application. The authors conclued PDT is a novel candidate for canine oral papillomatosis treatment, and further studies are warranted to elucidate its use as a veterinary oncological treatment and to understand the pathophysiology of this disease.

Equine

Squamous cell carcinomas in equine (SCC) is the most common tumor affecting the nictitating membrane, eyelids, conjunctiva and limbus and the second most common tumor in horses eyeball (Gelatt et al., 1974; Gelatt, 1975; Lavach, Severin, 1977). Correlation between etiological development of this malignancy and exposure to ultraviolet light is suggested. Squamous cell carcinoma periocular equine is typically invasive, resulting in ocular discomfort and blindness if not treated (Fischer et al., 2002). The therapeutic strategies include surgery to reduce (Koch, Cowles, 1971) with or without auxiliary cryotherapy (Hilbert et al., 1977), radiofrequency hyperthermia (Grier et al., 1980), beta-irradiation (Joyce, 1976; Frauenfelder et al., 1982), intralesional chemotherapy (Theon et al., 1993), and immunotherapy (Hendrix, 2005). However, it reported a high recurrence rate using these therapeutic modalities and the esthetic after surgery is deficient. There are reports of natural occurrence of this disease successfully treated with surgical cytoreduction followed by PDT-verteporfin in the center tumor (Giuliano et al., 2008).

Bird

There are few reports in veterinary literature about the treatment of birds with photodynamic therapy. The frequency and location of tumors in these species are little known. However, survey of nearly 1,500 tumors of birds, suggests that the parakeets are commonly affected among the bird species studied (Leach, 1992) and the integument the most affected place. As PDT is ideal for treating minor cutaneous lesions, there is enormous potential for application of this therapy in the treatment of birds. However, more extensive studies of the safety and pharmacokinetics of various photosensitizers are still needed to optimize the use of PDT in birds (Lucroy, 2005).

Suedmeyer et al. (2001) applied PDT in Great hornbill (*Buceris bicornis*), 33 years old, using 5-(pyropheophorbide-a-hexylether) (HPPH) to treat squamous cell carcinoma (SCC) of casque. It was administered 0.3 mg / kg of pyropheophorbide-a-hexylether intravenously 24 hours before exposure to light. Initially there was a good response, but it was noted recurrence and another session of therapy was performed eight weeks later. SCC recurrent was observed after a week of the second session of PDT and the animal was euthanized shortly thereafter. The failure was attributed to the size of the initial lesion. Experiments with the same photosensitizer in cats suggest an association between tumor size and effectiveness.

Reptile

Due to ability to destroy microorganisms such as bacteria, PDT can also be a useful treatment for infectious ulcerative stomatitis, disease potentially devastating of snake raised in captivity. However, more studies about on the application of PDT in snakes and other reptiles must be done to determine if this form of treatment should be applied in cancer and superficial infections that affect these species (Lucroy, 2005).

Others Animals Species

Lucroy (2005) treated 4-year-old castrated male ferret with oral squamous cell carcinoma involving the right cheek applying PDT with pyropheophorbide-a-hexylether. The ferret was given 0.3 mg/kg of the photosensitizer by intravenous injection 24 hours before tumor irradiation with 665 nm of light. Partial response was observed 4 weeks after treatment, and PDT repeated 8 weeks after initial treatment. After a brief partial response, the tumor grew beyond its original size. The owner refused to continue treatment. According to the author, the lack of complete response in this ferret was attributed to the thickness of the tumor (>2 cm) and the possibility of rapid clearance of the photosensitizer.

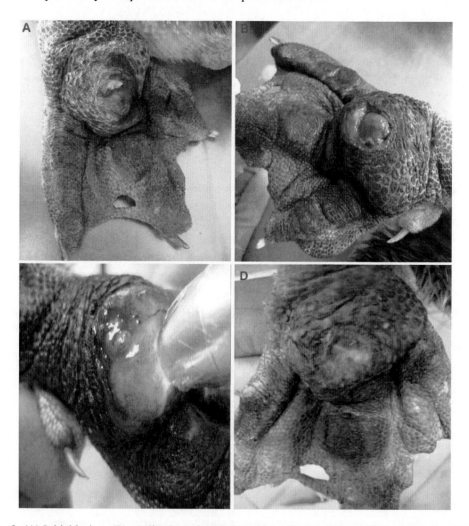

Figura 3. (A) Initial lesion, (B) application of methylene blue, (C) irradiation, (D) 1 month after PDT treatment. Image courtesy of Dr. Fábio Parra Sellera, University of São Paulo.

Sellera et al. (2014a) studied the effects of photodynamic therapy with methylene blue as photosensitizer and red diode laser as light source in the treatment of five Magellanic penguins, *Spheniscus magellanicus*, with pododermatitis lesions, as known bumblefoot, currently one of the most frequent clinical and important complications in birds kept in captivity or rehabilitation centers. All treated lesions successfully regressed and no recurrence was observed during the 6 months follow-up period. According to the authors, PDT seems to be an inexpensive and effective alternative treatment for pododermatitis in Magellanic penguins encouraging further research on this topic.

Sellera and colleagues (2013b) evaluated the effect of PDT as an alternative to conventional treatment of digital diseases of cattle, usually performed with topical antimicrobial on the lesion. Two bovines with hoof lesions diagnosed as toe ulcer were treated with methylene blue (300 mM) as a photosensitizer, followed by irradiation with laser diode with 660nm wavelength and energy of 8J/point, as a light source, twice a week until the complete resolution of the lesion. The autors could conclude that the therapy proved being effective for wound healing, with an average period of 30 days for complete recovery.

Experimental Model

Pires et al. (2013) evaluated the effect of PDT on *Pythium insidiosum* growth in vitro and in vivo for cutaneous pythiosis treatment. For in vitro studies, two photosensitizers were evaluated: hematoporphyrin derivative (Photogem®) and chlorine (Photodithazine®). Amphotericin B was also evaluated and the control group treated with sterile saline solution. All experiments (PDT, porphyrin, chlorine and light, amphotericin B and saline solution) were repeated 5 times. To in vivo studies, six rabbits were inoculated with 20,000 zoospores of *P. insidiosum* and 1 cm^3 of area was treated with the same sensitizers. In the irradiation was used diode light emitting at 660 nm for chlorine and 530 nm for hematoporphyrin. The animals were evaluated clinically and, 72 hours after PDT, histopathological analysis. In vitro results showed the inhibition rates for PDT ranged from 60 to 100% and had better results in comparison with amphotericin B. To in vivo testing, after PDT, histological analysis of the lesions showed no infection until 1 cm depth. The authors concluded that studies in vitro and in vivo demonstrated the efficacy of PDT in the inactivation of *P. insidiosum* suggesting new approach for treatment of pythiosis.

In studies by Barnes et al. (2009), successful treatment of naturally occurring periocular squamous cell carcinoma (SCC) in horses with photodynamic therapy was performed by topical application of verteporfin and laser irradiation immediately after photosensitizer administration. According to the authors, the intravenous injection (IV) of photosensitizing agents in horses is not a viable method of administration. Studies on pharmacokinetics, distribution drug and toxicity are scarce and the amount of drug to be delivered (500-1000 mg) would be excessive in volume and expense. Furthermore, IV application of photosensitizer may result in photosensitization skin induced by sunlight, requiring that animals be confined for several weeks, predisposing the development of potential diseases that threaten the patient's life, such as colic, laminitis and respiratory infection. For these reasons, the authors investigated the intralesional administration of the photosensitizer verteporfin in horses with SCC. The authors used the experimental model murine to evaluate the influence of the time between the application of verteporfin intralesional and laser irradiation in inhibition of tumor growth following PDT. The animals were randomly divided into six groups (n = 10). In each tumor 0.1 mg / cm^3 of verteporfin (Tx) or 5% dextrose in water (C) was injected. Tx and C groups 1, 2 and 3 were irradiated at 1, 30 and 180 minutes after injection. The Wilcoxonrank sum test (p = 0.05) was conducted to determine the relative change in tumor volume (RCTV) between the groups and statistical significance was demonstrated between treatment groups. Although PDT-verteporfin treated mice, Tx1 and Tx2 showed less RCTV compared to C1 and C2 mice, the differences were not statistically significant.

Vilensky et al. (2005) evaluated the effect of local vascular-targeted photodynamic therapy (VTP) using Pd-bacteriopheophorbide (WST09), alternative photosensitizing substance to conventional chemotherapy, and laser diode in the treatment of canine-transmissible venereal tumor, (CTVT). Male CD1 nude mice were subcutaneously grafted with the xenograft-transmissible canine venereal tumour (XTVT). The VTP protocol delivered once consisted of intravenous administration of WST09 (10 mg kg^{-1}) followed by immediate local illumination with a diode laser (763 nm). Controls included animals treated with light or WST09 alone. The macroscopic and microscopic evaluations of tumor remission were performed 10, 24 and 48 hours after treatment. Upon VTP, tumours underwent necrosis that lasted 8–10 days and exhibited complete healing by 25–35 days, reaching an overall long-term cure rate (83%) by 90 days after treatment. According to the authors, this study suggests that VTP with WST09 can efficiently treat CTVT in a single session, as compared with 4–6 sessions of chemotherapy and thus may be feasible for common veterinary practice, particularly under ambulatory conditions.

COMMENTS

Studies show be promising in relation to PDT, a safe and effective modality for treatment of various diseases affecting different animal species. However, more research to better understand the pharmacokinetics of photosensitizers, biodistribution in the affected tissues, as well as light sources capable of being absorbed by these agents without causing damage to patient and professional responsible, encourage the emergence of treatment protocols more optimized.

Over the years, several studies were designed to investigate the effects of PDT on prevention and treatment of infectious diseases using animals as models of infection, including mouse, rat, dog and pig. The purpose of these studies is the establishment an infection resembling disease affecting the species of interest, usually humans. To reproduce the disease as closely as possible the clinical infection, the cause of the infection can be researched and developed new treatments (Lewis, 2008; Jain et al., 2007; Wood, 2009; Dai et al., 2009).

The enormous biological complexity of human cancer has stimulated the development of more appropriate animal models that resemble a natural and spontaneous form to pathophysiological aspects of biology cancer (Pinho et al., 2012).

Mammary gland tumors are among the most common malignancies in humans and dogs. The mechanism underlying the occurrence of the tumor has developed similarly in both mammals (Klopfleisch et al., 2011; Li et al., 2013). Mammary tumors in canines and humans share several important epidemiological, morphological, clinical, biochemical and pathological aspects (Kumaraguruparan et al., 2006; Li et al., 2013). The spontaneous canine mammary tumor has been increasingly used as model more powerful study in the treatment of human breast cancer (Pinho et al., 2012; Li et al., 2013), because the tumors that occur naturally in dogs have many clinical and biological similarities with the development of cancer in humans which have difficult to reproduce in other models of experimental systems (MacEwen, 1990; Pinho et al., 2012). Many other types of spontaneous tumors in companion animals, such as osteosarcoma, hemangiosarcoma, lung cancer, skin cancer, prostate cancer and gastrointestinal demonstrated application in human cancer models (MacEwen, 1990; Hahn et al., 1994; De Vico et al., 2005; Porrello et al., 2006).

So, the growing interest in research on cancer treatments of animal model and the increase in the number of publications in oncology veterinary mark oncologic comparisons of extreme importance in translational medicine, allowing the fast and valid flow of data on clinical application in humans providing the identification of novel cancer-associated genes, study of environmental risk factors, understanding of the molecular biology of tumor development and evaluation of new diagnostic, prognostic and therapeutic applications that will benefit patients of both species (Pinho et al., 2012).

However, studies to develop therapeutic protocols in animals for later possible use in humans go far beyond oncology. So, not only the similarity of the pathogenesis of diseases, but also the development in searching for ideal photosensitizers, efficient light sources, evaluation of adverse effects and post-therapeutic protocol in two species are extremely necessary for treatments in human and veterinary medicine.

Therefore, it so much important to investigate and evaluate the possibility of better and less painful treatment regardless of the disease and species studied, concerned with the welfare of all and minimizing the incidence of cases.

CONCLUSION

Describe the use of photodynamic therapy in veterinary medicine is interesting not only for reporting the importance of this treatment, but their advance beyond human medicine. We have the way of documenting knowledge about human and animal universe separately. However, they are worlds that walk, not in parallel, but intrinsically linked and dependent.

Whereas in human medicine, photodynamic therapy is a treatment option recognized for several indications, in veterinary medicine, unfortunately, little known about this therapy and exist few application as a treatment option for pets (Buchholz, Walt, 2013). Furthermore, there is currently still a limited number of clinics, hospitals and veterinary professionals performing specialized treatment in PDT.

The use of PDT in veterinary medicine is still the subject of considerable research in clinical application of various diseases. The use of effective photosensitizing agents and light sources would become this technique an important tool in the practice of veterinary medicine (Lucroy, 2002; Wardlaw et al., 2012; Buchholz, Walt, 2013; Sellera et al., 2014a). Some of the advantages of PDT compared with surgery, chemotherapy or radiationtherapy include reduction in long-term morbidity and the fact not compromise future treatment options for patients with residual or recurrent disease. The uniqueness interdisciplinary of PDT inspires experts in physics, chemistry, biology and medicine, and its development and new applications become limited only by the imagination of those enormous researchers (Agostinis et al., 2011).

The development on PDT research will be increasingly dependent on combinations of different fields, resulting in a sophisticated, modern and advanced treatment protocols. It is tempting to suppose that such therapies are so complex that they can only be modeled empirically and, thus, the physical role decline. As we explore our growing knowledge of photochemistry, biology and physiology of PDT for the development of new and better treatments, it becomes more important to understand and optimize the treatment parameters that properly direct control. In the future, as in the past, will be the understanding PDT physics will allow us to harness scientific knowledge and translate it into improved clinical treatments (Zhu, Finlay, 2008).

This chapter aimed to provide the reader a general knowledge of PDT in animals as a form of application (topical or local), types of photosensitizers and light sources, clinical indication with case reports, animal species already treated with PDT, completed and development studies in this area, and comparison the use of PDT between humans and animals.

ACKNOWLEDGMENT

The authors would like to sincerely thank Dr. Fabio Parra Sellera, University of São Paulo, for providing photographs to this chapter.

REFERENCES

Ackroyd R, Kelty C, Brown N, Reed M. The history of photodetection and photodynamic therapy. *Photochem Photobiol.* 2001 Nov;74(5):656-69.

Agostinis P, Berg K, Cengel KA, Foster TH, Girotti AW, Gollnick SO, et al. Photodynamic therapy of cancer: an update. *CA Cancer J Clin.* 2011 Jul-Aug;61(4):250-81.

Allen CM, Sharman WM, Van Lier JE. Current Status of phthalocyanines in the photodynamic therapy of cancer. *J Porphyrins Phthalocyan.* 2001;5:161-9.

Allison BA, Pritchard PH, Hsiang YN, et al. Low density lipoprotein as a delivery vehicle in various applications of photodynamic therapy. *Clin Invest Med.* 1993;16:B9.

Allison BA, Pritchard PH, Levy JG. Evidence for low-density lipoprotein receptor-mediated uptake of benzoporphyrin derivative. *Br J Cancer.* 1994 May;69(5):833-9.

Allison RR, Sibata CH. Oncologic photodynamic therapy photosensitizers: a clinical review. *Photodiagnosis Photodyn Ther.* 2010 Jun;7(2):61-75.

Andrejevic-Blant S, Hadjur C, Ballini JP, Wagnières G, Fontolliet C, van den Bergh H, et al. Photodynamic therapy of early squamous cell carcinoma with tetra(m-hydroxyphenyl)chlorin: optimal drug-light interval. *Br J Cancer.* 1997;76(8):1021-8.

Barnes LD, Giuliano EA, Ota J, Cohn LA, Moore CP. The effect of photodynamic therapy on squamous cell carcinoma in a murine model: evaluation of time between intralesional injection to laser irradiation. *Vet J.* 2009 Apr;180(1):60-5.

Barnes LD, Giuliano EA, Ota J. Cellular localization of Visudyne as a function of time after local injection in an in vivo model of squamous cell carcinoma: an investigation into tumor cell death. *Vet Ophthalmol.* 2010 May;13(3):158-65.

Bellnier DA, Henderson BW, Pandey RK, Potter WR, Dougherty TJ. Murine pharmacokinetics and antitumor efficacy of the photodynamic sensitizer 2-[1-hexyloxyethyl]-2-devinyl pyropheophorbide-a. *J Photochem Photobiol B.* 1993 Sep;20(1):55-61.

Bernstein EF, Thomas GF, Smith PD, Mitchell JB, Glatstein E, Kantor GR, et al. Response of black and white guinea pig skin to photodynamic treatment using 514-nm light and dihematoporphyrin ether. *Arch Dermatol.* 1990 Oct;126(10):1303-7.

Berryessa NA, Marks SL, Pesavento PA, Krasnansky T, Yoshimoto SK, Johnson EG, et al. Gastrointestinal pythiosis in 10 dogs from California. *J Vet Intern Med.* 2008 Jul-Aug;22(4):1065-9.

Bexfield NH, Stell AJ, Gear RN, Dobson JM. Photodynamic therapy of superficial nasal planum squamous cell carcinomas in cats: 55 cases. *J Vet Intern Med.* 2008 Nov-Dec;22(6):1385-9.

Bonsor SJ, Nichol R, Reid TM, Pearson GJ. An alternative regimen for root canal disinfection. *Br Dent J.* 2006 Jul 22;201(2):101-5.

Brancaleon L, Moseley H. Laser and non-laser light sources for photodynamic therapy. *Lasers Med Sci.* 2002;17(3):173-86.

Brown SB, Mellish KJ. Verteporfin: a milestone in opthalmology and photodynamic therapy. *Expert Opin Pharmacother.* 2001 Feb;2(2):351-61.

Buchholz J, Walt H. Veterinary photodynamic therapy: a review. *Photodiagnosis Photodyn Ther.* 2013 Dec;10(4):342-7.

Buchholz J, Wergin M, Walt H, Gräfe S, Bley CR, Kaser-Hotz B. Photodynamic therapy of feline cutaneous squamous cell carcinoma using a newly developed liposomal photosensitizer: preliminary results concerning drug safety and efficacy. *J Vet Intern Med.* 2007 Jul-Aug;21(4):770-5.

Burch S, London C, Seguin B, Rodriguez C, Wilson BC, Bisland SK. Treatment of canine osseous tumors with photodynamic therapy: a pilot study. *Clin Orthop Relat Res.* 2009 Apr;467(4):1028-34.

Calista D, Coccia L. Photodynamic therapy for the treatment of in situ squamous cell carcinoma of the left eyelid. *Int J Dermatol.* 2008 Dec;47(12):1319-21.

Campbell GA, Bartels KE, Arnold C, Healey T, Cowell RL, Lucroy MD, et al. Tissue levels, histologic changes and plasma pharmacokinetics of meta-Tetra (hydroxyphenyl) chlorin (mTHPC) in the cat. *Lasers Med Sci.* 2002;17(2):79-85.

Chen B, Pogue BW, Goodwin IA, O'Hara JA, Wilmot CM, Hutchins JE, et al. Blood flow dynamics after photodynamic therapy with verteporfin in the RIF-1 tumor. *Radiat Res.* 2003 Oct;160(4):452-9.

Chen B, Pogue BW, Hoopes PJ, Hasan T. Combining vascular and cellular targeting regimens enhances the efficacy of photodynamic therapy. *Int J Radiat Oncol Biol Phys.* 2005 Mar 15;61(4):1216-26.

Chen Q, Huang Z, Luck D, Beckers J, Brun PH, Wilson BC, et al. Preclinical studies in normal canine prostate of a novel palladium-bacteriopheophorbide (WST09) photosensitizer for photodynamic therapy of prostate cancers. *Photochem Photobiol.* 2002 Oct;76(4):438-45.

Cheng J, Liang H, Li Q, Peng C, Li Z, Shi S, et al. Hematoporphyrin monomethyl ether-mediated photodynamic effects on THP-1 cell-derived macrophages. *J Photochem Photobiol B.* 2010 Oct 5;101(1):9-15.

Chowdhary RK, Shariff I, Dolphin D. Drug release characteristics of lipid based benzoporphyrin derivative. *J Pharm Pharm Sci.* 2003 Jan-Apr;6(1):13-9.

Dai T, Huang YY, Hamblin MR. Photodynamic therapy for localized infections--state of the art. *Photodiagnosis Photodyn Ther.* 2009 Sep-Dec;6(3-4):170-88.

Daniell MD, Hill JS. A history of photodynamic therapy. *Aust N Z J Surg.* 1991 May;61(5):340-8.

De Vico G, Maiolino P, Restucci B, Passantino A. Spontaneous tumours of pet dog as models for human cancers: searching for adequate guidelines. *Riv Biol.* 2005 May-Aug;98(2):279-96.

Dougherty TJ, Gomer CJ, Henderson BW, Jori G, Kessel D, Korbelik M, et al. Photodynamic therapy. *J Natl Cancer Inst.* 1998 Jun 17;90(12):889-905.

Dougherty TJ. An update on photodynamic therapy applications. *J Clin Laser Med Surg.* 2002 Feb;20(1):3-7.

Dougherty TJ. Photodynamic therapy. *Photochem Photobiol.* 1993 Dec;58(6):895-900.

Durand RE, Aquino-Parsons C. Non-constant tumour blood flow--implications for therapy. *Acta Oncol.* 2001;40(7):862-9.

Dykstra MJ, Sharp NJ, Olivry T, Hillier A, Murphy KM, Kaufman L, et al. A description of cutaneous-subcutaneous pythiosis in fifteen dogs. *Med Mycol.* 1999 Dec;37(6):427-33.

Faustino MA, Neves MG, Cavaleiro JA, Neumann M, Brauer HD, Jori G. Meso-tetraphenylporphyrin dimer derivatives as potential photosensitizers in photodynamic therapy. Part 2. *Photochem Photobiol.* 2000 Aug;72(2):217-25.

Ferreira I, Rahal SC, Rocha NS, Gouveia AH, Corrêa TP, Carvalho YK, et al. Hematoporphyrin-based photodynamic therapy for cutaneous squamous cell carcinoma in cats. *Vet Dermatol.* 2009 Jun;20(3):174-8.

Fischer C, Lindley D, Carlton W, Van Hecke H. Tumors of the Cornea and Sclera. In: Peiffer R, Simmons K editors. *Ocular Tumors in Animals and Humans.* Ames IA, USA: Iowa State Press; 2002; 149-51.

Frauenfelder HC, Blevins WE, Page EH. 90Sr for treatment of periocular squamous cell carcinoma in the horse. *J Am Vet Med Assoc.* 1982 Feb 1;180(3):307-9.

Friedberg JS, Skema C, Baum ED, Burdick J, Vinogradov SA, Wilson DF, et al. In vitro effects of photodynamic therapy on *Aspergillus fumigatus*. *J Antimicrob Chemother.* 2001 Jul;48(1):105-7.

Garcia-Zuazaga J, Cooper KD, Baron ED. Photodynamic therapy in dermatology: current concepts in the treatment of skin cancer. *Expert Rev Anticancer Ther.* 2005 Oct;5(5):791-800.

Gelatt KN, Myers VS Jr, Perman V, Jessen C. Conjunctival squamous cell carcinoma in the horse. *J Am Vet Med Assoc.* 1974 Oct 1;165(7):617-20.

Gelatt KN. Corneolombal squamous cell carcinoma in a horse. *Vet Med Small Anim Clin.* 1975 Jan;70(1):53.

Giuliano EA, MacDonald I, McCaw DL, Dougherty TJ, Klauss G, Ota J, et al. Photodynamic therapy for the treatment of periocular squamous cell carcinoma in horses: a pilot study. *Vet Ophthalmol.* 2008 Sep;11 Suppl 1:27-34.

Giuliano EA, Ota J, Tucker SA. Photodynamic therapy: basic principles and potential uses for the veterinary ophthalmologist. *Vet Ophthalmol.* 2007 Nov-Dec;10(6):337-43.

Grier RL, Brewer WG Jr, Paul SR, Theilen GH. Treatment of bovine and equine ocular squamous cell carcinoma by radiofrequency hyperthermia. *J Am Vet Med Assoc.* 1980 Jul 1;177(1):55-61.

Grosjean P, Savary JF, Mizeret J, Wagnieres G, Woodtli A, Theumann JF, et al. Photodynamic therapy for cancer of the upper aerodigestive tract using tetra(m-hydroxyphenyl)chlorin. *J Clin Laser Med Surg.* 1996 Oct;14(5):281-7.

Hahn KA, Bravo L, Adams WH, Frazier DL. Naturally occurring tumors in dogs as comparative models for cancer therapy research. *In Vivo.* 1994 Jan-Feb;8(1):133-43.

Hamblin MR, Hasan T. Photodynamic therapy: a new antimicrobial approach to infectious disease? *Photochem Photobiol Sci.* 2004 May;3(5):436-50.

Henderson BW, Dougherty TJ. How does photodynamic therapy work? *Photochem Photobiol.* 1992 Jan;55(1):145-57.

Hendrix D. Equine ocular squamous cell carcinoma. *Clin Tech Equine Pract.* 2005 Mar;4(1):87-94.

Hilbert BJ, Farrell RK, Grant BD. Cryotherapy of periocular squamous cell carcinoma in the horse. *J Am Vet Med Assoc.* 1977 Jun 1;170(11):1305-8.

Houle JM, Strong A. Clinical pharmacokinetics of verteporfin. *J Clin Pharmacol.* 2002 May;42(5):547-57.

Jain A, Gupta Y, Agrawal R, Khare P, Jain SK. Biofilms--a microbial life perspective: a critical review. *Crit Rev Ther Drug Carrier Syst.* 2007;24(5):393-443.

Jori G, Magaraggia M, Fabris C, Soncin M, Camerin M, Tallandini L, et al. Photodynamic inactivation of microbial pathogens: disinfection of water and prevention of water-borne diseases. *J Environ Pathol Toxicol Oncol.* 2011;30(3):261-71.

Joyce JR. Cryosurgical treatment of tumors of horses and cattle. *J Am Vet Med Assoc.* 1976 Feb 1;168(3):226-9.

Kanai M, Obana A, Gohto Y, Nagata S, Miki T, Kaneda K, et al. Long-term effectiveness of photodynamic therapy by using a hydrophilic photosensitizer ATX-S10(Na) against experimental choroidal neovascularization in rats. *Lasers Surg Med.* 2000;26(1):48-57.

Kato IT, Prates RA, Sabino CP, Fuchs BB, Tegos GP, Mylonakis E, et al. Antimicrobial photodynamic inactivation inhibits Candida albicans virulence factors and reduces in vivo pathogenicity. *Antimicrob Agents Chemother.* 2013 Jan;57(1):445-51.

Keijzer M, Jacques SL, Prahl SA, Welch AJ. Light distributions in artery tissue: Monte Carlo simulations for finite-diameter laser beams. *Lasers Surg Med.* 1989;9(2):148-54.

Kelleher DK, Thews O, Rzeznik J, Scherz A, Salomon Y, Vaupel P. Water-filtered infrared-A radiation: a novel technique for localized hyperthermia in combination with bacteriochlorophyll-based photodynamic therapy. *Int J Hyperthermia.* 1999 Nov-Dec;15(6):467-74.

Kelleher DK, Thews O, Scherz A, Salomon Y, Vaupel P. Combined hyperthermia and chlorophyll-based photodynamic therapy: tumour growth and metabolic microenvironment. *Br J Cancer.* 2003 Dec 15;89(12):2333-9.

Kennedy JC, Pottier RH, Pross DC. Photodynamic therapy with endogenous protoporphyrin IX: basic principles and present clinical experience. *J Photochem Photobiol B.* 1990 Jun;6(1-2):143-8.

Klein MK, Roberts WG. Recent advances in photodynamic therapy. *Comp Cont Educ.* 1993; 15:809-17.

Klopfleisch R, Lenze D, Hummel M, Gruber AD. The metastatic cascade is reflected in the transcriptome of metastatic canine mammary carcinomas. *Vet J.* 2011 Nov;190(2):236-43.

Koch SA, Cowles RR Jr. Surgical removal of squamous cell carcinoma of the equine eye. *Vet Med Small Anim Clin.* 1971 Apr;66(4):327-9.

Konopka K, Goslinski T. Photodynamic therapy in dentistry. *J Dent Res.* 2007 Aug;86(8):694-707.

Kumaraguruparan R, Karunagaran D, Balachandran C, Manohar BM, Nagini S. Of humans and canines: a comparative evaluation of heat shock and apoptosis-associated proteins in mammary tumors. *Clin Chim Acta.* 2006 Mar;365(1-2):168-76.

Lavach JD, Severin GA. Neoplasia of the equine eye, adnexa, and orbit: a review of 68 cases. *J Am Vet Med Assoc.* 1977 Jan 15;170(2):202-3.

Leach MW, Peaston AE. Adverse drug reaction attributable to aluminum phthalocyanine tetrasulphonate administration in domestic cats. *Vet Pathol.* 1994 Mar;31(2):283-7.

Leach MW. A survey of neoplasia in pet birds. *Semin Avian Exotic Pet.* 1992;1:52-64.

Lewis K. Multidrug tolerance of biofilms and persister cells. *Curr Top Microbiol Immunol.* 2008;322:107-31.

Li HT, Song XY, Yang C, Li Q, Tang D, Tian WR, et al. Effect of hematoporphyrin monomethyl ether-mediated PDT on the mitochondria of canine breast cancer cells. *Photodiagnosis Photodyn Ther.* 2013 Dec;10(4):414-21.

Lim EJ, Oak CH, Heo J, Kim YH. Methylene blue-mediated photodynamic therapy enhances apoptosis in lung cancer cells. *Oncol Rep.* 2013 Aug;30(2):856-62.

Liu Y, Ma XQ, Jin P, Li HT, Zhang RR, Ren XL, et al. Apoptosis induced by hematoporphyrin monomethyl ether combined with He-Ne laser irradiation in vitro on canine breast cancer cells. *Vet J.* 2011 Jun;188(3):325-30.

Liu-Chittenden Y, Huang B, Shim JS, Chen Q, Lee SJ, Anders RA, et al. Genetic and pharmacological disruption of the TEAD-YAP complex suppresses the oncogenic activity of YAP. *Genes Dev.* 2012 Jun 15;26(12):1300-5.

Lofgren LA, Ronn AM, Abramson AL, Shikowitz MJ, Nouri M, Lee CJ, et al. Photodynamic therapy using m-tetra(hydroxyphenyl) chlorin. An animal model. *Arch Otolaryngol Head Neck Surg.* 1994 Dec;120(12):1355-62.

Lucroy MD, Edwards BF, Madewell BR. Veterinary photodynamic therapy. *J Am Vet Med Assoc.* 2000 Jun 1;216(11):1745-51.

Lucroy MD, Edwards BF, Peavy GM, Krasieva TB, Griffey SM, Stiles JB. et al. Preclinical study in cats of the pro-photosensitizer 5-aminolevulinic acid. *Am J Vet Res.* 1999 Nov;60(11):1364-70.

Lucroy MD, Magne ML, Peavy GM, Madewell BR, Edwards BF. Photodynamic therapy in veterinary medicine: current status and implications for applications in human disease. *J Clin Laser Med Surg.* 1996 Oct;14(5):305-10.

Lucroy MD, Ridgway TD, Peavy GM, Krasieva TB, Higbee RG, Campbell GA, et al. Preclinical evaluation of 5-aminolevulinic acid-based photodynamic therapy for canine transitional cell carcinoma. *Vet Comp Oncol.* 2003 Jun;1(2):76-85.

Lucroy MD. Miscellaneous treatments for solid tumors: Photodynamic therapy. In: Withrow S, Vail D, editors. *Small Animal Clinical Oncology.* Philadelphia: WB Saunders; 2007; 283-90.

Lucroy MD. Photodynamic therapy for companion animals with cancer. *Vet Clin North Am Small Anim Pract.* 2002 May;32(3):693-702.

Lucroy MD. Photodynamic Therapy: Potential Applications for Exotic Animal Oncology. Topics in Medicine and Surgery. *Semin Avian Exotic Pet.* 2005 Jul;14(3):205-11.

Lui H, Hobbs L, Tope WD, Lee PK, Elmets C, Provost N, et al. Photodynamic therapy of multiple nonmelanoma skin cancers with verteporfin and red light-emitting diodes: two-year results evaluating tumor response and cosmetic outcomes. *Arch Dermatol.* 2004 Jan;140(1):26-32.

MacDonald IJ, Dougherty TJ. Basic principles of photodynamic therapy. *J Porphyr Phthalocya.* 2001;5(2):105-29.

MacEwen EG. Spontaneous tumors in dogs and cats: models for the study of cancer biology and treatment. *Cancer Metastasis Rev.* 1990 Sep;9(2):125-36.

Magne ML, Rodriguez CO, Autry SA, Edwards BF, Theon AP, Madewell BR. Photodynamic therapy of facial squamous cell carcinoma in cats using a new photosensitizer. *Lasers Surg Med. 1997*;20(2):202-9.

Marcus J, Glassberg E, Dimino-Emme L, Yamamoto R, Moy RL, Vari SG, et al. Photodynamic therapy for the treatment of squamous cell carcinoma using benzoporphyrin derivative. *J Dermatol Surg Oncol.* 1994 Jun;20(6):375-82.

Marcus SL, Sobel RS, Golub AL, Carroll RL, Lundahl S, Shulman DG. Photodynamic therapy (PDT) and photodiagnosis (PD) using endogenous photosensitization induced by 5-aminolevulinic acid (ALA): current clinical and development status. *J Clin Laser Med Surg.* 1996 Apr;14(2):59-66.

Mendoza L, Mandy W, Glass R. An improved Pythium insidiosum-vaccine formulation with enhanced immunotherapeutic properties in horses and dogs with pythiosis. *Vaccine.* 2003 Jun 20;21(21-22):2797-804.

Mendoza L, Newton JC. Immunology and immunotherapy of the infections caused by Pythium insidiosum. *Med Mycol.* 2005 Sep;43(6):477-86.

Messmer KJ, Abel SR. Verteporfin for age-related macular degeneration. *Ann Pharmacother.* 2001 Dec;35(12):1593-8.

Mohr H, Lambrecht B, Selz A. Photodynamic virus inactivation of blood components. *Immunol Invest.* 1995 Jan-Feb;24(1-2):73-85.

Moore AS, Ogilvie GK. Skin tumors. In: Ogilvie GK, Moore AS editors. *Feline Oncology.* Trenton, NJ: Veterinary Learning Systems; 2001; 398-428.

Morton C, Horn M, Leman J, Tack B, Bedane C, Tjioe M, et al. Comparison of topical methyl aminolevulinate photodynamic therapy with cryotherapy or Fluorouracil for treatment of squamous cell carcinoma in situ: Results of a multicenter randomized trial. *Arch Dermatol.* 2006 Jun;142(6):729-35.

Nagata JY, Hioka N, Kimura E, Batistela VR, Terada RS, Graciano AX, et al. Antibacterial photodynamic therapy for dental caries: evaluation of the photosensitizers used and light source properties. *Photodiagnosis Photodyn Ther.* 2012 Jun;9(2):122-31.

O'Riordan K, Akilov OE, Hasan T. The potential for photodynamic therapy in the treatment of localized infections. *Photodiagnosis Photodyn Ther.* 2005 Dec;2(4):247-62.

Osaki T, Hoshino S, Hoshino Y, Takagi S, Okumura M, Kadosawa T, et al. Clinical pharmacokinetics of anti-angiogenic photodynamic therapy with benzoporphyrin derivative monoacid ring-A in dogs having naturally occurring neoplasms. *J Vet Med A Physiol Pathol Clin Med.* 2006 Mar;53(2):108-12.

Osaki T, Takagi S, Hoshino Y, Aoki Y, Sunden Y, Ochiai K, et al. Temporary regression of locally invasive polypoid rhinosinusitis in a dog after photodynamic therapy. *Aust Vet J.* 2012 Nov;90(11):442-7.

Osaki T, Takagi S, Hoshino Y, Okumura M, Kadosawa T, Fujinaga T. Efficacy of antivascular photodynamic therapy using benzoporphyrin derivative monoacid ring A (BPD-MA) in 14 dogs with oral and nasal tumors. *J Vet Med Sci.* 2009 Feb;71(2):125-32.

Panjehpour M, DeNovo RC, Petersen MG, Overholt BF, Bower R, Rubinchik V, et al. Photodynamic therapy using Verteporfin (benzoporphyrin derivative monoacid ring A, BPD-MA) and 630 nm laser light in canine esophagus. *Lasers Surg Med.* 2002;30(1):26-30.

Peaston AE, Leach MW, Higgins RJ. Photodynamic therapy for nasal and aural squamous cell carcinoma in cats. *J Am Vet Med Assoc.* 1993 Apr 15;202(8):1261-5.

Pereira-Gonzales F, Maisch T. Photodynamic inactivation for controlling *Candida albicans* infections. *Fungal Biol.* 2012 Jan;116(1):1-10.

Pérez RC, Luis-León JJ, Vivas JL, Mendoza L. Epizootic cutaneous pythiosis in beef calves. *Vet Microbiol.* 2005 Aug 10;109(1-2):121-8.

Pesavento PA, Barr B, Riggs SM, Eigenheer AL, Pamma R, Walker RL. Cutaneous pythiosis in a nestling white-faced ibis. *Vet Pathol.* 2008 Jul;45(4):538-41.

Pinho SS, Carvalho S, Cabral J, Reis CA, Gärtner F. Canine tumors: a spontaneous animal model of human carcinogenesis. *Transl Res.* 2012 Mar;159(3):165-72.

Pires L, Bosco Sde M, da Silva NF Jr, Kurachi C. Photodynamic therapy for pythiosis. *Vet Dermatol.* 2013 Feb;24(1):130-6.e30.

Pogue BW, Chen B, Zhou X, Hoopes PJ. Analysis of sampling volume and tissue heterogeneity on the in vivo detection of fluorescence. *J Biomed Opt.* 2005 Jul-Aug;10(4):41206.

Porrello A, Cardelli P, Spugnini EP. Oncology of companion animals as a model for humans. an overview of tumor histotypes. *J Exp Clin Cancer Res.* 2006 Mar;25(1):97-105.

Puizina-Ivić N, Zorc H, Vanjaka-Rogosić L, Mirić L, Persin A. Fractionated illumination improves the outcome in the treatment of precancerous lesions with photodynamic therapy. *Coll Antropol.* 2008 Oct;32 Suppl 2:67-73.

Pupaibool J, Chindamporn A, Patrakul K, Suankratay C, Sindhuphak W, Kulwichit W. Human pythiosis. *Emerg Infect Dis.* 2006 Mar;12(3):517-8.

Rakich PM, Grooters AM, Tang KN. Gastrointestinal pythiosis in two cats. *J Vet Diagn Invest.* 2005 May;17(3):262-9.

Reeds KB, Ridgway TD, Higbee RG, Lucroy MD. Non-coherent light for photodynamic therapy of superficial tumours in animals. *Vet Comp Oncol.* 2004 Sep;2(3):157-63.

Ridgway TD, Lucroy MD. Phototoxic effects of 635-nm light on canine transitional cell carcinoma cells incubated with 5-aminolevulinic acid. *Am J Vet Res.* 2003 Feb;64(2):131-6.

Roberts WG, Klein MK, Loomis M, Weldy S, Berns MW. Photodynamic therapy of spontaneous cancers in felines, canines, and snakes with chloro-aluminum sulfonated phthalocyanine. *J Natl Cancer Inst.* 1991 Jan 2;83(1):18-23.

Romanova NA, Brovko LY, Moore L, Pometun E, Savitsky AP, Ugarova NN, et al. Assessment of photodynamic destruction of *Escherichia coli* O157:H7 and Listeria monocytogenes by using ATP bioluminescence. *Appl Environ Microbiol.* 2003 Nov;69(11):6393-8.

Ronn AM, Batti J, Lee CJ, Yoo D, Siegel ME, Nouri M, et al. Comparative biodistribution of meta-Tetra(Hydroxyphenyl) chlorin in multiple species: clinical implications for photodynamic therapy. *Lasers Surg Med.* 1997;20(4):437-42.

Rosenkranz AA, Jans DA, Sobolev AS. Targeted intracellular delivery of photosensitizers to enhance photodynamic efficiency. *Immunol Cell Biol.* 2000 Aug;78(4):452-64.

Rossi R, Assad GB, Buggiani G, Lotti T. Photodynamic therapy: treatment of choice for actinic cheilitis? *Dermatol Ther.* 2008 Sep-Oct;21(5):412-5.

Rousset N, Vonarx V, Eléouet S, Carré J, Bourré L, Lajat Y, et al. Cellular distribution and phototoxicity of benzoporphyrin derivative and Photofrin. *Res Exp Med (Berl).* 2000 Jun;199(6):341-57.

Rowe EA, Mathews KG, Linder KE, Tate LP. The effect of photodynamic therapy on cisterna chyli patency in rats. *Vet Surg.* 2014 Aug;43(6):642-9.

Ruslander D, Kaser-Hotz B, Sardinas JC. Cutaneous squamous cell carcinoma in cats. *Comp Cont Educ Pract.* 1997;19:1119–29.

Sallis ES, Pereira DI, Raffi MB. [Cutaneous pythiosis in horses: 14 cases]. *Cienc. Rural.* 2003;33: 899-903. [Portuguese]

Santurio JM, Leal AT, Leal AB, Festugatto R, Lubeck I, Sallis ES, et al. Three types of immunotherapics against pythiosis insidiosi developed and evaluated. *Vaccine.* 2003 Jun 2;21(19-20):2535-40.

Santurio JM, Monteiro AB, Leal AT, Kommers GD, de Sousa RS, Catto JB. Cutaneous Pythiosis insidiosi in calves from the Pantanal region of Brazil. *Mycopathologia.* 1998;141(3):123-5.

Savary JF, Grosjean P, Monnier P, Fontolliet C, Wagnieres G, Braichotte D, et al. Photodynamic therapy of early squamous cell carcinomas of the esophagus: a review of 31 cases. *Endoscopy.* 1998 Mar;30(3):258-65.

Scherz A, Feodor L, Salomon Y. US Patent No.#5,650,292, 1997.

Scherz A, Salomon Y, Scheer H and Brandis A. USPatent No. #6,569,846, 2003.

Sellera FP, Gargano RG, Azedo MR, Benesi FJ, Lopes LA, Pogliani FC. Antimicrobial photodynamic therapy as an adjuvant treatment of toe ulcer in cattle. *Eur Int J Sci Technol.* 2013b Dec;2(10):98-104.

Sellera FP, Gargano RG, Pogliani FC. [Photodynamic therapy: a review]. *Journal of Continuing Education in Animal Science of CRMV-SP.* 2014b;12(1):6-13. [Portuguese]

Sellera FP, Nascimento CL, Azedo MR, Pogliani FC, Sellera DP, Aranha AC. Photodynamic therapy in the treatment of canine oral papillomatosis. *Int J Sci Comm Hum.* 2013a Dec;1(8):23-7.

Sellera FP, Sabino CP, Ribeiro MS, Fernandes LT, Pogliani FC, Teixeira CR, et al. Photodynamic therapy for pododermatitis in penguins. *Zoo Biol.* 2014a Jul-Aug;33(4):353-6.

Smijs TG, Schuitmaker HJ. Photodynamic inactivation of the dermatophyte *Trichophyton rubrum.* Photochem Photobiol. 2003 May;77(5):556-60.

Soukos NS, Goodson JM. Photodynamic therapy in the control of oral biofilms. *Periodontol 2000.* 2011 Feb;55(1):143-66.

Soukos NS, Wilson M, Burns T, Speight PM. Photodynamic effects of toluidine blue on human oral keratinocytes and fibroblasts and Streptococcus sanguis evaluated in vitro. *Lasers Surg Med.* 1996;18(3):253-9.

Suedmeyer WK, McCaw DL, Turnquist S. Attempted photodynamic therapy of squamous cell carcinoma in the casque of a Great Hornbill (*Buceros bicornis*). *J Avian Med Surg.* 2001;15:44-49.

Svaasand LO, Wyss P, Wyss MT, Tadir Y, Tromberg BJ, Berns MW. Dosimetry model for photodynamic therapy with topically administered photosensitizers. *Lasers Surg Med.* 1996;18(2):139-49.

Tanaka M, Mroz P, Dai T, Huang L, Morimoto Y, Kinoshita M, et al. Photodynamic therapy can induce a protective innate immune response against murine bacterial arthritis via neutrophil accumulation. *PLoS One.* 2012;7(6):e39823.

Théon AP, Pascoe JR, Carlson GP, Krag DN. Intratumoral chemotherapy with cisplatin in oily emulsion in horses. *J Am Vet Med Assoc.* 1993 Jan 15;202(2):261-7.

Thomas RC, Fox LE. Tumors of the skin and subcutis. In: Morrison WB, editor. *Cancer in Dogs and Cats: Medical and Surgical Management.* Jackson,WY: Teton NewMedia; 2002; 469-88.

Tierney E, Barker A, Ahdout J, Hanke CW, Moy RL, Kouba DJ. Photodynamic therapy for the treatment of cutaneous neoplasia, inflammatory disorders, and photoaging. *Dermatol Surg.* 2009 May;35(5):725-46.

Triesscheijn M, Baas P, Schellens JH, Stewart FA. Photodynamic therapy in oncology. *Oncologist.* 2006 Oct;11(9):1034-44.

Videla R, van Amstel S, O'neill SH, Frank LA, Newman SJ, Vilela R, et al. Vulvar pythiosis in two captive camels (*Camelus dromedarius*). *Med Mycol.* 2012 Feb;50(2):219-24.

Vilensky J, Koudinova NV, Harmelin A, Scherz A, Salomon Y. Vascular-targeted photodynamic therapy (VTP) of a canine-transmissible venereal tumour in a murine model with Pd-bacteriopheophorbide (WST09). *Vet Comp Oncol.* 2005 Dec;3(4):182-93.

Vrouenraets MB, Visser GW, Loup C, Meunier B, Stigter M, Oppelaar H, et al. Targeting of a hydrophilic photosensitizer by use of internalizing monoclonal antibodies: A new possibility for use in photodynamic therapy. *Int J Cancer.* 2000 Oct 1;88(1):108-14.

Vrouenraets MB, Visser GW, Snow GB, van Dongen GA. Basic principles, applications in oncology and improved selectivity of photodynamic therapy. *Anticancer Res.* 2003 Jan-Feb;23(1B):505-22.

Wainwright M, Crossley KB. Photosensitizing agents circumventing resistance and breaking down biofilms: a review. *Int Biodeterior Biodegrad.* 2004;53(2):119-26.

Wainwright M. Photoinactivation of viruses. *Photochem Photobiol Sci.* 2004 May;3(5):406-11.

Wang XL, Wang HW, Guo MX, Xu SZ. Treatment of skin cancer and pre-cancer using topical ALA-PDT--a single hospital experience. *Photodiagnosis Photodyn Ther.* 2008 Jun;5(2):127-33.

Wardlaw JL, Sullivan TJ, Lux CN, Austin FW. Photodynamic therapy against common bacteria causing wound and skin infections. *Vet J.* 2012 Jun;192(3):374-7.

Whitacre CM, Feyes DK, Satoh T, Grossmann J, Mulvihill JW, Mukhtar H, et al. Photodynamic therapy with the phthalocyanine photosensitizer Pc 4 of SW480 human colon cancer xenografts in athymic mice. *Clin Cancer Res.* 2000 May;6(5):2021-7.

Wolfsen HC, Ng CS. Cutaneous consequences of photodynamic therapy. *Cutis.* 2002 Feb;69(2):140-2.

Wong TW, Wang YY, Sheu HM, Chuang YC. Bactericidal effects of toluidine blue-mediated photodynamic action on *Vibrio vulnificus*. *Antimicrob Agents Chemother.* 2005 Mar;49(3):895-902.

Wood TK. Insights on *Escherichia coli* biofilm formation and inhibition from whole-transcriptome profiling. *Environ Microbiol.* 2009 Jan;11(1):1-15.

Zeina B, Greenman J, Purcell WM, Das B. Killing of cutaneous microbial species by photodynamic therapy. *Br J Dermatol.* 2001 Feb;144(2):274-8.

Zelickson BD. Mechanism of action of topical aminolevulinic acid. In: Goldman MP, editor. *Photodynamic therapy.* Philadelphia: Elsevier Saunders; 2005; 1-12.

Zellweger M, Grosjean P, Monnier P, van den Bergh H, Wagnières G. Stability of the fluorescence measurement of Foscan in the normal human oral cavity as an indicator of its content in early cancers of the esophagus and the bronchi. *Photochem Photobiol.* 1999 May;69(5):605-10.

Zhou X, Chen B, Hoopes PJ, Hasan T, Pogue BW. Tumor vascular area correlates with photosensitizer uptake: analysis of verteporfin microvascular delivery in the Dunning rat prostate tumor. *Photochem Photobiol.* 2006 Sep-Oct;82(5):1348-57.

Zhu TC, Finlay JC. The role of photodynamic therapy (PDT) physics. *Med Phys.* 2008 Jul;35(7):3127-36.

Zilberstein J, Schreiber S, Bloemers MC, Bendel P, Neeman M, Schechtman E, et al. Antivascular treatment of solid melanoma tumors with bacteriochlorophyll-serine-based photodynamic therapy. *Photochem Photobiol.* 2001 Mar;73(3):257-66.

In: Photodynamic Therapy
Editor: Adrian G. Hugo

ISBN: 978-1-63463-857-9
© 2015 Nova Science Publishers, Inc.

Chapter 6

THE USE OF PHOTOSENSITIZERS IN PHOTODYNAMIC THERAPY

Michelle Peneluppi Silva and Antonio Olavo Cardoso Jorge*

Department of Biosciences and Oral Diagnosis, Institute of Science and Technology,
UNESP – Univ Estadual Paulista, São José dos Campos, SP, Brazil

ABSTRACT

Number of studies and advances in health has been made in the discovery of new photosensitizers (PS) proposed as potentially useful in photodynamic therapy (PDT) for the treatment of various diseases. Photodynamic therapy has been known and applied for over a hundred years, and it is used in the treatment of malignant and nonmalignant diseases, through the interaction of three factors: photosensitizer, light source and oxygen. These factors act intrinsically, so photodynamic effect not occurring separately. The photosensitizer administered to the patient, topically or systemically, plays a key role in the development of PDT. The photosensitizer agent is responsible for capturing light and its transformation into energy, resulting in factors capable of destroying the target, it's cannot exert toxicity beyond the affected area. Thus, researches are presented in constant development to find the photosensitizer as close to optimal. In this chapter, the reader will have access to information concerning the photosensitizer in PDT.

INTRODUCTION

Photodynamic therapy was discovered over 100 years ago by observing the killing of microorganisms when harmless dyes and visible light were combined in vitro. Since then it has primarily been developed as a treatment for cancer, ophthalmologic disorders and in dermatology (Dai et al., 2009). However, in recent years interest the effects of PDT has revived and it has been proposed as a therapy for a large variety of diseases.

---

* M.P. Silva (corresponding author): michellepeneluppi@gmail.com.

There has been progress made in the last 2 decades in new technologies and in understanding of the basic biophysical mechanisms of PDT, inherently a dynamic process. The most important question to be answered is: "What determines PDT efficacy for a particular patient, photosensitizer, and treatment protocol?" Answering this question will require a unified understanding of the interactions of the three basic components: light, photosensitizer, and tissue oxygenation (Zhu, Finlay, 2008).

Photosensitizers are compounds able to absorb light of a specific wavelength and turn it into useful energy (Sharman et al., 1999). The distribution of light is determined by the characteristics of the light source and optical properties of the tissue. These are influenced by the concentration of photosensitizer and blood oxygenation. The oxygen distribution is modified by the photodynamic process, through its consumption. Finally, the distribution of the photosensitizer can change as a result of photobleaching and photodynamic destruction of the agent itself. For these interactions, a dynamic model of photodynamic process is required (Zhu, Finlay, 2008).

HISTORY OF THE PHOTOSENSITIZER

Substances with photosensitizing properties in combination with sunlight were used for decades to treat some diseases without knowing exactly the basic principles of action and properties.

Reports of photodynamic therapy were dated from the time of egyptian civilization through the ingestion of plants containing psoralens, furo [3,2-g] -coumarin or 6-hydroxy-5-benzofuran-acrylic acid δ-lactone, and sunlight for treatment of diseases such as vitiligo (Simplício et al., 2002) and psoriasis. In 1900s, Oscar Raab, Ludwig-Maximillian University, Munich, described the lethal action of the acridine dye and light on paramecium, unicellular organism causes malaria (Sternberg et al., 1998; Kübler et al., 2001; Pervaiz, 2001; Malik et al., 2010).

The german physician Friedrich Meyer-Betz has pioneered the development of studies on Photo Radiation Therapy with porphyrin, in 1913s, and observed the effects of PRT-hematoporphyrin on your skin by injection of 200 mg of hematoporphyrin. None of effect was observed, but when exposing to the light, local photosensitivity appeared for a few months (Simplício et al., 2002).

PHOTOSENSITIZER

Several photosensitizing drugs have been developed over the years, most of which were introduced between 1980s and 1990s. Photosensitizer can be classified in various ways, all with limitations, such as generation, targeting (Allison, Sibata, 2010), synthetic Purity, chemical structure (Moser, 1997; Huang, 2005; Allison, Sibata, 2010). In general, they can be divided into non-porphyrins and porphyrin. Porphyrin-based photosensitizer are often classified into first, second and third generation (Moser, 1997; Huang, 2005).

Porphyrins and photosensitizing developed in the 1970s and early 1980s are called first generation photosensitizers, Photofrin. Porphyrin derivatives or synthetic in the late 1980s are second-generation photosensitizers, such as ALA. The third generation, generally, refers to changes, such as biological conjugates of antibody, liposome and built-in photo quenching or bleaching capability (Moser, 1997; Huang, 2005).

In 1841s, the agent hematoporphyrin first generation was isolated from hemoglobin during research on the nature of the blood (Calzavara-Pinton et al., 2007; O'Connor et al., 2009). Unfortunately, this first photosensitizer demonstrated several limitations that resulted in the investigation of new agents, second-generation photosensitizers with better properties and lower toxic side effects (O'Connor et al., 2009).

Second generation photosensitizers, chemically synthesized as pure compounds of constant composition, show higher absorption in the range of 650 to 800 nm, with an optimum penetration of tissue and have higher extinction coefficients of absorption in the red than first generation compounds (Chen et al., 2005). The accumulation in the tissue is lower and thus the treatment can be performed on the same day as the administration of the drug. In addition, the second-generation photosensitizers have lower toxicity, but most of these agents still remains very hydrophobic and demonstrate poor selectivity for the tumor (Josefsen, Boyle, 2008).

Currently, extensive research on third generation photosensitizers are in development and new drugs are characterized by conjugation to carriers molecules or stages of converting the pro-drug which specifically direct the photosensitizer to the target cells, resulting in minimal accumulation in healthy tissues (Josefsen, Boyle, 2008).

Photosensitizers can make the skin vulnerable to ultraviolet light exposure, causing symptoms such as erythema, itching, scaling, rashes or inflammation. These substances combined with ultraviolet light also may contribute to other health problems, including skin cancer, photoaging and allergic reactions. Thus, photosensitizers can be further divided into the following groups: photodynamic agents, photosensitizing agents, substance-induced photosensitivity and photosensitivity management (Jain et al., 2011).

The photodynamic agents are naturally occurring or pigments and synthetic dyes that require oxygen to act, as erythrosine, rhodamin, hypericine, rose bengal, anthracene, acridine dye, methylene blue, quinine, buckwheat and porphyrin. In the case of photosensitizing agents, no need oxygen for reaction. These are represented by furanocoumarins and its derivatives psoralen, xanthotoxin, bergapten, imperatorin and isobergapten (Jain et al., 2011; Sen et al., 1992). The rash caused by drugs is one of the most common types of adverse reactions to drug treatment (Breathnach, Hintner, 1992; Wolkenstein, Revuz, 1995; Crowson et al., 2003; Jain et al., 2011). Any drug may induce skin reactions and certain classes of drugs such as non-steroidal anti-inflammatory, antibiotics and antiepileptics at rates from 1 to 5% of incidence (Bigby, 2001; Jain et al., 2011). Photosensitivity management corresponds to prevent photosensitivity reactions, mainly by guiding the patient to minimal sun exposure (Moore, 2002; Jain et al., 2011).

The chemical natures of photosensitizers, including size, charge, amphiphilicity, and partition coefficients, are important parameters that influence the subcellular localization. Furthermore, it was shown that the subcellular localization of photosensitizers determined the therapeutic efficacy in the PDT (Fabris et al., 2001; Yow et al., 2000; Rosenkranz et al., 2000; Kim et al., 2014). Thus, the subcellular location of photosensitizers delivered to the cells during the irradiation period becomes an important variable and can lead to enhancement of therapeutic outcome in the PDT. However, most of photosensitizers are insoluble or easily aggregated in physiological conditions due to their hydrophobicity, restricting the selective delivery to target cells and subsequent subcellular compartments (Kim et al., 2014).

Photophysics and Photochemistry

Most of photosensitizers in PDT have a structure heterocyclic ring similar of chlorophyll or heme in hemoglobin. After the light energy captured by the photosensitizer, chemical reactions of transfer and translation of light energy occur in the presence of molecular oxygen producing singlet oxygen and superoxide and inducing cellular damage through direct and indirect cytotoxicity. Therefore, the photosensitizer is considered critical element in PDT (Huang, 2005; Moser, 1997).

The activated photosensitizer leads to type II photo-oxidative reactions, in which it reacts directly with oxygen to form the very toxic singlet oxygen that damages lipids, proteins and/or nucleic acids (Moan, Berg, 1991; Heukers et al., 2014). Type I reactions can also occur, in which reactive oxygen species are formed via intermediate reaction of photosensitizer with substrates other than oxygen. As these transient oxygen species are short-lived molecules and have very short diffusion distances (O'Connor et al., 2009; Heukers et al., 2014), their toxicity is confined to the photosensitizer localization upon light application. Subsequently, cells die through necrosis and/or apoptosis and tumor destruction occurs through microvasculature damage and involvement of both immune and inflammatory systems (Dougherty et al., 1998; Heukers et al., 2014).

In general, most photosensitizers in their ground singlet state have two electrons with opposite spins located in an energetically most favorable molecular orbital. Absorption of light leads to a transfer of one electron to a higher energy orbital. This excited photosensitizer is very unstable and emits this excess energy as fluorescence and/or heat. Alternatively, an excited photosensitizer may undergo an intersystem crossing to form a more stable triplet state with inverted spin of one electron. The photosensitizer in triplet state can either decay radiationlessly to the ground state or transfer its energy to molecular oxygen (O_2), which is unique in being a triplet in its ground state. This step leads to the formation of $^1O_2$, and the reaction is referred to as a Type II process (Agostinis et al., 2011).

A Type I process can also occur whereby the photosensitizer reacts directly with an organic molecule in a cellular microenvironment, acquiring a hydrogen atom or electron to form a radical. Subsequent autoxidation of the reduced photosensitizer produces a superoxide anion radical. Dismutation or one electron reduction of O_2 gives hydrogen peroxide, which in turn can undergo one electron reduction to a powerful and virtually indiscriminate oxidant hydroxyl radical. Reactive oxygen species (ROS) generation via Type II chemistry is mechanistically much simpler than via Type I, and most photosensitizers are believed to operate via a Type II rather than Type I mechanism (Agostinis et al.,2011).

Properties of Photosensitizer

There are hundreds of substances, such as natural and synthetic dyes, that can act as photosensitizers in PDT, ranging from plant abstracts to complex synthetic macrocyclesque (Sharman et al., 1999).

The photosensitizer to be considered ideal must present numerous properties, including:

- Be chemically pure and of known and constant composition (Sharman et al., 1999; Allison, Sibata, 2010; Agostinis et al., 2011; Paszko et al., 2011; Jiang et al., 2014);
- Allow analysis of quality control with low production costs (Allison, Sibata, 2010; Agostinis et al., 2011);
- Provide good storage stability (Allison, Sibata, 2010; Agostinis et al., 2011; Jiang et al., 2014);
- High absorption peak between 600 and 800 nm, because the absorption of photons with wavelengths greater than 800 nm does not provide enough energy to excite oxygen in singlet state and generate reactive oxygen species, ROS (Sharman et al., 1999; Allison, Sibata, 2010; Agostinis et al., 2011; Paszko et al., 2011), with minimal absorption between 400 and 600 nm (Jiang et al., 2014);
- Solubility in water (Paszko et al., 2011);
- Selective for target cell or tissue (Sharman et al., 1999; Paszko et al., 2011);
- Safe, without causing side effects such as mutagenic changes, carcinogenic or allergic reactions (Paszko et al., 2011);
- Must not be toxic at therapeutic doses (Paszko et al., 2011);
- Have a minimal dark toxicity and only be cytotoxic in the presence of light (Sharman et al., 1999);
- Not damage the normal and healthy cells (Paszko et al., 2011);
- Provide rapid metabolism and excretion after the administration to minimize systemic toxicity and photosensitivity (Sharman et al., 1999; Paszko et al., 2011);
- Must be low cost (Paszko et al., 2011);
- Easy to synthesize (Paszko et al., 2011);
- Commercially available (Paszko et al., 2011).

To improve the selectivity of PDT, photosensitizers should be delivered by a drug-delivery system (DDS). A DDS is a technology designed to optimize drug therapy by controlling drug disposition and selectively transporting the drug to a target sit eat a preferred density or time. An ideal DDS also effectively reduces the side effects and improves the safety of a given drug (Yamauchi et al., 2014).

Various photosensitizers have been clinically approved for use in PDT of malignant and non-malignant diseases treatments. Currently, each photosensitizing commercially available has specific characteristics, but none is ideal agent. Most photosensitizers are hydrophobic and can easily aggregate in aqueous medium, affecting photophysical, chemical and biological properties (Paszko et al., 2011).

Types of Photosensitizers

Below are some types of photosensitizers, their properties and applications:

Benzoporphyrin Derivative

Verteporfin, benzoporphyrin derivative, belongs to the porphyrin family, which contains aromatic heterocyclic cyclic molecules composed of four modified pyrrole units which are interconnected at their carbon atoms via methine bridges (Liu-Chittenden et al., 2012) has been developed for the treatment of macular degeneration (Brown, Mellish, 2001; Messmer, Abel, 2001). Although not indicated for cancer, this drug is one of the most useful ophthalmology drugs ever developed and thus might have lessons for the development of PDT drugs for cancer. Verteporfin is cleared rapidly and does not induce a generalised skin photosensitivity that lasts longer than 24 h. In 2000s, it was approved in the US under the commercial name Visudyne® for treatment of choroidal neovascularization by acting preferentially target neovascularization (Brown et al., 2004).

Photodynamic therapy using verteporfin is a clinically approved, minimally invasive therapeutic procedure that involves administration of a photosensitizing agent followed by irradiation at a wavelength of 693 nm corresponding to an absorbance band of the sensitizer (Agostinis et al., 2011; Brodowska et al., 2014). In wet age related macular degeneration, liposomal Verteporfin accumulates in abnormal blood vessels, where it is activated by nonthermal laser at 693 nm generating reactive oxygen radicals. This results in local damage to the endothelium as well as blockage, and potential elimination of the vessels. It has been clinically used worldwide resulting in vision preservation in many patients (Brodowska et al., 2014).

Verteporfin has also been tested but not yet approved as a light based therapeutic modality for several human cancers (Pogue et al., 2003; Harbour, 2004; Isola et al., 2006; Celli et al., 2011; Tripursky et al., 2011; Tamella et al., 2011; Brodowska et al., 2014). In human cancers, PDT with visudyne® may act not only at the cancer vasculature but also directly on the cancer cells and act as an inducer of apoptosis or autophagy (Kessel et al., 2006; Brodowska et al., 2014).

5,10,15,20-Tetrakis(3-Hydroxyphenyl)Chlorin

5,10,15,20-Tetrakis(3-hydroxyphenyl)chlorine, Foscan®, Temoporfin, is a second-generation photosensitizer that accumulates at high levels in tumors and that has excellent photocytotoxicity (Yano et al., 2011). It is a very active photosensitizer and thus requires a much lower dose of both the drug and light than does porfimer sodium (Sharman et al., 1999; Brown et al., 2004). Furthermore, temoporfin is a pure compound with a very strong absorption at 652 nm (Ris et al., 1991; Mitra, Foster, 2005; Dragicevic-Curic et al., 2008; Brown et al., 2004). However, like porfimer sodium, the drug is also associated with a pronounced and lengthy generalised skin photosensitivity and can show little initial selectivity, with the selective benefits arising later from selective healing of healthy tissue (Brown et al., 2004).

To avoid skin photosensitization, however, temoporfin requires a long clearance time of 4–6 weeks from human plasma after injection, which is almost same as that of Photofrin® (Ronn et al., 1996; Yano et al., 2011). Temoporfin has been investigated for use against esophageal cancer (Lovat et al., 2005; Etienne et al., 2004; Yano et al., 2011), lung cancer, gastric cancer, prostate cancer (Nathan et al., 2002; Moore et al., 2006; Yano et al., 2011) and skin cancer and has been approved for clinical use against had head cancer and neck cancer (Sharman et al., 1999; Rauschning et al., 2004; Biel, 2006; Brown et al., 2004; Yano et al., 2011). In addition, this photosensitizer has been investigated in phase II clinical trials against head cancer, neck cancer, nasopharyngeal carcinoma and bile duct carcinoma in Europe, the USA and Canada (Yano et al., 2011).

Photofrin® (Porfimer Sodium)

Hematoporphyrin derivatives were the first photosensitizers studied in detail and reported in the literature (Castano et al., 2005; Stylli et al., 2005) and Photofrin® was the first photosensitizer approved for use in clinical, in 1993, in Canada (Henderson, Dougherty, 1992; Paszko et al., 2011). Belonging to the first generation, it is a mixture of dimers and oligomers of hematoporphyrin in which porphyrin units are linked by ether, ester and C-C bonds (Sharman et al., 1999; Yano et al., 2011).

Photofrin®, porfimer sodium, was approved in most countries for treatment of various indications of cancer, such as esophageal cancer, superficial bladder cancer and lung cancer in initial and final stages, as well as malignant and non-malignant skin disease (Leung et al., 2002; O'Connor et al., 2009; Yano et al., 2011).

The applicability of this photosensitizing agent in PDT has been limited to factors, such as low water solubility (Chen et al., 2005), long wavelength absorption (Henderson, Dougherty, 1992; Leung et al., 2002; Agostinis et al., 2011), long skin photosensitivity lasting up to six weeks with low rate of excretion (Paszko et al., 2011; Tetard et al., 2014; Stummer et al., 1993; Hebeda et al., 1995; Agostinis et al., 2011) and low selectivity tumor (Tetard et al., 2014; Stummer et al., 1993; Hebeda et al., 1995).

5-Aminolevulinic Acid

Another development in research is prodrug 5-aminolevulinic acid (ALA), the second generation, with authorized use in the European Union in fluorescence-guided resection (Kostron, 2010; Eljamel, 2010). Unlike other substances used in PDT, ALA is not photosensitizer by itself. Is a precursor and when absorbed by cells, is converted, naturally, by biosynthetic process, as part endogenous heme pathway, in protoporphyrin IX photosensitizer (PpIX) (Rimington, 1966; Zhu, Finlay, 2008; Tetard et al., 2014).

Under physiological conditions, the next phase of the cycle is the insertion of iron to convert PpIX to heme, which controls endogenous production of 5-ALA through feedback inhibition (Rimington, 1966). Various mechanisms, including low expression quelatase iron in malignant tumors are correlated with higher concentrations of PpIX in the tumor tissue than in healthy brain (Peng et al., 1997; Collaud et al., 2004; Greenbaum et al., 2002; Ennis et al., 2003). Thus, exogenous administration of 5-ALA controls the feedback inhibition intracellular resulting in accumulation of PpIX (Peng et al., 1997; Tetard et al., 2014).

The use of 5-ALA in PDT shows rapid elimination of PpIX from the body, limiting the risk of skin photosensitization in 48 hours (Webber et al., 1997) and high tumor selectivity (Tetard et al., 2014). The adverse effects caused with 5-ALA have been reported rarely, including abnormal liver function, nausea and anecdotally generalized edema (Stummer et al., 2006; Webber et al., 1997; Stepp et al., 2007; Hennig et al., 2011; Hefti et al., 2008).

Topical PDT with ALA has proved to be successful in the treatment of non-melanoma skin cancers, including superficial basal cell carcinoma and Bowen's disease, and associated pre-cancers actinic keratosis (Babilas et al., 2005; Krammer, Plaetzer, 2008; Foley, 2003; Morton et al., 2006; Szeimies et al., 2008).

In 1999, it was approved by the Food and Drug Administration for treatment of actinic keratosis (Zhu, Finlay, 2008), and other therapies such as basal cell carcinoma, Paget's disease, squamous cell carcinoma, T-cell lymphomas and other cancers such as in lung, bladder, oral cavity, esophagus and brain tumors. ALA is effective in dermatology for treating neoplastic cutaneous tissues (Fukuda et al., 2005).

Hematoporphyrin Monomethyl Ether

Hematoporphyrin monomethyl ether (HMME) consists of a mixture of two positional isomers of 7(12)-(1-methoxyethyl)-12(7)-(1-hydroxyethyl)-3,8,13,17-tetramethyl-21H,23H-porphyrin-2,18-dipropionic acid (Li et al., 2008). In the late 1980s, it was first described in the literature the use of Hemoporfin® as a photosensitizer in photodynamic therapy (Huang, 2006; Xu, 2007).

Several in vivo studies suggest that HMME may be useful in PDT ocular, as well as anti-tumor (Song et al., 2007; Lei et al., 2012.). Furthermore, HMME has potential when applied in photodynamic therapy in viral and bacterial infections. Similar to other photosensitizers based on hematoporphyrin (Lei et al., 2012), HMME exhibits strong absorption in the Soret band and four distinct peaks Q-band in the range of 500-800 nm. Molar extinction coefficients of HMME are similar to those reported by Photofrin® (Andreoni, Cubeddu, 1984). The multiple peaks Q-band HMME allows selection of the wavelength of excitation according target lesion type, thickness and location (Lei et al., 2012).

Tetra-Methylthionine Chloride

The photosensitizer methylene blue, phenothiazinium class of compounds, is a histological dye and its photomicrobial action is known since 1928s (Schultz, Krueger, 1928; Wainwright, Baptista, 2011; Tuite, Kelly, 1993). It having been used as an antimalarial drug as early as 1890s (Wainwright, Baptista, 2011) and was in many cases the primary example used to investigate photoantimicrobial action until the 1960s (Wainwright, Crossley, 2002). The characteristic color of methylene blue is caused by the strong absorption band in the 550 a 700 nm region with maximum molar absorptivity of $85,000M^{-1}$ cm^{-1} at 664 nm (Junqueira et al., 2002; Tardivo et al., 2005).

Despite the efficiency as photo antimicrobial agent broad spectrum, their use in blood products is limited to photo disinfecting plasma (Wainwright et al., 2007) because its hydrophilic origin located on external cell membranes, causing lack of activity against intracellular targets (Skripchenko et al., 1997; Wainwright, Baptista, 2011) and photodamage membrane (Wainwright, Baptista, 2011).

In addition to the effects presented against HIV, methylene blue has been shown photoinactivation other RNA viruses such as West Nile virus (Papin et al., 2005), dengue virus (Huang et al., 2004) and yellow fever virus (Findlay, 1934; Wainwright, Baptista, 2011). Regarding antiprotozoal activity, including African and American trypanosomiasis (T'ung, 1938; Gironés et al., 2006) and leishmaniasis (Mauel, 1984; Wainwright, Baptista, 2011).

Methylene blue has interesting characteristics conferring to this molecule a great potential for application in PDT. It absorbs light intensively in the therapeutic window; it has a well-characterized and effective photochemistry that triggers both photosensitization mechanisms type I and type II; it damages biomolecules and efficiently induces death in several target cells, tissues and organisms. Therefore, upon irradiation it can be used to treat a variety of cancerous and non-cancerous diseases (Tardivo et al., 2005).

Riboflavin

The use of riboflavin as a photosensitizer in combination with long-wave ultraviolet light has been shown (Goodrich et al., 2006), due to essential nature, shows less toxicity problems with riboflavin than completely synthetic xenobiotics (Reddy et al., 2008). Photochemical associated riboflavin, dissociates into lumiflavin and lumichrome (Hardwick et al., 2004) and photoproducts, each of them is also a photosensitizer, is nontoxic to humans (Seghatchian, de Sousa, 2006). Riboflavin and its degradation products interact with DNA, making this system possible to photodisinfecting blood and products (Dardare, Platz, 2002).

There are reports in the literature about the significant photo antimicrobial activity riboflavin in Gram positive and negative bacteria, virus in blood derivatives products, such as HIV-1, cytomegalovirus and West Nile Virus (Goodrich et al., 2006), and protozoan, *Leishmania donovani infantum*, *Tripanossoma cruzi* e *Plasmodia* spp.(Cardo et al., 2006; Cardo et al., 2007; Reddy, Goodrich, 2003).

4,5,6,7-Tetrachloro-20,40,50,70- Traiodofluoresceindisodium

Rose bengal is a xanthene dye and actually it is the most popular sensitizer used in water solutions. This chomophore is a water soluble nontoxic dye and is capable of absorbing light in the visible spectral region. Its excited triplet state is efficiently quenched by oxygen showing high quantum yield of singlet oxygen formation (Wilkinson et al., 1993; Ferreira et al., 2013). Rose bengal has been used as photodynamic inactivator of different bacterial species (Kim et al., 2008; Dahl et al., 1988; Ferreira et al., 2013).

It has been used as a photodynamic sensitizer for cancer chemotherapy (Ito, Kobayashi, 1977; Theodossiou et al., 2003; Delprat et al., 1924; Nordyke, 1965) as well as a topical ophthalmic diagnostic (Argueso et al., 2006) suggests rose bengal should have minimal side effects (Wachter et al., 2003). It operates via the Type II photosensitization mechanism, in which produced singlet oxygen is the main responsible species for bacterial inactivation (Luksiene, 2005; Ferreira et al., 2013).

However, rose bengal application is strongly limited by the fact that it tends to aggregate in aqueous solution. More over it is well known that positively charged photosensitizers are generally more efficient than anionic ones as they are able to bind and penetrate the microbial permeability barrier (Jori, Brown, 2004; Ferreira et al., 2013).

3-(1-Hexyloxyethyl)-3-Divinylpyropheophorbide

3-(1-Hexyloxyethyl)-3-divinylpyropheophorbide, Photochlor®, a highly lipophilic second-generation photosensitizer, was designed for cellular membrane penetration. Photochlor® has a higher level of tumor-accumulation than either Photofrin® or Temoporfin (Marchal et al., 2007; Yow et al., 2000). Similar to Photofrin®, Photochlor® is not metabolized but is instead removed from human plasma and excreted slowly (Bellnier et al., 2006; Yano et al., 2011). Photochlor® has been investigated in phase I/II clinical trials against Barrett's esophagus, esophageal cancer, non-small cell lung cancer, basal cell carcinoma and early and late stage lung cancer. When esophageal cancer was treated with Photochlor®-PDT, severe skin photosensitization did not occur, in contrast to Photofrin® (Pandey et al., 1991; Yano et al., 2011).

Mono-l-Aspartylchlorin-e_6

Mono-l-aspartylchlorin-e_6, Laserphyrin®, Talaporfin, is a water-soluble second-generation photosensitizer with a short tumor accumulation time, more rapid clearance and better availability for deeper cells in comparison with Photofrin® (Yano et al., 2011).

The very short clearance time, 3–7 days after injection, and low accumulation in skin of Laserphyrin® efficiently reduce serious skin photosensitization. The primary mechanism of Laserphyrin® mediated PDT is cell death triggered by vascular stasis and direct tumor cytotoxicity (Spikes, Bommer, 1993). Laserphyrin® was approved for clinical use against early-stage lung cancer in 2003 in Japan, and phase III studies are underway for liver cancer and recurrent neck cancer and head cancer (Yano et al., 2011).

Lutetium Texaphyrin

Lutetium texaphyrin, Lutrin®, a water-soluble second generation photosensitizer, has a high tumor-selectivity and is excreted at almost the same rate as Visudyne®. Lutrin® has been approved for clinical use against recurrent prostate cancer and cervical cancer and has been investigated in phase I/II/III clinical trials against breast cancer including recurrent breast cancer, melanoma and Kaposi's sarcoma (Sessler et al., 1994; Yano et al., 2011).

Palladium Bacteriopheophorbide a

The palladium bacteriopheophorbide *a*, Tookad®, WST09, is a lipophilic photosensitizer and has the advantage of rapid clearance from circulation without skin photocytotoxicity in comparison with Visudyne™ and Lutrin®. Tookad® clears from the blood stream within less than 20 minutes, and in addition, the skin photocytotoxicity is negligible at approximately 1.3 hours after injection (Josefsen, Boyle, 2008; Yano et al., 2011).

Phthalocyanines

Phthalocyanines are tetrapyrrolic macrocycles that, unlike the porphyrins, have nitrogen atoms linking the individual pyrrole units instead of methine bridges. The periphery of the macrocycle is extended by benzene rings, which strengthens the absorption at longer wavelengths compared to porphyrins such as Photofrin. Phthalocyanines have long been used as dyes and colouring agents (Philips, 1997; Sharman et al., 1999; Van Lier, Spikes, 1989).

Naphthalocyanines

Napthalocyanines are macrocycles with a second benzene ring added on the periphery of the phthalocyanine ring. This additional conjugation leads to the absorption of longer wavelength light than the phthalocyanines, 770 compared with 680 nm, that could prove useful in the treatment of highly pigmented tumors in PDT (Sharman et al., 1999; Soncin, 1998; DeRosa, Crutchley, 2002).

OTHERS PHOTOSENSITIZERS

Today, the development of third generation photosensitizers, which have high accumulation in tumor tissue, is challenging field in PDT study. One promising approach in study is conjugation of a photosensitizer with a biologically active element (Yano et al., 2011) to carry the drug for the appropriated local in each established protocol.

CONCLUSION

Nowadays, the development of safe and highly selective photosensitizers is the main topic of many research programs and a challenging course in the study of PDT. There are several factors that influence the effectiveness of the functioning of the photosensitizer. Many researchers focus, mainly, on improving drug delivery, and in spite of several clinically approved photosensitizers, there is no an ideal, safe and selective agent yet (Chatterjee et al., 2008).

A long-standing dream in the field of cancer therapy is ability to treat subcutaneous tumors noninvasively. Many new second-generation photosensitizers have been developed and a few of them are already in clinical trials. Future photosensitizers, third generation photosensitizers, are still in the initial stages of research (Yano, et al., 2011).

While no photosensitizer can be deemed ideal for every possible application, a number of others photosensitizers have been developed to overcome the shortcomings and to take advantage of their more ideal properties.

This chapter aimed to provide the reader a description about the use of photosensitizers in photodynamic therapy through the concept and properties of the photosensitizer and its action mechanism in the development of PDT.

REFERENCES

Agostinis P, Berg K, Cengel KA, Foster TH, Girotti AW, Gollnick SO, et al., Photodynamic therapy of cancer: an update. *CA Cancer J. Clin.* 2011 Jul-Aug;61(4):250-81.

Allison RR, Sibata CH. Oncologic photodynamic therapy photosensitizers: a clinical review. *Photodiagnosis Photodyn Ther.* 2010 Jun;7(2):61-75.

Andreoni A, Cubeddu R. Photophysical properties of Photofrin II in different solvents. *Chem. Phys. Lett.* 1984;108(2):141-4.

Argüeso P, Tisdale A, Spurr-Michaud S, Sumiyoshi M, Gipson IK. Mucin characteristics of human corneal-limbal epithelial cells that exclude the rose bengal anionic dye. *Invest Ophthalmol. Vis. Sci.* 2006 Jan;47(1):113-9.

Babilas P, Karrer S, Sidoroff A, Landthaler M, Szeimies RM. Photodynamic therapy in dermatology--an update. *Photodermatol. Photoimmunol. Photomed.* 2005 Jun;21(3):142-9.

Bellnier DA, Greco WR, Nava H, Loewen GM, Oseroff AR, Dougherty TJ. Mild skin photosensitivity in cancer patients following injection of Photochlor (2-[1-hexyloxyethyl]-2-devinyl pyropheophorbide-a; HPPH) for photodynamic therapy. *Cancer Chemother Pharmacol.* 2006 Jan;57(1):40-5.

Biel M. Advances in photodynamic therapy for the treatment of head and neck cancers. *Lasers Surg. Med.* 2006 Jun;38(5):349-55.

Bigby M. Rates of cutaneous reactions to drugs. *Arch Dermatol.* 2001 Jun;137(6):765-70.

Breathnach SM, Hintner H. *Adverse drug reactions and the skin*. Oxford, UK: Blackwell Scientific; 1992.

Brodowska K, Al-Moujahed A, Marmalidou A, Meyer Zu Horste M, Cichy J, Miller JW, et al., The clinically used photosensitizer Verteporfin (VP) inhibits YAP-TEAD and human retinoblastoma cell growth in vitro without light activation. *Exp. Eye Res.* 2014 Jul;124:67-73.

Brown SB, Brown EA, Walker I. The present and future role of photodynamic therapy in cancer treatment. *Lancet Oncol.* 2004 Aug;5(8):497-508.

Brown SB, Mellish KJ. Verteporfin: a milestone in opthalmology and photodynamic therapy. *Expert Opin Pharmacother*. 2001 Feb;2(2):351-61.

Calzavara-Pinton PG, Venturini M, Sala R. Photodynamic therapy: update 2006. Part 1: Photochemistry and photobiology. *J. Eur. Acad. Dermatol. Venereol.* 2007 Mar;21(3):293-302.

Cardo LJ, Rentas FJ, Ketchum L, Salata J, Harman R, Melvin W, et al., Pathogen inactivation of *Leishmania donovani infantum* in plasma and platelet concentrates using riboflavin and ultraviolet light. *Vox Sang.* 2006 Feb;90(2):85-91.

Cardo LJ, Salata J, Mendez J, Reddy H, Goodrich R. Pathogen inactivation of *Trypanosoma cruzi* in plasma and platelet concentrates using riboflavin and ultraviolet light. *Transfus Apher Sci.* 2007 Oct;37(2):131-7.

Castano AP, Demidova TN, Hamblin MR. Mechanisms in photodynamic therapy: Part three-Photosensitizer pharmacokinetics, biodistribution, tumor localization and modes of tumor destruction. *Photodiagnosis Photodyn Ther.* 2005 Jun;2(2):91-106.

Celli JP, Solban N, Liang A, Pereira SP, Hasan T. Verteporfin-based photodynamic therapy overcomes gemcitabine insensitivity in a panel of pancreatic cancer cell lines. *Lasers Surg. Med.* 2011 Sep;43(7):565-74.

Chatterjee DK, Fong LS, Zhang Y. Nanoparticles in photodynamic therapy: an emerging paradigm. *Adv. Drug Deliv. Rev.* 2008 Dec 14;60(15):1627-37.

Chen B, Pogue BW, Hasan T. Liposomal delivery of photosensitising agents. *Expert Opin Drug Deliv.* 2005 May;2(3):477-87.

Collaud S, Juzeniene A, Moan J, Lange N. On the selectivity of 5-aminolevulinic acid-induced protoporphyrin IX formation. *Curr. Med. Chem. Anticancer Agents*. 2004 May;4(3):301-16.

Crowson AN, Brown TJ, Magro CM. Progress in the understanding of the pathology and pathogenesis of cutaneous drug eruptions: implications for management. *Am. J. Clin. Dermatol.* 2003;4(6):407-28.

Dahl TA, Midden WR, Neckers DC. Comparison of photodynamic action by Rose Bengal in gram-positive and gram-negative bacteria. *Photochem. Photobiol.* 1988 Nov;48(5):607-12.

Dai T, Huang YY, Hamblin MR. Photodynamic therapy for localized infections--state of the art. *Photodiagnosis Photodyn Ther.* 2009 Sep-Dec;6(3-4):170-88.

Dardare N, Platz MS. Binding affinities of commonly employed sensitizers of viral inactivation. *Photochem. Photobiol.* 2002 Jun;75(6):561-4.

Delprat GD, Epstein NN, Kerr WJ. A new liver function test: the elimination of Rose Bengal when injected into the circulation of human subjects. *Arch. Intern Med.* 1924;34:533-41.

DeRosa MC, Crutchley RJ. Photosensitized singlet oxygen and its applications. *Coordin. Chem. Rev.* 2002;233-234;351-71.

Dougherty TJ, Gomer CJ, Henderson BW, Jori G, Kessel D, Korbelik M, et al., Photodynamic therapy. *J Natl Cancer Inst.* 1998 Jun 17;90(12):889-905.

Dragicevic-Curic N, Scheglmann D, Albrecht V, Fahr A. Temoporfin-loaded invasomes: development, characterization and in vitro skin penetration studies. *J. Control Release.* 2008 Apr 7;127(1):59-69.

Eljamel S. Photodynamic applications in brain tumors: a comprehensive review of the literature. *Photodiagnosis Photodyn Ther.* 2010 Jun;7(2):76-85.

Ennis SR, Novotny A, Xiang J, Shakui P, Masada T, Stummer W, et al., Transport of 5-aminolevulinic acid between blood and brain. *Brain Res.* 2003 Jan 10;959(2):226-34.

Etienne J, Dorme N, Bourg-Heckly G, Raimbert P, Fléjou JF. Photodynamic therapy with green light and m-tetrahydroxyphenyl chlorin for intramucosal adenocarcinoma and high-grade dysplasia in Barrett's esophagus. *Gastrointest Endosc.* 2004 Jun;59(7):880-9.

Fabris C, Valduga G, Miotto G, Borsetto L, Jori G, Garbisa S, et al., Photosensitization with zinc (II) phthalocyanine as a switch in the decision between apoptosis and necrosis. *Cancer Res.* 2001 Oct 15;61(20):7495-500.

Ferreira AM, Carmagnola I, Chiono V, Gentile P, Fracchia L, Ceresa C, et al., Surface modification of poly(dimethylsiloxane) by two-step plasma treatment for further grafting with chitosan–Rose Bengal photosensitizer. *Surf Coat Tech.* 2013 May;223:92-7.

Findlay GM. Immunization against yellow fever. *Trans R. Soc. Trop Med. Hyg.* 1934;27:437-69.

Foley P. Clinical efficacy of methyl aminolevulinate (Metvix) photodynamic therapy. *J. Dermatolog. Treat.* 2003;14 Suppl 3:15-22.

Fukuda H, Casas A, Batlle A. Aminolevulinic acid: from its unique biological function to its star role in photodynamic therapy. *Int. J. Biochem. Cell Biol.* 2005 Feb;37(2):272-6.

Gironés N, Bueno JL, Carrión J, Fresno M, Castro E. The efficacy of photochemical treatment with methylene blue and light for the reduction of *Trypanosoma cruzi* in infected plasma. *Vox Sang.* 2006 Nov;91(4):285-91.

Goodrich RP, Edrich RA, Li J, Seghatchian J. The Mirasol PRT system for pathogen reduction of platelets and plasma: an overview of current status and future trends. *Transfus Apher Sci.* 2006 Aug;35(1):5-17.

Greenbaum L, Gozlan Y, Schwartz D, Katcoff DJ, Malik Z. Nuclear distribution of porphobilinogen deaminase (PBGD) in glioma cells: a regulatory role in cancer transformation? *Br. J. Cancer.* 2002 Mar 18;86(6):1006-11.

Harbour JW. Photodynamic therapy for choroidal metastasis from carcinoid tumor. *Am. J. Ophthalmol.* 2004 Jun;137(6):1143-5.

Hardwick CC, Herivel TR, Hernandez SC, Ruane PH, Goodrich RP. Separation, identification and quantification of riboflavin and its photoproducts in blood products using high-performance liquid chromatography with fluorescence detection: a method to support pathogen reduction technology. *Photochem. Photobiol.* 2004 Nov-Dec;80(3):609-15.

Hebeda KM, Wolbers JG, Sterenborg HJ, Kamphorst W, van Gemert MJ, van Alphen HA. Fluorescence localization in tumour and normal brain after intratumoral injection of haematoporphyrin derivative into rat brain tumour. *J. Photochem. Photobiol. B.* 1995 Jan;27(1):85-92.

Hefti M, von Campe G, Moschopulos M, Siegner A, Looser H, Landolt H. 5-aminolevulinic acid induced protoporphyrin IX fluorescence in high-grade glioma surgery: a one-year experience at a single institutuion. *Swiss Med. Wkly.* 2008 Mar 22;138(11-12):180-5.

Henderson BW, Dougherty TJ. How does photodynamic therapy work? *Photochem. Photobiol.* 1992 Jan;55(1):145-57.

Hennig G, Stepp H, Johansson A. Photobleaching-based method to individualize irradiation time during interstitial 5-aminolevulinic acid photodynamic therapy. *Photodiagnosis Photodyn Ther.* 2011 Sep;8(3):275-81.

Heukers R, van Bergen En Henegouwen PM, Oliveira S. Nanobody-photosensitizer conjugates for targeted photodynamic therapy. *Nanomedicine.* 2014 Oct;10(7):1441-51.

Huang Q, Fu WL, Chen B, Huang JF, Zhang X, Xue Q. Inactivation of dengue virus by methylene blue/narrow bandwidth light system. *J. Photochem. Photobiol. B.* 2004 Dec 2;77(1-3):39-43.

Huang Z. A review of progress in clinical photodynamic therapy. *Technol Cancer Res. Treat.* 2005 Jun;4(3):283-93.

Huang Z. Photodynamic therapy in China: Over 25 years of unique clinical experience Part One-History and domestic photosensitizers. *Photodiagnosis Photodyn Ther.* 2006 Mar;3(1):3-10.

Isola V, Pece A, Pierro L. Photodynamic therapy with verteporfin of choroidal malignancy from breast cancer. *Am. J. Ophthalmol.* 2006 Nov;142(5):885-7.

Ito T, Kobayashi K. A survey of in vivo photodynamic activity of xanthenes, thiazines, and acridines in yeast cells. *Photochem. Photobiol.* 1977 Jan;26(6):581-7.

Jain N, Sharma PK, Banik A, Bhardwaj V. Applications of Photosensitizer in Therapy. *Pharmacogn J.* 2011 Jun;3(22):11-7.

Jiang Z, Shao J, Yang T, Wang J, Jia L. Pharmaceutical development, composition and quantitative analysis of phthalocyanine as the photosensitizer for cancer photodynamic therapy. *J. Pharm Biomed. Anal.* 2014 Jan;87:98-104.

Jori G, Brown SB. Photosensitized inactivation of microorganisms. *Photochem. Photobiol. Sci.* 2004 May;3(5):403-5.

Josefsen LB, Boyle RW. Photodynamic therapy: novel third-generation photosensitizers one step closer? *Br. J. Pharmacol.* 2008 May;154(1):1-3.

Junqueira HC, Severino D, Dias LG, Gugliotti M, Baptista MS. Modulation of the methylene blue photochemical properties based on the adsorption at aqueous micelle interfaces. *Phys. Chem. Chem. Phys..* 2002;4:2320-8.

Kessel D, Vicente MG, Reiners JJ Jr. Initiation of apoptosis and autophagy by photodynamic therapy. *Lasers Surg. Med.* 2006 Jun;38(5):482-8.

Kim J, Santos OA, Park JH. Selective photosensitizer delivery into plasma membrane for effective photodynamic therapy. *J. Control Release.* 2014 Oct 10;191:98-104.

Kim YS, Park SJ, Lee EJ, Cerbo RM, Lee SM, Ryu CH, et al., Antibacterial compounds from Rose Bengal-sensitized photooxidation of beta-caryophyllene. *J. Food Sci.* 2008 Sep;73(7):C540-5.

Kostron H. Photodynamic diagnosis and therapy and the brain. *Methods Mol. Biol.* 2010;635:261-80.

Krammer B, Plaetzer K. ALA and its clinical impact, from bench to bedside. *Photochem. Photobiol. Sci.* 2008 Mar;7(3):283-9.

Kübler AC, Scheer M, Zöller JE. Photodynamic therapy of head and neck cancer. *Onkologie*. 2001 Jun;24(3):230-7.

Lei TC, Glazner GF, Duffy M, Scherrer L, Pendyala S, Li B, et al., Optical properties of hematoporphyrin monomethyl ether (HMME), a PDT photosensitizer. *Photodiagnosis Photodyn Ther*. 2012 Sep;9(3):232-42.

Leung WN, Sun X, Mak NK, Yow CM. Photodynamic effects of mTHPC on human colon adenocarcinoma cells: photocytotoxicity, subcellular localization and apoptosis. *Photochem. Photobiol*. 2002 Apr;75(4):406-11.

Li BH, Lin LS, Lin HY, Xie SS. Singlet oxygen quantum yields of porphyrin-based photosensitizers for photodynamic therapy. *J. Innov. Opt. Health Sci*. 2008;1(1):141-9.

Liu-Chittenden Y, Huang B, Shim JS, Chen Q, Lee SJ, Anders RA, et al., Genetic and pharmacological disruption of the TEAD-YAP complex suppresses the oncogenic activity of YAP. *Genes Dev*. 2012 Jun 15;26(12):1300-5.

Lovat LB, Jamieson NF, Novelli MR, Mosse CA, Selvasekar C, Mackenzie GD, et al., Photodynamic therapy with m-tetrahydroxyphenyl chlorin for high-grade dysplasia and early cancer in Barrett's columnar lined esophagus. *Gastrointest Endosc*. 2005 Oct;62(4):617-23.

Luksiene Z. New approach to inactivation of harmful and pathogenic microorganisms by photosensitization. *Food Technol Biotech*. 2005;43(4):411-18.

Malik R, Manocha A, Suresh DK. Photodynamic therapy--a strategic review. *Indian J. Dent Res*. 2010 Apr-Jun;21(2):285-91.

Marchal S, François A, Dumas D, Guillemin F, Bezdetnaya L. Relationship between subcellular localisation of Foscan and caspase activation in photosensitised MCF-7 cells. *Br. J. Cancer*. 2007 Mar 26;96(6):944-51.

Mauel J. Intracellular parasite killing induced by electron carriers. I. Effect of electron carriers on intracellular *Leishmania* spp. in macrophages from different genetic backgrounds. *Mol Biochem Parasitol*. 1984 Sep;13(1):83-96.

Messmer KJ, Abel SR. Verteporfin for age-related macular degeneration. *Ann. Pharmacother*. 2001 Dec;35(12):1593-8.

Mitra S, Foster TH. Photophysical parameters, photosensitizer retention and tissue optical properties completely account for the higher photodynamic efficacy of meso-tetra-hydroxyphenyl-chlorin vs Photofrin. *Photochem. Photobiol*. 2005 Jul-Aug;81(4):849-59.

Moan J, Berg K. The photodegradation of porphyrins in cells can be used to estimate the lifetime of singlet oxygen. *Photochem. Photobiol*. 1991 Apr;53(4):549-53.

Moore CM, Nathan TR, Lees WR, Mosse CA, Freeman A, Emberton M, et al., Photodynamic therapy using meso tetra hydroxy phenyl chlorin (mTHPC) in early prostate cancer. *Lasers Surg. Med*. 2006 Jun;38(5):356-63.

Moore DE. Drug-induced cutaneous photosensitivity: incidence, mechanism, prevention and management. *Drug Saf*. 2002;25(5):345-72.

Morton C, Horn M, Leman J, Tack B, Bedane C, Tjioe M, et al., Comparison of topical methyl aminolevulinate photodynamic therapy with cryotherapy or Fluorouracil for treatment of squamous cell carcinoma in situ: Results of a multicenter randomized trial. *Arch. Dermatol*. 2006 Jun;142(6):729-35.

Moser JG. Definitions and General Properties of 2nd & 3rd Generation Photosensitizers. In: Moser JG, editor. *Photodynamic Tumor Therapy-2nd & 3rd Generation Photosensitizers*. London, UK: Harwood Academic Publishers; 1997; 3-8.

Nathan TR, Whitelaw DE, Chang SC, Lees WR, Ripley PM, Payne H, et al., Photodynamic therapy for prostate cancer recurrence after radiotherapy: a phase I study. *J. Urol.* 2002 Oct;168(4 Pt 1):1427-32.

Nordyke RA. Surgical vs nonsurgical jaundice. Differentiation by a combination of rose bengal I-131 and standard liver-function tests. *JAMA.* 1965 Nov 29;194(9):949-53.

O'Connor AE, Gallagher WM, Byrne AT. Porphyrin and nonporphyrin photosensitizers in oncology: preclinical and clinical advances in photodynamic therapy. *Photochem. Photobiol.* 2009 Sep-Oct;85(5):1053-74.

Pandey RK, Bellnier DA, Smith KM, Dougherty TJ. Chlorin and porphyrin derivatives as potential photosensitizers in photodynamic therapy. *Photochem. Photobiol.* 1991 Jan;53(1):65-72.

Papin JF, Floyd RA, Dittmer DP. Methylene blue photoinactivation abolishes West Nile virus infectivity in vivo. *Antiviral Res.* 2005 Nov;68(2):84-7.

Paszko E, Ehrhardt C, Senge MO, Kelleher DP, Reynolds JV. Nanodrug applications in photodynamic therapy. *Photodiagnosis Photodyn Ther.* 2011 Mar;8(1):14-29.

Peng Q, Warloe T, Berg K, Moan J, Kongshaug M, Giercksky KE, et al., 5-Aminolevulinic acid-based photodynamic therapy. Clinical research and future challenges. *Cancer.* 1997 Jun 15;79(12):2282-308.

Pervaiz S. Reactive oxygen-dependent production of novel photochemotherapeutic agents. *FASEB J.* 2001 Mar;15(3):612-7.

Phillips D. Chemical mechanisms in photodynamic therapy with phthalocyanines. *Prog Reaction Kinetics.* 1997;22:175-300.

Pogue BW, O'Hara JA, Demidenko E, Wilmot CM, Goodwin IA, Chen B, et al., Photodynamic therapy with verteporfin in the radiation-induced fibrosarcoma-1 tumor causes enhanced radiation sensitivity. *Cancer Res.* 2003 Mar 1;63(5):1025-33.

Rauschning W, Tan IB, Dolivet G. Photodynamic therapy (PDT) with mTHPC in the palliation of advanced head and neck cancer in patients who have failed prior therapies and are unsuitable for radiatiotherapy, surgery or systemic chemotherapy. *J. Clin. Oncol.* 2004 Jul;22(14 Suppl):5596.

Reddy H, Goodrich RP. Inactivation of West Nile virus and malaria using photosensitizers. *Vox Sang* 2003. WO2003063902.

Reddy HL, Dayan AD, Cavagnaro J, Gad S, Li J, Goodrich RP. Toxicity testing of a novel riboflavin-based technology for pathogen reduction and white blood cell inactivation. *Transfus Med. Rev.* 2008 Apr;22(2):133-53.

Rimington C. Porphyrin and haem biosynthesis and its control. *Acta Med. Scand. Suppl.* 1966;445:11-24.

Ris HB, Altermatt HJ, Inderbitzi R, Hess R, Nachbur B, Stewart JC, et al., Photodynamic therapy with chlorins for diffuse malignant mesothelioma: initial clinical results. *Br. J. Cancer.* 1991 Dec;64(6):1116-20.

Ronn AM, Nouri M, Lofgren LA, Steinberg BM, Westerborn A, Windal T, Shikowitz MJ. Human tissue levels and plasma pharmacokinetics of temoporfin (Foscan®, mTHPC). *Lasers Med. Sci.* 1996;11(4):267-72.

Rosenkranz AA, Jans DA, Sobolev AS. Targeted intracellular delivery of photosensitizers to enhance photodynamic efficiency. *Immunol. Cell Biol.* 2000 Aug;78(4):452-64.

Schmidt-Erfurth U, Miller JW, Sickenberg M, Laqua H, Barbazetto I, Gragoudas ES, et al., Photodynamic therapy with verteporfin for choroidal neovascularization caused by age-related macular degeneration. *Arch. Ophthalmol.* 1999;117:1177-87.

Schultz EW, Krueger AP. Inactivation of *Staphylococcus* bacteriophage by methylene blue. *Proc. Soc. Exp. Biol. Med.* 1928;26:100-1.

Seghatchian J, de Sousa G. Pathogen-reduction systems for blood components: the current position and future trends. *Transfus Apher Sci.* 2006 Dec;35(3):189-96.

Sen P, Mediratta PK, Bhaduri J. Light, skin and drugs. *Indian J. Pharmacol.* 1992:24(2):82-9.

Sessler JL, Hemmi G, Mody TD, Murai T, Burrell A, Young SW, Texaphyrins: synthesis and applications. *Acc. Chem. Res.* 1994 Feb;27(2):43-50.

Sharman WM, Allen CM, van Lier JE. Photodynamic therapeutics: basic principles and clinical applications. *Drug Discov. Today.* 1999 Nov;4(11):507-517.

Simplício FI, Maionchi F, Hioka N. [Photodynamic therapy: pharmacological aspects, applications and recent advances in drug development]. *Quim Nova.* 2002;25(5):801-7. [Portuguese].

Skripchenko A, Robinette D, Wagner SJ. Comparison of methylene blue and methylene violet for photoinactivation of intracellular and extracellular virus in red cell suspensions. *Photochem Photobiol.* 1997 Mar;65(3):451-5.

Soncin M, Busetti A, Biolo R, Jori G, Kwag G, Li YS, et al., Photoinactivation of amelanotic and melanotic melanoma cells sensitized by axially substituted Si-naphthalocyanines. *J. Photochem. Photobiol. B.* 1998 Mar;42(3):202-10.

Song K, Kong B, Li L, Yang Q, Wei Y, Qu X. Intraperitoneal photodynamic therapy for an ovarian cancer ascite model in Fischer 344 rat using hematoporphyrin monomethyl ether. *Cancer Sci.* 2007 Dec;98(12):1959-64.

Spikes JD, Bommer JC. Photosensitizing properties of mono-L-aspartyl chlorin e6 (NPe6): a candidate sensitizer for the photodynamic therapy of tumors. *J. Photochem. Photobiol. B.* 1993 Feb;17(2):135-43.

Stepp H, Beck T, Pongratz T, Meinel T, Kreth FW, Tonn JCh, et al., ALA and malignant glioma: fluorescence-guided resection and photodynamic treatment. *J. Environ. Pathol. Toxicol. Oncol.* 2007;26(2):157-64.

Sternberg ED, Dolphin D, Brückner C. Porphyrin-based photosensitizers for use in photodynamic therapy. *Tetrahedron.* 1998 Apr;54(17):4151-202.

Stummer W, Götz C, Hassan A, Heimann A, Kempski O. Kinetics of Photofrin II in perifocal brain edema. *Neurosurgery.* 1993 Dec;33(6):1075-81; discussion 1081-2.

Stummer W, Pichlmeier U, Meinel T, Wiestler OD, Zanella F, Reulen HJ, et al., Fluorescence-guided surgery with 5-aminolevulinic acid for resection of malignant glioma: a randomised controlled multicentre phase III trial. *Lancet Oncol.* 2006 May;7(5):392-401.

Stylli SS, Kaye AH, MacGregor L, Howes M, Rajendra P. Photodynamic therapy of high grade glioma - long term survival. *J. Clin. Neurosci.* 2005 May;12(4):389-98.

Szeimies RM, Ibbotson S, Murrell DF, Rubel D, Frambach Y, de Berker D, et al., A clinical study comparing methyl aminolevulinate photodynamic therapy and surgery in small superficial basal cell carcinoma (8-20 mm), with a 12-month follow-up. *J. Eur. Acad. Dermatol. Venereol.* 2008 Nov;22(11):1302-11.

T'ung T. In vitro photodynamic action of methylene blue on *Trypanosoma brucei. Proc. Soc. Exp. Biol. Med.* 1938;38:29-31.

Tammela T, Saaristo A, Holopainen T, Ylä-Herttuala S, Andersson LC, Virolainen S, et al., Photodynamic ablation of lymphatic vessels and intralymphatic cancer cells prevents metastasis. *Sci. Transl. Med.* 2011 Feb 9;3(69):69ra11.

Tardivo JP, Del Giglio A, de Oliveira CS, Gabrielli DS, Junqueira HC, Tada DB, et al., Methylene blue in photodynamic therapy: From basic mechanisms to clinical applications. *Photodiagnosis Photodyn Ther.* 2005 Sep;2(3):175-91.

Tetard MC, Vermandel M, Mordon S, Lejeune JP, Reyns N. Experimental use of photodynamic therapy in high grade gliomas: a review focused on 5-aminolevulinic acid. *Photodiagnosis Photodyn Ther.* 2014 Sep;11(3):319-30.

Theodossiou T, Hothersall JS, Woods EA, Okkenhaug K, Jacobson J, MacRobert AJ. Firefly luciferin-activated rose bengal: in vitro photodynamic therapy by intracellular chemiluminescence in transgenic NIH 3T3 cells. *Cancer Res.* 2003 Apr 15;63(8):1818-21.

Tripursky MS, Churgin DS, Conway MD, Peyman GA. A review of photodynamic therapy for intraocular tumors. *J. Anal. Bioanal. Tech.* 2011;S1:001.

Tuite EM, Kelly JM. Photochemical interactions of methylene blue and analogues with DNA and other biological substrates. *J. Photochem. Photobiol. B.* 1993 Dec;21(2-3):103-24.

van Lier JE, Spikes JD. The chemistry, photophysics and photosensitizing properties of phthalocyanines. In: Bock G, Harnett S, editors. *Photosensitizing Compounds: Their Chemistry, Biology and Clinical Use.* Chichester, UK: John Wiley & Sons Ltd; 1989; 17-32.

Wachter E, Dees C, Harkins J, Scott T, Petersen M, Rush RE, et al., Topical rose bengal: pre-clinical evaluation of pharmacokinetics and safety. *Lasers Surg. Med.* 2003;32(2):101-10.

Wainwright M, Baptista MS. The application of photosensitisers to tropical pathogens in the blood supply. *Photodiagnosis Photodyn Ther.* 2011 Sep;8(3):240-8.

Wainwright M, Crossley KB. Methylene Blue--a therapeutic dye for all seasons? *J. Chemother.* 2002 Oct;14(5):431-43.

Wainwright M, Mohr H, Walker WH. Phenothiazinium derivatives for pathogen inactivation in blood products. *J. Photochem. Photobiol. B.* 2007 Jan 3;86(1):45-58.

Webber J, Kessel D, Fromm D. Side effects and photosensitization of human tissues after aminolevulinic acid. *J. Surg Res.* 1997 Feb 15;68(1):31-7.

Wilkinson F, Helman WP, Ross AB. Quantum Yields for the Photosensitized Formation of the Lowest Electronically Excited Singlet State of Molecular Oxygen in Solution. *J. Phys. Chem.* 1993;22(1):113-262.

Wolkenstein P, Revuz J. Drug-induced severe skin reactions. Incidence, management and prevention. *Drug Saf.* 1995 Jul;13(1):56-68.

Xu DY. Research and development of photodynamic therapy photosensitizers in China. *Photodiagnosis Photodyn Ther.* 2007 Mar;4(1):13-25.

Yamauchi M, Honda N, Hazama H, Tachikawa S, Nakamura H, Kaneda Y, et al., A novel photodynamic therapy for drug-resistant prostate cancer cells using porphyrus envelope as a novel photosensitizer. *Photodiagnosis Photodyn Ther.* 2014 Mar;11(1):48-54.

Yano S, Hirohara S, Obata M, Hagiya Y, Ogura S, Ikeda A, et al., Current states and future views in photodynamic therapy. *J. Photoch. Photobio C.* 2011;12:46-67.

Yow CM, Chen JY, Mak NK, Cheung NH, Leung AW. Cellular uptake, subcellular localization and photodamaging effect of temoporfin (mTHPC) in nasopharyngeal carcinoma cells: comparison with hematoporphyrin derivative. *Cancer Lett*. 2000 Sep 1;157(2):123-31.

Zhu TC, Finlay JC. The role of photodynamic therapy (PDT) physics. *Med. Phys*. 2008 Jul;35(7):3127-36.

In: Photodynamic Therapy
Editor: Adrian G. Hugo

ISBN: 978-1-63463-857-9
© 2015 Nova Science Publishers, Inc.

Chapter 7

IN VITRO AND *IN VIVO* 5-AMINOLEVULINIC ACID-BASED PHOTODYNAMIC THERAPY IN SENSITIVE AND DRUG RESISTANT LEUKEMIC MURINE CELLS

Berenice Diez[1,2], Silvia Hajos[3], Roberto Meiss[4], Glenda Ernst[3], Maria Julieta Teijo[1,2], Alcira Batlle[2] and Haydée Fukuda[1,2,]*

[1]Departamento de Química Biológica, Facultad de Ciencias Exactas y Naturales, Universidad de Buenos Aires, Argentina
[2]Centro de Investigaciones sobre Porfirias y Porfirinas (CIPYP), CONICET, Hospital de Clínicas, UBA, Argentina
[3]Cátedra de Inmunología, IDEHU, Facultad de Farmacia y Bioquímica, UBA and CONICET, Argentina
[4]Instituto de Estudios Oncológicos, Sección Patología, Academia Nacional de Medicina, Argentina

ABSTRACT

The effects of combined administration of doxorubicin (DOX) and vincristine (VCR), with 5-aminolevulinic acid photodynamic treatment (ALA-PDT), were analyzed in sensitive murine leukemic cell lines (LBR-) and DOX and VCR chemoresistant LBR-D160 and LBR-V160 cell lines. Low doses of DOX and VCR increased anti-cancer effect of ALA-PDT in LBR-cells. Decrease in cell survival was higher when the combination VCR + ALA-PDT was used compared to DOX + ALA-PDT. Resistant cell lines LBR-D160 and LBR-V160 were sensitive to ALA-PDT; however, no changes occured when combining therapies. Thus, ALA-PDT can overcome drug resistance and is a good candidate for using treating multidrug resistant (MDR) cells.

This combined treatment were evaluated in a murine model. For this purpose, BALB/c mice were inoculated with LBR-cells previously treated with DOX or VCR plus ALA-PDT. 30 days after treatment animals were sacrificed and tumoral infiltration

---

[*] Corresponding author: Haydée Fukuda, PhD. Porphyirins and Porphyrias Research Center (CIPYP), Viamonte 1881-10 A, Buenos Aires (1056) Argentina. Tel: 54 11 4812 3357 / 54 11 5950 8346; Fax: 54 11 4811 7447 / 54 11 5950 8347; E-mail: hfukuda@qb.fcen.uba.ar.

analyzed in many tissues: liver, kidney, spleen, lung, brain, timus, lymph nodes. Histologic studies revealed that in control animals inoculated with LBR-cells without any treatment, infiltration reached 87% in all the tissues analyzed. Animals inoculated with LBR-cells treated with only ALA-PDT, showed 50% of organs infiltrated. When animals were inoculated with cells treated with DOX or VCR, tumor infiltration was found in 87.5% and 75% of organs, respectively. In the case of inoculation with LBR- cells treated with DOX or VCR plus ALA-PDT, no evidence of tumor infiltration was observed in any of the tissues. These results show the beneficial effect of combining therapies, suggesting the potential therapeutic alternative in leukemic patients, additionaly bringing the possibility of diminishing chemotherapy dose, thus minimizing undesirable drug side effects.

Keywords: Photodynamic therapy; chemotherapy resistance; 5-aminolevulinic acid; leukemic cells

INTRODUCTION

Chemotherapy resistance represents a major problem for the treatment of patients with cancer, including hematologic malignancies, and contributes to the recurrence of the disease and high mortality rates [1, 2, 3]. For the management of hematologic malignancies and also a number of solid tumors, autologous bone marrow transplantation (ABMT) is one of the accepted therapeutic modality [4, 5]. However, contamination of the autograft with remaining leukemic cells and persistence of minimal residual disease despite the administration of a high-dose drug therapy contributes to limit the success of the treatment [6, 7, 8]. In an attempt to decrease or eliminate leukemia cells, *in vitro* treatment of the marrow autograft (bone marrow purging) using chemotherapeutic agents such as 4-Hydroxi cyclophosfamide (4-HC) or mafosfamide (ASTA-Z), are also performed [9].

Doxorubicin (DOX) and vincristine (VCR) are chemotherapeutic drugs commonly used for the treatment of hematologic malignances [10, 11]. Although the mechanism of action is not fully understood, it is well accepted that DOX cytotoxic activity is associated with DNA adducts formation and inhibition of the nuclear enzyme topoisomerase II. Other biological effects include free radicals formation and interaction with components of cell membrane [12]. On the other hand, VCR exerts its anti-cancer effect binding to the building blocks of microtubules. In this way, VCR disables the cell's mechanism for aligning and moving the chromosomes, and stops the separation of the duplicated chromosomes preventing cell division [13].

Another cancer treatment modality is the so called Photodynamic therapy (PDT). It is based on the administration of a photosensitizing agent (PS), which is selectively accumulated in malignant tissue and the subsequent activation by light of appropriate wavelength. The photochemical interaction between the excited PS and molecular oxygen produces singlet oxygen as well as other reactive oxygen species (ROS), causing the death of the target cells [14, 15].

Among the many sensitizers known, porphyrins are the only endogenously generated PS by the administration of the biological precursor, 5-aminolevulinic acid (ALA), inducing the accumulation of Protoporphyrin IX (PpIX), a highly photosensitive compound [16]. ALA-induced PDT (ALA-PDT) has received increased attention during the last years and it has been successfully applied in various medical fields, such as dermatology, urology and gastroenterology, also in the photodiagnosis of tumors by means of the fluorescence detection [17].

PDT has been used to eradicate residual tumor cells in autografts and to reduce contamination of tumor cells producing minimal toxicity to progenitor or stem cells [18]. Due to the localized effect of PDT, its combination with other therapies such as radiotherapy or chemotherapy has become an active subject of research. The development of new PSs and improved laser instrumentation also contributes to propose clinical protocols incorporating PDT into multi-treatment modalities [19, 20].

The use of PDT in addition to conventional chemotherapy in the treatment of hematological malignancies could be useful not only to optimize the purging process in ABTM, but also to reach a desirable death proportion of malignant cells with lower doses of chemotherapeutic drugs. In this way, it is possible to minimize side effects of these agents and the acquisition of a drug resistance phenotype.

In this chapter, studies on the *in vitro* and *in vivo* effects of ALA-PDT in combination with the administration of chemotherapeutic drugs doxorubicine (DOX) and vincristine (VCR), in sensitive and chemoresistant murine leukemic cell lines, are presented.

MATERIALS AND METHODS

Chemicals. ALA, hydroethidine (HE), diehexyloxacarbocyanine iodide (DiOC6), 3-(4,5-dimethylthiazol-2-yl)-2,5-diphenyl-2H-tetrazolium bromide (MTT), acridine orange and ethidium bromide were obtained from Sigma Chem. Co. Annexin-V FITC and propidium iodide (PI) were obtained from Invitrogen, Argentina. VCR was kindly provided by Filaxis Pharmaceuticals S.A., Argentina and DOX by Gador Pharmaceuticals, Argentina.

In Vitro Experiments

Cell lines. Vincristine resistant (LBR-V160), doxorubicine resistant (LBR-D160) and senstitive (LBR-) murine leukemic cell lines [21], were cultured in RPMI 1640 medium (GIBCO, Gran Island, NY. USA), supplemented with 10% FCS, gentamycin and l-glutamine, at 37° C in a 5% CO_2 humidified atmosphere.

ALA incubation and porphyrin extraction. Cells grown in 15 ml Falcon tubes were incubated 4 h at 37° C with 1 mM ALA. At the end of incubation, they were centrifuged, resuspended in PBS, and intracellular porphyrins were extracted with 5% HCl. Porphyrin quantification were performed in a Perkin ElmerLS-55 luminescence spectrofluorometer. The excitation and emission wavelengths of light used were 406 and 604 nm respectively. PpIX from Porphyrin Products, Logan, Utah, USA was used as reference standard.

ALA-PDT and chemotherapy treatments. To perform combination of therapies, cells were incubated during 20 h with DOX/VCR, in RPMI complete medium. Afterwards, 1 mM ALA was added, and incubation was continued for 4 h. At the end of incubation, cells were resuspended in drug free medium and irradiated with two fluorescent lamps (Osram L

18W/765) located at 21 cm; the light spectrum was between 400 and 700 nm with the highest radiant power at 600 nm.

Intracellular PPIX fluorescence. After incubation with 1 mM ALA, cells were centrifuged and resuspended in fresh medium. They were incubated with 100 nM Mito Tracker Green and 100 nM Lyso Tracker Green (Invitrogen) 30 min at 37° C. Fluorescence were observed under confocal microscopy (Nikon D-Eclipse C1, IByME, Fundación Sales).

Cell survival analysis. Viability of cells was assessed by the MTT assay [22], performed at different times after treatments.

Oxidative stress At different times after PDT, cells were centrifuged, resuspended in PBS and loaded with the fluorescent probes for ROS, superoxide anion and mitocondrial damage detection. Stained cells were examined with a Partec PAS III flow cytometer. Superoxide anion production was detected by incubating the cells with 2 μM HE (λ excitation: 510 nm; λ emission: 590 nm) during 30 min at 37° C. To perform a positive control a cell suspension aliquot was incubated 1 h with 25 μM menadione prior to the probe addition. Mitochondrial damage was detected incubating the cells with 30 nM DiOC6 (λ excitation: 484 nm; λ emission: 511 nm) during 30 min at 37° C. For the positive control cells were incubated with 250 nM FCCP, 10 min prior to the probe addition [23].

Apoptosis detection. Nuclear changes and apoptotic body formation characteristic of apoptosis were identified by acridine orange/ethidium bromide (AO/EB) staining and fluorescence microscopy (Olympus); to quantify apoptosis and necrosis a minimum number of 200 cells were counted. The percentage of apoptotic cells (apoptotic index) was calculated as: Apoptotic cells (%) = (total number of cells with apoptotic nuclei/total number of cells counted) × 100 [24].

Morphological cell features were also analyzed by light scatter properties using a Partec PAS III flow cytometer [25]. The 3D scattergrams were obtained using WinMDI 2.9 software (Scripps Institute, La Jolla, CA).

In order to evaluate biochemical changes induced by DOX, VCR, ALA-PDT, and combined therapies, cells were collected at different times after treatments and the changes in phosphatidylserine localization in cellular membranes were analyzed using Annexin V-FITC/PI according to manufacturer's protocol. Samples were examined with a Partec PAS III flow cytometer and data obtained were analyzed using WinMDI 2.9 software (Scripps Institute, La Jolla, CA).

In Vivo Experiments

Animals. Male Balb/c strain mice, weighing 20-25 g and 2 month old were used (Bioterio FFyB,UBA). They were allowed free access to food and water, and received human care in accordance to guidelines established by the National Institute of Health Guide for the Care and Use of Laboratory Animals (AACyTAL). For each treatment, 3 to 6 animals per group were used. Mice were i.v. inoculated (200 ul) with 1×10^6 LBR- cells which have been previously subjected to the different treatments: LBR- cells without any treatment (control group), treated with only ALA-PDT, or DOX or VCR, and the combinations ALA-PDT + DOX, ALA-PDT + VCR. Control of vehicle (RPMI medium) was also performed.

Cytology studies. After the inoculations, blood extraction were performed once a week and the presence of leukemic blasts were analyzed by Giemsa staining and optical microscopy.

Histopathology. At day 30 after the inoculations, animals were sacrificed and different organs were extracted: thymus, kidney, spleen, heart, lungs, lymphatic nodes and brain; they were washed with PBS, fixed in 10% formol, paraffin included and cutted with microtome. After staining with H&E, they were analyzed under optical microscopy.

Statistics. The values in the figures are expressed as means ± standard error of the mean, and they are the average of three independent experiments run in triplicate. Data were analyzed with GraphPad Prism (GraphPad Software Inc., San Diego, CA, USA).

RESULTS

1. *In Vitro* Experiments

1.1. PPIX Production Induced by Incubation with ALA and ALA-PDT Treatment

Cells were incubated with 1 mM ALA during 4 h, afterwards, intracellular porphyrins were extracted and quantified. The amount of porphyrin accumulated in the LBR-, LBR-V160 and LBR-D160 cells was 22.5 pmol PpIX / 10^6 cells; 51.6 pmol PpIX / 10^6 cells and 27.5 pmol PpIX / 10^6 cells, respectively (Figure 1). These amount of porphyrins produced 31, 49.5 and 50.8 % of cell death when 10 min ALA-PDT was performed (Figure 2), were indicating that DOX and VCR resistant cell lines are sensitive to PDT treatment.

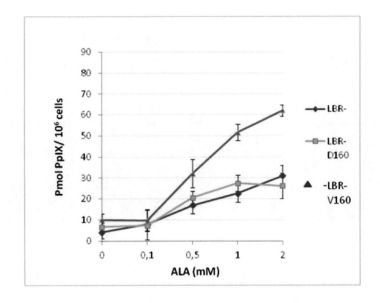

Figure 1. PpIX synthesis in LBR-, LBR-D160 and LBR-V160 cells. Cells were incubated with different concentrations of ALA during 4 h. Porphyrins were extracted and quantified as described in M&M. Data represent the mean ± SD of three independent experiments.

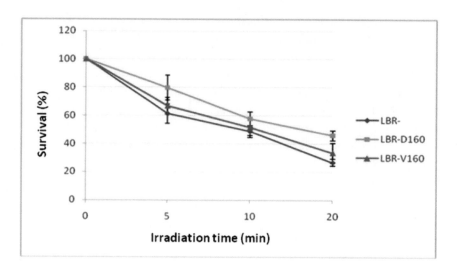

Figure 2. ALA-PDT in LBR-, LBR-D160 and LBR-V160 cells. Surviving cells were determined by the MTT assay. Data represent the mean ± SD of three independent experiments.

The typical red fluorescence of porphyrins was observed in the three cell lines under confocal fluorescence microscopy; it was confined at the mitochondria, according to the specific organelle markers. As incubation time increases, the fluorescence pattern diffuses to all the cytoplasm (Figure 3). This observation is consistent with the fact that PpIX is synthesized in the mitochondria and then diffuses to the cytosol [26] and even into the nucleus [27]. Similar results were reported by other authors in leukemic cells [28], adenocarcinoma cells [29] and hepatoma cells [30].

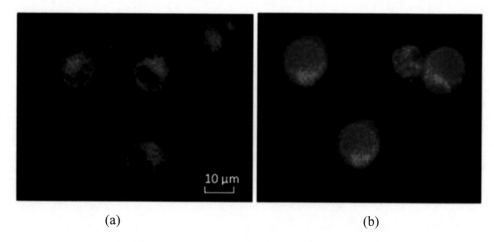

(a)   (b)

Figure 3. Intracellular PPIX fluorescence in LBR-D160 cells. Cells were incubated with 1 mM ALA during 4 h (a) and 20 h (b) 20, afterwards, observed under confocal microscopy.

1.2. Effects of ALA-PDT and Chemotherapy Agents in the LBR- Sensitive Cell Line

The sensitive LBR- cell line was treated with different doses of DOX and VCR during 24 h and LD50 for each drug was determined (Figure 4). Values obtained were 0.05 µg/ml and

0.01 µg/ml for DOX and VCR, respectively. These concentrations were used in the subsequent experiments.

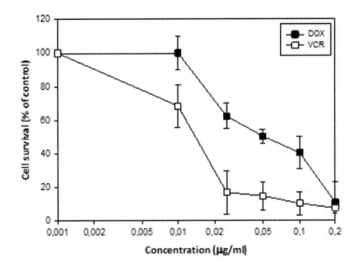

Figure 4. DOX and VCR dark toxicity. LBR- cells were incubated with different concentrations of DOX or VCR during 24 h; survival was measured by MTT assay. Control: non-treated cells. Results represent the mean ± SD of three independent experiments.

Cell viability significantly diminished when both therapies (chemotherapy + ALA-PDT) were used, in comparison with each therapy alone (Figure 5). Combination of VCR + ALA-PDT, produced higher decrease in cell survival with respect to DOX + ALA-PDT treatment.

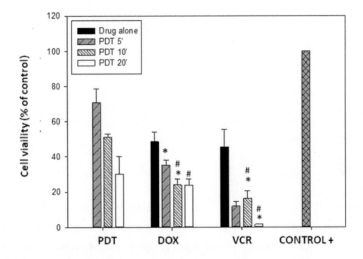

Figure 5. Survival of LBR- cells after PDT, DOX and VCR chemotherapy, and combined treatments. Survival was measured by the MTT assay after different irradiation times: 5, 10 or 20 min, in cells subjected to ALA-PDT alone, +DOX (A), +VCR (B) and combined therapies. Control: cells without any treatment. Data represent the mean ± SD of three independent experiments (* $P < 0.05$ vs. PDT, # $P < 0.05$ vs. chemotherapy drug).

Incubation of cells with DOX or VCR followed by 20 min ALA-PDT, induced cell death equivalent to that obtained with DOX or VCR doses higher than 0.1 µg/ml. These doses are twice higher than the amount of drug used in the standard chemotherapy treatment.

1.3. Effects of ALA-PDT and Chemotherapy Agents in LBR-D160 and LBR-V160 Drug Resistant Cell Lines

As indicated previously [31], drug resistant cell lines LBR-V160 and LBR-D160 were sensitive to ALA-PDT, showing a significant decrease in viability as the irradiation time increased. However, no significant differences were observed when combined therapies were used, compared to each therapy alone. These cell lines showed different responses to DOX or VCR treatment: while a 40% viability decrease was observed in LBR-D160 cells when treated with VCR, no response to any of the drugs occurred in the LBR-V160 cell line (Table I A, B).

Table I. Cell survival assessed by MTT assay after ALA-PDT (irradiation times: 5, 10 and 20 min), DOX, VCR treatment and combined therapies in LBR-D160 (A) and LBR-V160 (B) cell lines

A)

LBR-D160	Irradiation time			
Treatments	0 min	5 min	10 min	20 min
DOX	100 ± 0	98.7 ± 6.1	93.1 ± 3.7	94.1 ± 7.1
PDT + DOX		91.1 ± 3.4	78.3 ± 11	47.5 ± 7.4
VCR	60.1 ± 6.9	51.7 ± 10	57.8 ± 7.3	64.8 ± 9.1
PDT + VCR		61.03 ± 4.5	51.5 ± 2.9	22.6 ± 7.4

B)

LBR-V160	Irradiation time			
Treatments Tratamientos	0 min	5 min	10 min	20 min
VCR	100 ± 0	100 ± 0	100 ± 0	100 ± 0
PDT + VCR		69.0 ± 8.2	56.4 ± 1.5	25.4 ± 2.3
DOX	100 ± 0	97.1 ± 9.8	86.9 ± 2.8	91.5 ± 6
PDT + DOX		84.1 ± 5.4	60.4 ± 4.9	40.7 ± 2.3

Results are reported as a percentage of non-treated cells and represent the mean ± SD of three independent experiments.

1.4. Oxidative Stress Induced by ALA-PDT and Chemotherapy Agents in the LBR-Sensitive Cell Line

Superoxide anion production and changes in mitochondrial membrane potential were analyzed in order to evaluate the role of oxidative stress when combined ALA-PDT and chemotherapy agents were used. Superoxide anion was measured with the fluorescent probe HE; upon oxidation, an increase in the red fluorescence intensity of the probe is detected. The main responsible for this oxidation is oxygen free radical, with minimal oxidation by H_2O_2. [32].

We have previously demonstrated that, in the three cell lines, induction of superoxide anion (O_2^2) production and mitochondrial membrane depolarization by ALA-PDT treatment was dependent on the irradiation dose [33]. As shown in Figure 6A levels of superoxide anion increased with irradiation time in the LBR- cell line. When cells were treated with ALA-PDT in addition to DOX or VCR, production of superoxide anion was significantly higher compared to each therapy alone.

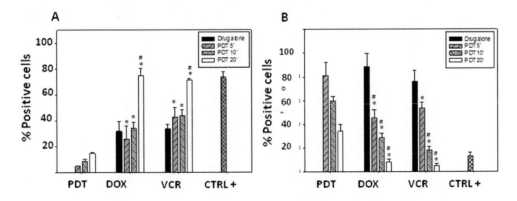

Figure 6. Superoxide anion production and mitochondrial membrane potential in the LBR- cells. Superoxide anion production was measured by HE staining (A) and changes in mitochondrial membrane potential assesed by DIOC6 staining (B), was performed 1 h after ALA-PDT with different irradiation times. Results are expressed as a percentage of stained cells relative to the control, and represent the mean ± SD of three independent experiments (* $P < 0.05$ vs PDT, # $P < 0.05$ vs chemotherapy drug).

The uptake of DiOC6, a lipophilic cationic probe commonly used for monitoring changes of the mitochondrial and/or the plasma membrane potential was also studied [33]. Results are represented in Figure 6B. It can be seen that fluorescence intensity decreased as irradiation time increased when ALA-PDT alone was performed, and diminution was higher when it was combined with DOX or VCR treatment.

1.5. Death Mechanisms Induced by ALA-PDT and Chemotherapy Agents in the LBR-Sensitive Cell Line

We evaluated the death mechanisms induced by DOX, VCR or the combination of them with ALA-PDT. Morphological changes induced by chemotherapy drugs and ALA-PDT were studied by flow cytometry analyzing the light-scattering properties of cells. It is known that cells undergoing apoptosis can be recognized by a lower intensity of forward light scatter (FSC) and a higher intensity of side light scatter (SSC), which is attributed to the cell shrinkage [25]. As can be seen in Figure 7A, cells presented a decrease in FSC and an increase in SSC, with the different treatments (DOX, VCR or ALA-PDT), as the irradiation time was longer. The effect was significantly higher when combination of therapies was used, compared to each therapy alone.

Morphological apoptotic and necrotic features were also studied by AO/EB staining. As shown in Figure 7B, an increase in apoptosis induction when combined therapies were used compared to each therapy alone, occurred in the LBR- cell line. When cells were treated with DOX (+) ALA-PDT, no significant differences in apoptotic index were observed at the different PDT light doses, while VCR (+) ALA-PDT combination exhibited a lower increase of apoptotic cells.

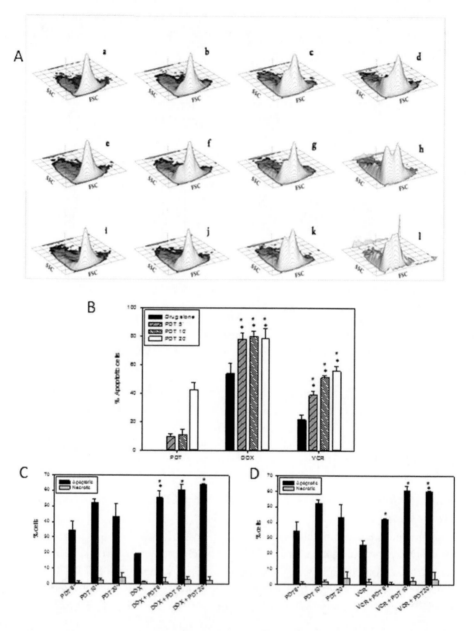

Figure 7. Three dimensional scattergrams of LBR- cells obtained by flow cytometry (A): negative control (a), treated with PDT 5 min(b), PDT 10 min (c), PDT 20 min (d), DOX (e), DOX + PDT 5 min (f), DOX + PDT 10 min (g), DOX + PDT 20 min (h), VCR (i), VCR + PDT 5 min (j), VCR + PDT 10 min (k), VCR + PDT 20 min (l). Apoptosis and necrosis induction measured by EB/OA staining (B) and Annexin V-FITC/PI staining for ALA-PDT, DOX, VCR and combined therapies (C and D). Data represent the mean ± SD of three independent experiments (* P < 0.05 vs. PDT, # P < 0.05 vs. chemotherapy drug).

Treatment with Annexin V-FITC and PI staining was used to evaluate the exposure of phosphatidylserine (PS) on the outer leaflet of the plasma membrane. The number of apoptotic cells increased with the irradiation time when ALA-PDT alone was performed. Combination of therapies using DOX (+) ALA-PDT or VCR (+) ALA-PDT, significantly increased the apoptotic cell fraction compared to each therapy alone (Figure 7 C,D). Induction of necrosis was low compared to apoptosis, suggesting that apoptosis is the major death pathway involved in these therapies. These results are consistent with those obtained with AO/EB staining.

2. *In Vivo* Experiments

2.1. Effects of ALA-PDT, Chemotherapy and the Combination of Both Therapies on Leukemic Infiltration in the Different Organs

Taking into account the results obtained in the *in vitro* model using the combination of ALA-PDT and chemotherapy, we decided to evaluate the effects in an *in vivo* model. For this purpose, Balb/c strain mice were i.v. inoculated with $1x10^6$ LBR- cells which has been previously subjected to the different treatments: LBR- cells without any treatment (control group), treated with only ALA-PDT, DOX or VCR, and ALA-PDT in addition to DOX or VCR.

As the level of blasts in blood reflects the total leukemic cells infiltrating the organs (IL), once inoculated with treated cells, animals were subjected to blood extraction once a week to evaluate blasts and undifferentiated cells with Giemsa staining.

Control group showed more undifferentiated cells compared to the groups inoculated with cells subjected to any of the treatments, and according to the results observed, we decided to sacrifice the animals 30 day after the inoculations. Then, different organs were extracted: thymus, kidney, spleen, heart, lungs, lymphatic nodes and brain; they were maintained in 10% formol until histology studies were performed, staining with H&E and analyzing under microscopy.

In the control group, IL were observed in all the animals, and in the 87.5% of the organs (Tables II and III). Animals inoculated with cells treated with ALA-PDT also showed IL, but only in the 50% of the organs.

In the case of animals inoculated with cells treated with DOX or VCR only, tumoral cells were observed in 25 and 75% of the organs respectively, and when the combination therapies: ALA-PDT + DOX or ALA-PDT + VCR were used, no IL were observed in any organ of the animals analyzed.

Table II. Leukemic infiltration (IL) in the different groups of treatment

	Animals with IL (%)	VS CONTROL	VS PDT	VS DOX	VS DOX + PDT	VS VCR
CONTROL	100					
PDT	100	NR				
DOX	50	0.1473 (NS)	0.3017 (NS)			
DOX + PDT	0	0.0047 (**)	0.0016 (**)	0.0528 (*)		
VCR	50	0.1473 (NS)	0.3017 (NS)	NR	0.0730 (NS)	
VCR + PDT	0	0.0027 (**)	0.0009 (**)	0.0730 (NS)	NR	0.0528 (NS)

P values are reported comparing the different groups according to Pearson's χ^2 test with Yates correction. Differences are not significant (NS), significant (*), highly significant (**), or not relevant (NR).

Table III. Leukemic infiltration (IL) in the organs of different groups of treatment

	Organs with IL (%)	VS CONTROL	VS PDT	VS DOX	VS DOX + PDT	VS VCR
CONTROL	87.5					
PDT	50	0.105 (NS)				
DOX	25	0.0209 (*)	0.1056 (NS)			
DOX + PDT	0	0.0004 (**)	0.0209 (*)	0.0209 (*)		
VCR	75	0.5218 (NS)	0.3017 (NS)	0.3029(NS)	0.0019 (**)	
VCR + PDT	0	0.0004 (**)	0.0209 (*)	0.1056 (NS)	NR	0.0019 (**)

P values are reported comparing the different groups, according to Pearson's χ^2 test with Yates correction. Differences are classified as not significant (NS), significant (*), highly significant (**), or not relevant (NR).

In the control group (animals inoculated with not-treated cells), all the organs analyzed except heart, were affected with IL (Table IV). In the animals inoculated with cells subjected to only ALA-PDT, or DOX, or VCR, the level of IL and the variety of organs affected were lesser than in the control group, and the organs principally affected were thymus, lungs and spleen.

Histology of the control group showed blasts focus in all the organs (Figure 8, A1 circles); in the brain, a broad peri-ventricular IL can be seen (Figure 8, B1, arrows). In the liver, leukemic cells are surrounded by vascular structures like liver arteria (AH) and central-lobulillar vein (VCL) (Figure 8 C1, arrows). The alveolar parenquima of the lung were also affected (Figure 8, D1, circle), and spleen showed alterations of the normal structure owing to the intense IL (Figure 8, E1).

Table IV. Leukemic infiltration (IL), in the different groups of treatment

	% of organs affected with IL							
LBR-	Thymus	Lung	Heart	Liver	Spleen	Kidney	Ganglion	Brain
CONTROL	100	100	0	100	100	33.3	33.3	33.3
PDT	40	60	0	0	60	0	100	0
DOX	0	0	0	0	50	0	25	0
DOX+PDT	0	0	0	0	0	0	0	0
VCR	50	25	0	25	50	0	33.3	25
VCR +PDT	0	0	0	0	0	0	0	0

Table V. Semi-quantitative evaluation of IL in each organ analyzed of the different treatment groups, determined by H&E and microscopy

	Thymus	Lung	Heart	Liver	Spleen	Kidney	Ganglion	CNS
CONTROL	+++	++	-	+	++	+++	+++	+++
PDT	+	+	-	-	+	-	+	-
DOX	-	-	-	-	+++	-	++	-
DOX + PDT	-	-	-	-	-	-	-	-
VCR	+++	+	-	+	++	-	++	+
VCR + PDT	-	-	-	-	-	-	-	-

Results represent an average of cases studied in each group. Level of IL: negative (-), mild (+), moderate (++) intense (+++).

CONTROL   **DOX + ALA-PDT**

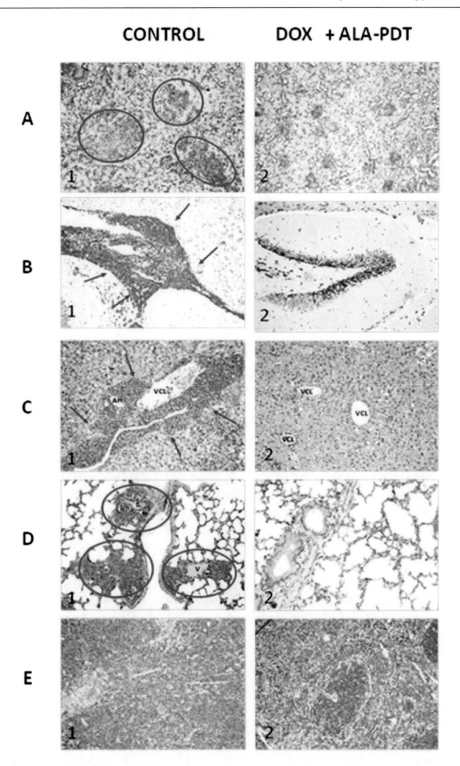

Figure 8. Histologic sections of kidney (A), brain (B), liver (C), lung (D) and spleen (E) of control group (left) and DOX + PDT treated animals (right), stained with H&E. Leukemic infiltration (IL) is indicated with circles and arrows. In the liver, central vein (VCL) and liver artery (AH) are marked.

CONCLUSION

The most common method to remove malignant cells from marrow involves a short-term *ex vivo* exposure to a variety of cytotoxic agents [34]. However, a major disadvantage of autologous bone marrow transplantation in the management of hematologic malignancies, is the contamination of the autograft with remaining leukemic cells which leads to recurrence of the disease [8]). Also, chemotherapeutic drugs do not appear to exhibit major selectivity to leukemic cells compared to normal cells; for this reason, methods to differentially protect hematopoietic progenitors from toxic chemotherapy effects using cytoprotective agents have been studied [35].

PDT is a minimally invasive therapeutic procedure based in the selective accumulation of a given PS in malignant cells and its subsequent activation with visible light and oxygen, resulting in the production of ROS, mainly singlet oxygen, which eventually produces cell death [15]. It was proposed as a method to reduce tumoral cell contamination when purging bone marrow with minimal toxicity toward hematopoietic progenitor cells [18], and combination of PDT with radiotherapy and chemotherapy was also studied [19, 20].

The complex nature of cancer disease leads to the fact that no single therapeutic modality is likely to be curative. It is becoming generally accepted that combined therapeutic modalities are important to eradicate malignant disease. Previously [31], we showed that ALA-PDT induces apoptosis in murine leukemic cells via ROS generation, a mechanism different from DOX and from VCR. Therefore, it would be expected that ALA-PDT may cooperate with DOX and VCR to increase killing of tumor cells.

There are some reports concerning the ability of chemotherapeutic drugs to enhance the effects of PDT in cell culture and transplantable mouse tumors. Using an *in vitro - in vivo* model of murine mammary adenocarcinoma, inhibition of tumor growth was significantly enhanced by the combined treatment of Adriamycin and ALA-PDT [36], and a 30% increased efficacy was observed when tumor explants were exposed to the alkylant drug Cyclophosphamide and ALA-PDT in comparison with ALA-PDT treatment alone [37]. Sinha et al. [38] found an improved overall outcome in terms of cell killing in LNcaP cells, when ALA-PDT was used in combination with methotrexate respect to each therapy alone. Peterson et al. [39] and Snyder et al. [40] reported that PDT in combination with DOX was more effective than using both therapies alone. Kirveliene et al. [41] studied the interaction between DOX and meta-tetra 3(hydrochlorin)-mediated PDT in the murine hepatoma model MH-22A; they found that DOX potentiates therapeutic efficacy of PDT and viceversa. Low dose gemcitabine increased the anticancer effect of photosan-mediated PDT evaluated in a model of human pancreatic cancer xenograft in nude mice, with no obvious adverse effects [20]. However, as far as we know, no studies about the effects of chemotherapy agents combined with ALA-PDT in leukemia cells had been reported yet.

In this chapter, we show that low doses of DOX and VCR (two times lower than the amount of drug used in the standard chemotherapy treatment) increased the anti cancer effect of ALA-PDT in LBR-cells. A significant cell viability decrease was observed in the LBR-cell line when both therapies: chemotherapy + ALA-PDT, were used in comparison with each therapy alone. The decrease in cell survival was higher when the combination VCR + ALA-PDT was used compared to DOX + ALA-PDT. When drug + PDT were used, apoptosis induction, evaluated by morphological and biochemical assays, was increased compared to each therapy alone, and similar results were observed concerning changes in the mitochondria/plasma membrane potential. The resistant cell lines LBR-V160 and LBR-D160 were sensitive to ALA-PDT, however, no significant differences were observed when combination of therapies was used.

The development of drug resistance is the major reason for failure in cancer treatment. PDT has been proposed as an alternative approach in overcoming multidrug resistance (MDR) phenotype [42]. In MCF-7 human breast cancer cells and derived doxorubicin resistant sublines, Teiten et al. [43] and Tsai et al. [44] found that PDT with Meta-tetra(hydroxyphenyl) chlorin (mTHPC) and ALA was able to killing cells expressing the MDR phenotype. More recently, it was reported that drug resistant MCF-7/DOX breast cancer cells were photodynamically killed by the pro-drug AlaAcBu, an effective ALA derivative [45]. ALA-PDT treatment was also effective in multidrug resistant leukemia cells NB4/MDR and NOMO-1/ADR but not in K562 and K562/ADR cell lines, which accumulated relatively low levels of PpIX [18], suggesting that multidrug resistant leukemia cells do not have cross-resistance to ALA-PDT. In this work we demonstrated the efficacy of ALA-PDT to overcome drug resistance on malignant cells, and we expect that apoptotic processes and oxidative stress induced by this therapy affects minimally normal cells.

The beneficial effects of using the combination of ALA-PDT with DOX or VCR in the *in vivo* model, are in concordance with the results obtained in the *in vitro* model. Canti et al. [46]. reported an additive antitumoral effect using the combination of phtalocyanine-PDT with ADR and cysplatine in mice inoculated with L1210 leukemic cells and P388 lymphoma cells. More recently, the same authors combined three therapies: m-THPC-based PDT, immunotherapy and chemotherapy with vinorelbin or cisplatine, and they found a synergic effect with both agents [47].

We realize that the inoculation of cells treated *ex-vivo* into healthy animals is not strictly comparable to bone marrow transplantation in the patients with leukemia who receive antineoplasic drugs systemically. However, the fact that leukemic infiltration were found in the brain (SNC) and kidney of the control group, suggests that the *in vitro-in vivo* model used in this research can be potentially extrapolated to humans, as this kind of IL can be observed in leukemic patients [48, 49].

Taking into account the results previously described, the benefits of ALA-PDT combined with DOX or VCR to eradicate malign cells during the bone marrow purging in leukemic patients is clear, with the addition that combined therapy allows the use of lower doses of chemotherapeutic drugs, thus minimizing undesirable drug side effects and reducing the possibility of drug resistance development. Also ALA-PDT may be a good candidate for using in the treatment of MDR cells.

ACKNOWLEDGEMENTS

This work was supported by grants from University of Buenos Aires (UBACyT X083 and 01/W521), the National Agency for Science and Technology (PICT-1806) and the National Research Council (CONICET). Authors are grateful to Gador Pharmaceuticals, Argentina and Filaxis Pharmaceuticals SA, Argentina for providing Doxorubicin and Vincristine sulfate.

REFERENCES

[1]   Gatti, L; Zunino, F. (2005). Overview of tumor cell chemoresistance mechanisms. *Methods Mol. Med.,* 111:127-148. Review.

[2]   Wilson, TR; Longley, DB; Johnston, PG. (2006). *Chemoresistance in solid tumours. Ann. Oncol.,* 17 (Suppl. 10):315-324. Review.

[3]   Fodale, V; Pierobon, M; Liotta, L; Petricoin, E. (2011). Mechanism of cell adaptation: when and how do cancer cells develop chemoresistance? *Cancer J.,* 17(2): 89-95. Review.

[4]   Hale, GA; Tong, X; Benaim, E; Cunningham, JM; Heslop, HE; Horwiz, EM et al. (2001). Allogeneic bone marrow transplantation in children failing prior autologous bone marrow transplantation. *Bone Marrow Transplant,* 27(2):155–162.

[5]   Lie, AK; Au, WY; Liang, R. (2009). Haematopoietic stem cell transplantation in Hong Kong. *Hong Kong Med. J.,* 15 (Suppl. 3):17–21.

[6]   Schultz, FW; Martens, ACM; Hagenbeek, A. (1989). The contribution of residual leukemia cells in the graft to leukemia relapse after autologous bone marrow transplantation: mathematical considerations. *Leukemia,* 3(7):530–534.

[7]   Imrie, K; Dicke, KA; Keating, A. (1996). Autologous bone marrow transplantation for acute myeloid leukemia. *Stem Cells,* 14(1):69–78. Review.

[8]   Devetten, M; Armitage, JO. (2007). Hematopoietic cell transplantation: progress and obstacles. *Ann Oncol.,* 18(9):1450–1456. Review.

[9]   Houtenbos, I; Bracho, F; Davenport, V; Slack, R; van de Ven, C; Suen, Y et al. (2001). Autologous bone marrow transplantation for childhood acute lymphoblastic leukemia: a novel combined approach consisting of *ex vivo* marrow purging, modulation of multi-drug resistance, induction of autograft vs. leukemia effect, and post-transplant immuno- and chemo-therapy (PTIC). *Bone Marrow Transplant,* 27(2):145–153.

[10]   Kostrzewa-Nowak, D; Paine, MJ; Wolf, CR; Tarasiuk, J. (2005). The role of bioreductive activation of doxorubicin in cytotoxic activity against leukaemia HL60-sensitive cell line and its multidrug-resistant sublines. *Br. J. Cancer.,* 93:89–97.

[11]   Eden, TO; Pieters, R; Richards, S. (2010). Systematic review of the addition of vincristine plus steroid pulses in maintenance treatment for childhood acute lymphoblastic leukemia – an individual patient data meta-analysis involving 5,659 children. *Br. J. Haematol.,* 149(5):722-733.

[12]   Cutts, SM; Swift, LP; Rephaeli, A; Nudelman, A; Phillips, DR. (2005). Recent advances in understanding and exploiting the activation of anthracyclines by formaldehyde. *Curr. Med. Chem. Anti-Cancer Agents,* 5:431–447.

[13]   Meininger, V; Binet, S; Chaineau, E; Fellous, A. (1990). *In situ* response to vinka alkaloids by microtubules in cultured post-implanted mouse embryos. *Biol. Cell,* 68(1):21–29.

[14]   Triesscheijn, M; Baas, P; Schellens, JH; Stewart, FA. (2006). Photodynamic therapy in oncology. *Oncologist,* 11(9):1034–1044.

[15]   Agostinis, P; Berg, K; Cengel, KA; Foster, TH; Girotti, AW; Gollnick, SO et al. (2011) Photodynamic therapy of cancer: an update. *CA Cancer J. Clin.,* 61(4):250–281.

[16] Fukuda, H; Casas, A; Batlle, A. (2005). Aminolevulinic acid: from its unique biological function to its star role in photodynamic therapy. *Int. J. Biochem. Cell Biol.,* 37:272-276.

[17] Krammer, B; Plaetzer, K. (2008). ALA and its clinical impact, from bench to bedside. *Photochem. Photobiol. Sci.,* 7(3):283–289. Review.

[18] Li, W; Zhang, WJ; Ohnishi, K; Yamada, I; Ohno, R; Hashimoto, K. (2001). 5-Aminolaevulinic acid-mediated photodynamic therapy in multidrug resistant leukemia cells. *J. Photochem. Photobiol.* B, 60(2–3):79–86.

[19] Zimmermann, A; Walt, H; Haller, U; Baas, P; Klein, SD. (2003). Effects of chlorin-mediated photodynamic therapy combined with fluoropyrimidines in vitro and in a patient. *Cancer Chemother. Pharmacol.,* 51(2):147–154.

[20] Xie, Q; Jia, L; Liu, YH; Wei, CG. (2009). Synergetic anticancer effect of combined gemcitabine and photodynamic therapy on pancreatic cancer in vivo. *World J. Gastroenterol.,* 15(6):737–741.

[21] Lopez, EL; Scolnik, M; Alvarez, E; Hajos, E. (2001). Modulatory activity of PSC 833 and cyclosporin-A in vincristine and doxorubicin-selected multidrug resistant murine leukemic cells. *Leuk. Res.,* 25:85–93.

[22] Merlin, JL; Azzi, S; Lignon, D; Ramacci, C; Zeghari, N; Guillemin, F. (1992). MTT assays allow quick and reliable measurement of the response of human tumour cells to photodynamic therapy. *Eur. J. Cancer,* 28:1452–1458.

[23] Paz, ML; González Maglio, DH; Weill, FS; Bustamante, J; Leoni, J. (2008). Mitochondrial dysfunction and cellular stress progression after ultraviolet B irradiation in human keratinocytes. *Photodermatol. Photoimmunol. Photomed.,* 24(3): 115–122.

[24] García, MG; Alaniz, L; Lopes, EC; Blanco, G; Hajos, SE; Alvarez, E. (2005). Inhibition of NF- kappaB activity by BAY 11-7082 increases apoptosis in multidrug resistant leukemic T-cell lines. *Leuk. Res.,* 29(12):1425–1434.

[25] Luksiene, Z; Eggen, I; Moan, J; Nesland, JM; Peng, Q. (2001). Evaluation of protoporphyrin IX production, phototoxicity and cell death pathway induced by hexylester of 5-aminolevulinic acid in Reh and HPB-ALL cells. *Cancer Lett.,* 169(1): 33–39.

[26] Peng, Q; Warloe, T; Berg, K; Moan, J; Kongshaug, M; Giercksky, KE; Nesland, JM. (1997) 5-Aminolevulinic acid-based photodynamic therapy: clinical research and future challenges. *Cancer,* 79:2282–2307.

[27] Chu, ES; Wu, RW; Yow, CM; Wong, TK; Chen, JY. (2006). The cytotoxic and genotoxic potential of 5-aminolevulinic acid on lymphocytes: a comet assay study. *Cancer Chemother. Pharmacol.,* 58(3):408-414.

[28] Chen, JY; Mak, NQ; Cheung, NH; Leung, RN; Peng, Q. (2001). Endogenous production of protoporphyrin IX induced by 5-aminolevulinic acid in leukemia cells. *Acta Pharmacol. Sin.,* 22(2):163-168.

[29] Gaullier, JM; Berg, K; Peng, Q; Anholt, H; Selbo, PK; Ma, LW; Moan, J. (1997). Use of 5-aminolevulinic acid esters to improve photodynamic therapy on cells in culture. *Cancer Res.,* 57:1481–86.

[30] Ren, QG; Wu, SM; Peng, Q; Chen, JY. (2002). Comparison of 5-aminolevulinic acid and its hexyl ester mediated photodynamic action on human hepatoma cells. *Acta Biochem. Biophys. Sin.,* 34(5): 650–654.

[31] Diez, B; Ernst, G; Teijo, MJ; Batlle, A; Hajos, S; Fukuda, H. (2012). Combined Chemotherapy and ALA-based Photodynamic Therapy in leukemic murine cells. *Leukemia Res.,* 36:1179-1184.

[32] Carter, W0; Narayanan, PK; Robinson, JP. (1994). Intracellular hydrogen peroxide and superoxide anion detection in endothelial cells. *J. Leukoc. Biol.,* 55:253–258.

[33] Diez, B; Cordo Russo, R; Teijo, MJ; Hajos, S; Batlle, A; Fukuda, H. (2009). Ros production by endogenously generated Protoporphyrin IX in murine leukemia cells. *Cell. Mol. Biol.,* (Noisy-le-grand) 55(2):15–19.

[34] Gorin, NC; Aegerter, P; Auvert, B; Meloni, G; Goldstone, AH; Burnett, A, et al. (1990). Autologous bone marrow transplantation for acute myelocytic leukemia in first remission: a European survey of the role of marrow purging. *Blood,* 75:1606–1614.

[35] Peters, W; Hamm, C; Baynes, R. (2000). Principles of bone marrow transplantation. In: Bast Jr RC, Kufe DW, Pollock RE, editors. *Cancer Medicine,* 18 (67), 5th edition Hamilton (ON) BC Decker; 2000. p. 890–910.

[36] Casas, A; Fukuda, H; Riley, PA; Batlle, AM del C. (1997). Enhancement of aminolevulinic acid based photodynamic therapy by adriamycin. *Cancer Lett.,* 121:105–113.

[37]] Casas, A; Fukuda, H; Batlle, AM del C. (1998). Potentiation of the 5-aminolevulinic acid-based photodynamic therapy with cyclophosphamide. *Cancer Biochem. Biophys.,* 16:183–196.

[38] Sinha, AK; Anand, S; Ortel, BJ; Chang, Y; Mai, Z; Hasan, T; et al. (2006). Methotrexate used in combination with aminolaevulinic acid for photodynamic killing of prostate cancer cells. *Br. J. Cancer,* 95(4):485–495.

[39] Peterson, CM; Shiah, JG; Sun, Y; Kopecková, P; Minko, T; Straight, RC; et al. (2003). HPMA copolymer delivery of chemotherapy and photodynamic therapy in ovarian cancer. *Adv. Exp. Med. Biol.,* 519:101–123.

[40] Snyder, JW; Greco, WR; Bellnier, DA; Vaughan, L; Henderson, BW. (2003). Photodynamic therapy: a means to enhanced drug delivery to tumors. *Cancer Res.,* 63(23):8126–8131.

[41] Kirveliene, V; Grazeliene, G; Dabkeviciene, D; Micke, I; Kirvelis, D; Juodka, B; et al. (2006). Schedule-dependent interaction between Doxorubicin and mTHPC-mediated photodynamic therapy in murine hepatoma *in vitro* and *in vivo*. *Cancer Chemother. Pharmacol.,* 57(1):65–72.

[42] Capella, MA; Capella, LS. (2003). A light in multidrug resistance: photodynamic treatment of multidrug-resistant tumors. *J. Biomed. Sci.,* 10(4):361–366. Review.

[43] Teiten, MH; Bezdetnaya, L; Merlin, JL; Bour-Dill, C; Pauly, ME; Dicato, M; et al. (2001). Effect of meta-tetra(hydroxyphenyl)chlorin (mTHPC)-mediated photodynamic therapy on sensitive and multidrug-resistant human breast cancer cells. *J. Photochem. Photobiol.* B, 62(3):146–152.

[44] Tsai, T; Hong, RL; Tsai, JC; Lou, PJ; Ling, IF; Chen, CT. (2004). Effect of 5-aminolevulinic acid mediated photodynamic therapy on MCF-7 and MCF-7/ADR cells. *Lasers Surg. Med.,* 34(1):62–72.

[45] Feuerstein, T; Berkovitch-Luria, G; Nudelman, A; Rephaeli, A; Malik, Z. (2011). Modulating ALA-PDT efficacy of mutlidrug resistant MCF-7 breast cancer cells using ALA prodrug. *Photochem. Photobiol. Sci.,* 10(12):1926–1933.

[46] Canti, B; Nicolin, A; Cubeddu, R; Taroni, P; Bandieramonte, G; Valentini, G. (1998) Antitumor efficacy of the combination of photodynamic therapy and chemotherapy in murine tumors. *Cancer Lett.,* 125: 39–44.

[47] Canti, G; Calastretti, A; Bevilacqua, A; Reddi, E; Palumbo, G; Nicolin, A. (2010). Combination of photodynamic therapy + immunotherapy + chemotherapy in murine leukemia. *Neoplasma,* 57(2):184-188.

[48] Barcos, M; Lane, W; Gomez, GA; Han, T; Freeman, A; Preisler, H; Henderson, E. (1987). An autopsy study of 1206 acute and chronic leukemias (1958 to 1982). *Cancer.* 60: 827–837.

[49] Crazzolara, R; Kreczy, A; Mann, G; Heitger, A; Eibl, G; Fink, FM; Möhle, R; Meister, B. (2001). High expression of the chemokine receptor CXCR4 predicts extramedullary organ infiltration in childhood acute lymphoblastic leukaemia. *Br. J. Haematol.,* 115(3):545-553.

Reviewed by:

  Prof. Viviana Rivarola
    Laboratorio de Biología Molecular, Facultad de Ciencias Exactas, Fisico-Químicas y Naturales, Universidad Nacional de Río Cuarto, Córdoba, Argentina. Tel: 54 0358-4676437; Email: vrivarola@exa.unrc.edu.ar

  Prof. Dr. Rafael Enríquez de Salamanca
    Research Center, Hospital 12 de Octubre, Francisco Gervás 9, Madrid 28020, Spain,
    Tel: +34 91 556 1828 S 91 556 1828 Fax: +34 91 556 9857
    Email: salamanca@med.ucm.es, enriquez@h12o.es

In: Photodynamic Therapy
Editor: Adrian G. Hugo

ISBN: 978-1-63463-857-9
© 2015 Nova Science Publishers, Inc.

Chapter 8

4-THIOTHYMIDINE AND ITS ANALOGUES AS UVA-ACTIVATED PHOTOSENSITIZERS

Giuseppe Trigiante[1,2] and Dr. Yao-Zhong Xu[1]
[1]LHCS Department, The Open University, Milton Keynes, UK
[2]Centre for Cutaneous Research, Queen Mary University, London, UK

ABSTRACT

Classical photodynamic therapy, as it has evolved in the span of nearly a century, is based on the interaction between red light and a macrocycle resulting in the subsequent activation of molecular oxygen to a highly reactive and cytotoxic singlet species. This approach has the fundamental clinical drawbacks of nonspecific bystander tissue effects and local inflammation due to necrosis. Over the last two decades an alternative approach has emerged with the potential to overcome both these limitations and it involves the use of thiated nucleoside mimics of thymidine which promise tumour selective localization and exclusive apoptotic cell killing. In this chapter we survey the development of this technology from synthesis to clinical applications.

The Open University is incorporated by Royal Charter (RC 000391), an exempt charity in England & Wales and a charity registered in Scotland(SC 038302). The Open University is authorised and regulated by the Financial Conduct Authority.

1. LIMITATIONS OF CLASSICAL PHOTODYNAMIC THERAPY

Since its beginning due to the seminal discoveries of Raab and Tappeiner (Raab 1904; Tappeiner 1904) on the toxic effects of light activated dyes, photodynamic therapy (PDT) has undergone a long evolution in terms of techniques, applications and results, some of which are extensively being discussed in other chapters in the book. As of today, PDT consists of a range of photosensitizers (porphyrins, phtalocyanins, chlorins and texaphyrins) which are clinically licensed for the treatment of some pre-malignant conditions (Actinic keratosis, Bowen's disease) and early stage basal cell carcinomas(Basset-Seguin 2013). Of these, the treatment of choice is topical aminolevulinic acid (ALA), marketed as Metvix[TM]. The main side effects reported with topical ALA treatment instead are pain and local inflammation (Lehmann 2007).

Systemic treatment using porphyrins such as Photofrin^{TM} has been largely discontinued due to the requirement of shielding the patient from ambient light for days following treatment in order to avoid unpleasant side effects on the skin due to photoactivation of the agent still in circulation. Taken together, these observations point to the weaknesses of the "classical" photosensitizers, all of which are based on the same fundamental biochemical mechanism. This core mechanism, exemplified by the archetype photosensitizer Protoporphyrin IX (PpIX, Figure 1), entails the activation of ground state "triplet" molecular oxygen to the highly reactive "singlet" species and underlies all the agents presently in use. The main reasons for the observed side effects can be thus summarized:

1. Systemic: incidental activation of the uncleared photosensitizer by ambient light following the therapeutic session
2. Local pain: diffusion of either the sensitizer itself or singlet oxygen into "bystander" cells present in the treatment area such as neurons
3. Inflammation: death occurring via necrosis of the target cells with concomitant release of cellular components able to trigger the inflammatory response(Iyer, Pulskens et al. 2009)

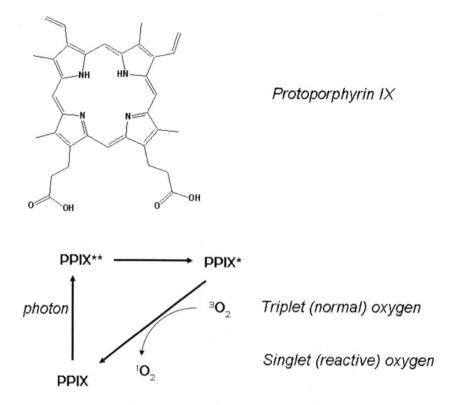

Figure 1. The structure of Protoporphyrin IX and its photodynamic reaction mechanism.

These side effects are one of the main obstacles to a more widespread application of photodynamic therapy, but there are also intrinsic requirements which by themselves prevent application of the technique to a larger set of cancers and pre-malignant conditions:

1. The lesion must be well oxygenated: As shown in Figure 1, PDT requires oxygen as a component and consumes it during the course of treatment so oxygen must be locally abundant and easily replenished
2. The lesion cannot be set more than about 10 mm deep into the body as this is the limit of red light penetration into tissues and obviously light is an essential component of the treatment itself.
3. The photosensitizer itself must diffuse into the lesion in sufficient quantities as to achieve a working concentration.

With these considerations in mind it is possible to draft a "wish-list" of the characteristics which the "ideal" photosensitizer would possess(Allison, Downie et al. 2004). The essential are:

- No intrinsic toxicity/mutagenicity
- Selective accumulation in the target tissue for selective activity
- Selective activation by a certain wavelength only to avoid unwanted activation by ambient light
- Suitable half life to allow multiple light treatments but not unwanted persistence in the body
- No side effects, either systemic or on local bystander cells
- Ease of administration

It is apparent that classical PDT agents fall short of a number of these requirements. While the "ideal" photosensitizer is an abstraction, there are other molecules which, moving away from the "singlet oxygen" paradigm as shown in Figure 1, offer an alternative better approximation to it.

The present chapter deals with one such class, the thiated thymidine nucleosides, and explores the rationale behind their possible employment in PDT and the history of their development.

2. 4-THIOTHYMIDINE

2.1. 4-Thiothymidine as a Thymidine Mimic

The nucleoside analog 4-thiothymidine (S^4dT) is a very simple derivative of its cognate nucleoside thymidine, differing from it in the simple substitution of the oxygen atom in position 4 on the pyrimidine ring by a sulfur atom (Figure 2).

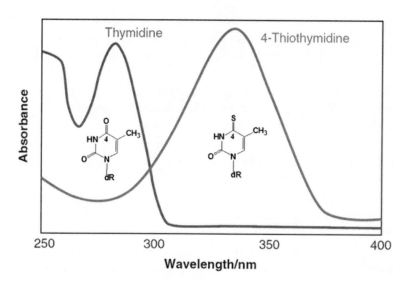

Figure 2. The structures of thymidine and 4-thiothymidine with their respective UV absorbance spectra.

In contrast to the photosensitizers in use today, which, as remarked, all share structural and functional similarity to porphyrins, the origins and history of S⁴dT are quite different. It was first synthesized in 1959 by Fox et al. (Jack J. Fox 1959) and later by Scheit (Scheit 1968) as its 5'-triphosphate. A number of studies subsequently showed the suitability of this nucleotide for DNA incorporation as a mimic of thymidine by *E.coli* DNA polymerase I, resulting in dsDNA albeit with apparently altered physical properties (Hofer and Koster 1981). Chemical synthesis of oligonucleotides containing S⁴dT by the cyanoethyl phosphoramidite method was demonstrated by Connolly and Newman (Connolly and Newman 1989) and the oligonucleotide based study approach has since been the most productive source of information about this thiobase.

One remarkable finding soon followed (Nikiforov and Connolly 1992) describing the most peculiar feature of S⁴dT: the ability to undergo photoactivation and subsequent crosslinking reactions under UV-A light (340-360 nm) wavelengths. Photoactivation of normal bases is a known phenomenon but it only occurs under UV-C and UV-B (100-280 and 280-315 nm respectively) irradiation, because of the intrinsic absorbance maxima of pyrimidines and purines in this region (around 260 nm). Photoactivation of thymine (the base of thymidine) in particular gives rise to a photochemical reaction called Diels-Alder resulting in intermolecular crosslinks within DNA among which the "thymine dimer" product is the most common (Setlow 1966). This is a lesion which is normally recognized and repaired by a dedicated DNA repair system, the nucleotide excision repair pathway (Friedberg 2003).

The reason for the different behaviour of S⁴dT lies in its molecular orbital energy levels. The C=S double bond in 4-thiothymidine is weaker than the ketone C=O bond in thymidine, resulting in a smaller energy gap between the two molecular orbitals involved in the electronic transition, therefore increasing the excitation wavelength. Moreover, the steric repulsion between the larger sulfur atom and the neighboring 5-methyl group further increases the orbital energy by distorting its shape (Yosuke Harada 2010). The net result is a substantial shift in absorbance maximum from 260 to 340 nm

The ability to undergo photoreactivity under UV-A irradiation is by no means peculiar to S^4dT. Another thiobase, 6-thioguanine, like S^4dT, also displays an important shift in its absorbance maximum to 340 nm and an increased photoreactivity following UV-A irradiation, which mostly results in DNA oxidation products (Brem and Karran 2012). What makes S^4dT unique, though, is its ability to mimic the nucleoside thymidine with little negative consequences for cells in the absence of UV-A irradiation. The thio-base in S^4dT, like thymine (T), can base-pair very well with adenine (Massey, Xu et al. 2002). The ability of S^4dT to undergo biological incorporation into eukaryotic synthesized DNA was initially shown by Domi et al. (Domi, Siromachkova et al. 1995) who successfully inactivated vaccinia virus produced in mouse cells by irradiation at 364 nm. Their study also proved that S^4dT exposure is not toxic to cells but instead only slows down proliferation, and, crucially, that DNA incorporation is conditional to the presence of the enzyme Thymidine Kinase (TK).

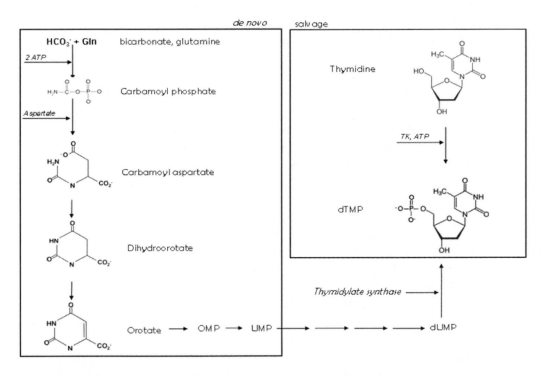

Figure 3. The *de novo* and salvage biosynthesic pathways for thymine monophosphate (dTMP). Abbreviations: OMP, orotidine 5' monophosphate; UMP, uridine 5' monophosphate; dUMP, deoxyuridine monophosphate; ATP, adenosine 5' triphosphate; TK, thymidine kinase.

Thymidine kinase is the key enzyme in the "salvage" pyrimidine biosynthesis pathway (Figure 3) and catalyzes the 5'-monophosphorylation of thymidine to form TMP, which then feeds into the normal nucleotide metabolism. It exists in two isoforms, TK1 and TK2. While the latter is constitutively expressed and localized in mitochondria, the former is cell cycle dependent and only expressed at significant levels during the G1/S phases of cellular division and hence only in actively proliferating cells (Aufderklamm, Todenhofer et al. 2011); for this reason it has been considered as a possible cancer biomarker.

2.2. 4-Thiothymidine as a Photosensitizer

By comparing the properties of S^4dT outlined above to the list of requirements of an "ideal" photosensitizer in Section 1, it becomes apparent that this molecule could play a role in photodynamic therapy. These properties of S^4dT can be summarized as below:

- It is not toxic to cells in the absence of radiation
- As a nucleoside of deoxyribose, it can only be taken up by proliferating tissues for DNA incorporation
- It is highly sensitive to the light of 320-350 nm (within UV-A range)
- It is not absorbed by non-proliferating cells (bystander tissues) such as neurons, keratinocytes
- It is a small, uncharged molecule with good water solubility and easy cellular permeation.
- It does not require any other molecule (e.g. molecular oxygen) to be activated

In fact, S^4dT fulfills more of those requirements than the classical singlet oxygen photosensitizers used in PDT as the latter easily damage non-proliferating cells such as neurons and cause considerable pain during treatment; moreover, tissue oxygenation is an absolute requirement for their function and solid cancer tissues are notoriously hypoxic, a circumstance which often hampers PDT treatments (McKeown 2014).

The investigation of the possible employment of S^4dT in photodynamic therapy was started by Karran's group at Cancer Research UK (Massey, Xu et al. 2001). They demonstrated the incorporation of S^4dT in human cells and subsequent enhancement of UV-A photosensitization by over 100 fold, a factor which was further increased (1000 fold) in xeroderma pigmentosum cells which are deficient for nucleotide excision repair pathway, proving that large adducts in DNA were responsible for the increased death rate. The fact that the observed cell death was mainly due to apoptosis was an additional welcome discovery.

Apoptosis, or programmed cell death, is an organized form of cellular death which, in contrast to necrosis, does not result in the release of cellular components in the extracellular milieu but instead causes a clean disgregation of the cell into vesicles which are then taken up by macrophages. The result is that whereas necrosis provokes intense inflammations, apoptosis doesn't and would therefore be much preferable as a means to cull cancerous cells.

The work on identifying and understanding the mechanism of action of S^4dT progressed with the identification of oligonucleotide DNA lesions induced by the drug/UV-A combination (Reelfs, Macpherson et al. 2011) and realization that such products are similar to the equivalent thymidine adducts formed following UV-B irradiation. Moreover, any role of singlet oxygen and radical oxygen species was ruled out.

This research formed the conceptual basis from which to move on to biological experiments. The first *in vivo* experiment on S^4dT was carried out by Alan Boddy and his co-workers at Newcastle University. In their 2011 article (Pridgeon, Heer et al. 2011) they injected S^4dT in rats which had been implanted with bladder cancer cells in an orthotopic fashion. Their key findings are that the drug was incorporated in the bladder cancer cells but not significantly in any other organ examined and no toxicity detected; the combination of drug and intra bladder UV-A resulted in tumour regression. Moreover, the sensitivity of cells to the drug/UV-A treatment was increased by the thymidine synthase inhibitor raltitrexed, a fact which underlines the importance of the salvage thymidine synthesis pathway in facilitating incorporation of S^4dT into DNA.

In a further move towards human cancer treatment, an experiment involving real life human cancers (basal and squamous cell carcinomas) biopsies was carried out at Queen Mary University, London, where Gemenetzidis et al., in one of the authors' (Trigiante) group, successfully demonstrated both the chemical penetration of S^4dT into the biopsies and the induced susceptibility of the cancers, even to millimeter depth, to UV-A irradiation (Gemenetzidis, Shavorskaya et al. 2013). This fact is of great clinical relevance because UV-A, unlike the red light of classical PDT, is not as penetrating into tissue (Meinhardt, Krebs et al. 2008) as red light (Stolik, Delgado et al. 2000) and the whole feasibility of S^4dT mediated cancer treatment is actually conditional to enough radiation reaching the entirety of the tumour as to activate the molecule.

Because of these results, work is now underway in our laboratory on the required preclinical studies which would eventually lead to a Phase I clinical trial on human subjects.

3. OTHER THIOBASES

3.1. 2-Thiopyrimidines

As discussed above 4-thiothymidine is UVA-sensitive due to the fact that one oxygen atom is replaced by a sulfur atom, forming an S=C double bond in the base. Besides 4-thiothymidine, it is possible to synthesize several thiobases by replacing other oxygen atoms in the nucleobases shown in Figure 4a, however not all replacements result in UVA-sensitive analogues.

2- and 4-thio pyrimidines are naturally occurring molecules. They have been found in minute amounts in the tRNA of *E. coli* and *P. aeruginosa* among the others. Their function however is the object of debate. Unlike 4-thiothymine, 2-thiothymine and 2-thiocytosine have a UV absorption maximum at 272 and 280 nm respectively (UV-B range) rather than UV-A, thus are not UV-A sensitive. In bacteria it has been suggested that they act as UV sensors (Ramabhadran, Fossum et al. 1976) used by the organisms to modulate their growth. It has also been argued that substitution of the 2-oxygen as opposed to the 4-oxygen with a sulfur atom imparts a higher stability to DNA duplexes and RNA secondary structure, and this is considered the main rationale for the observed presence of 2-thiothymidine and 2-thiouridine in the tRNA of thermophilic bacteria (Edmonds, Crain et al. 1991). The replication of 2-thiothymidine containing DNA appears to occur more efficiently than for 4-thiothymidine when bacterial DNA polymerase I is employed (Sintim and Kool 2006). However, in parallel to this 2-thiopyrimidines appear to have a light-independent deleterious effect on viral replication in eukaryotic cells (Shigeta, Mori et al. 1999) and cytotoxicity (Latosinska, Seliger et al. 2012) (Lozzio and Wigler 1971), a possible indication of a less efficient incorporation operated by eukaryotic DNA polymerases, although research in this field is very limited.

A

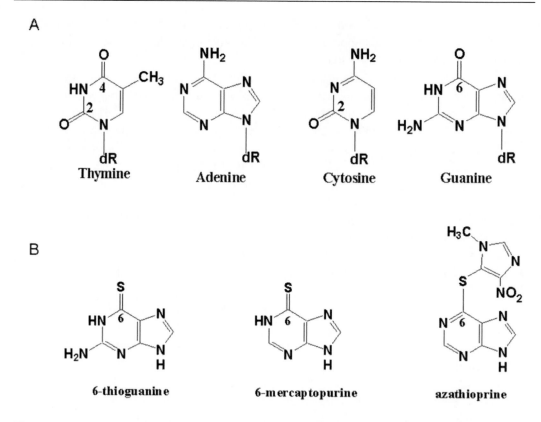

B

Figure 4. Structure of the four nucleobases (A) and of the 6-thiopurine base analogues (B).

3.2. 6-Thiopurines

Of all thiobases, the 6-thiopurines receive the most attention as they have been in clinical use for a long time. The family comprises three compounds: 6-thioguanine, 6-mercaptopurine and azathioprine, the latter being but a prodrug of mercaptopurine (Figure 4b).

Unlike 4-thiothymidine, 6-thioguanine and 6-mercaptopurine are antimetabolites which exhibit cytotoxic effects regardless of external radiation and are thus in widespread clinical use as immunosuppressants (Munshi, Lubin et al. 2014) in the treatment of conditions such as inflammatory bowel disease, Crohns disease and post-transplant immunosuppression. At higher doses they act as proper chemotherapics and are employed in the treatment of leukaemias.

The underlying mechanism of action of thiopurines is poorly understood (Fotoohi, Coulthard et al. 2010) but it involves substitution for genuine substrates in enzymes of the *de novo* biosynthesis pathway of purine nucleotides, which ultimately allows thiated guanine 5'-triphosphate into the DNA of replicating cells. The anomalous base is then methylated and either directs incorporation of the wrong complementary nucleotide (T instead of C) or engages the DNA mismatch repair system (MMR) in a futile repair attempt which leads to cell cycle arrest and apoptosis (Swann, Waters et al. 1996). In support of this fact, MMR deficiency leads to increased drug resistance.

Taken at face value, this would categorize the thiopurines as mere antimetabolites or chemotherapics whose activity is independent of external factors. However, the long standing observation that transplant recipients under azathioprine treatment are tens to hundreds of times more susceptible to late onset non melanoma skin cancers (Moloney, Comber et al. 2006) and that sun exposure is a risk factor (Fuente, Sabat et al. 2003) has led to the observation that 6-thioguanine incorporated in DNA behaves as a photosensitizer towards UV-A light like 4-thiothymidine, causing oxidative DNA lesions (Brem and Karran 2012) and to the speculation that this may ultimately be the causative agent behind the cancers (Attard and Karran 2012).

The main action of thiopurines is however the systemic, light-independent immunosuppression and chemotherapic one and although very useful as drugs in their present fields of use, it is unlikely that they can be used as pure photosensitizers unless perhaps administered topically, but so far no attempts have been made at this requalification of the molecules.

4. DERIVATIVES

4.1. 5'-Halo-4-Thiodeoxyuridines

Given the success of 4-thiothymidine as a potential photosensitizer drug, research has since gone into the synthesis of analogues and precursors with enhanced biological activity or more desirable pharmacokinetic properties. This work has been conducted mainly by Xu at the Open University and Zhang at Dalian University, China.

Taking the sulfur atom in position 4 as the necessary determinant of the UV absorbance shift and therefore of the UV-A sensitivity, modifications have been attempted on other parts of the molecule. The replacement of 2-oxygen with a sulfur atom, as previously seen, appears to impede DNA replication and does not shift the absorption of the base to the UV-A range, thus it has therefore been left unmodified. More attention was drawn by the methyl in position 5 in view of the fact that, in thymidine, replacement of it with bromine leads to 5-bromodeoxyuridine (5-BrdU). This is a viable thymidine analog which has been used for almost 40 years in immunologic quantification of cell proliferation (Gratzner, Leif et al. 1975). It is incorporated and retained in cells for many cell doublings and does not cause significant toxicity. It is therefore, just like 4-thiothymidine, a viable substrate for both thymidine kinase and human DNA polymerase II thus implying a certain tolerance of these enzymes for the 5-substituent of a pyrimidine. With this in mind, Xu and colleagues synthesized a series of 5-halogenated deoxyuridines (the term thymidine requires the presence of a 5 methyl group) and evaluated their physico-chemical properties(Zhang and Xu 2011; Zhang, Gu et al. 2014). A summary of these properties is outlined in Figure 5A.

The biological properties of these molecules, and in particular DNA incorporation efficiency and cytotoxicity in the presence and absence of UV-A light are being studied in Trigiante's lab at Queen Mary University, London. Preliminary results ascribe the strongest, even more than S^4dT itself, cytotoxic effect to the 5-Br derivative (Figure 5B, unpublished data). This could be linked to enzymatic compatibility of the bases, with the iodine atom's van der Waals radius around 0.21 nm (by comparison to that of bromine, 0.19 nm and the methyl group, 0.2 nm) (Batsanov 2001).

A

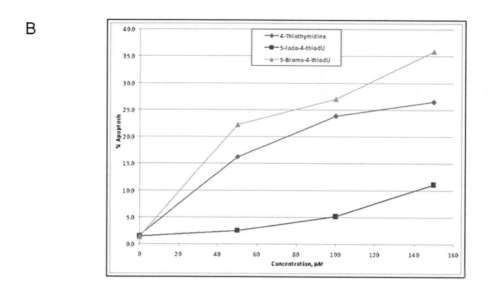

Group (X)	Electro-negativity	^{13}C NMR of 5-C (ppm)	UV absorption (maximum, nm)
CH_3	2.5 (C)	117.70	335
F	4.0	147.23	331
Cl	3.0	116.37	338
Br	2.8	106.63	340
I	2.5	82.99	345

B

Figure 5. Comparison of selected properties of 5-substituted 4-thiodeoxyuridines (A); compared photodynamic biological activity of 4-thiothymidine, 5-iodo and 5-bromo 4-thiodeoxyuridine (B).

4.2. 5'-Substituted 4-Thiodeoxyuridines

Synthesis of a series of 5-substituted 4-thiodeoxyuridines including 5-furanyl and 5-thien-2yl analogues have also been carried out in Zhang's lab, but their biological activity has not been evaluated yet. It is of note that a relatively new thymidine analogue has been described, 5-ethynyl deoxyuridine or EdU (Chehrehasa, Meedeniya et al. 2009) which is efficiently incorporated in DNA and therefore used as a proliferation marker. The biologic viability of EdU confirms the flexibility at position 5, opening synthetic possibilities for the future.

4.3. Other Possible Variations on 4-Thiothymidine

In view of the present knowledge about the molecule and its mechanism of action, it is possible to speculate on other potential activity enhancing modifications. For example, as the sulfur atom on the 4-position is crucial for its high UV-A sensitivity, a suitable masking of the sulfur atom, such as N-methyl-imidazole used at the drug azathioprine (see Fig 4b) is expected to increase the stability of the drug and possibly enhance the pharmacological properties. Similarly a phosphoramidate form of 4-thiothymidine would avoid the need for the phosphorylation step by thymidine kinase, thus increasing cellular uptake and potency of the drug.

CONCLUSION

The two remarkable properties of 4-thiothymidine, its ability to mimic thymidine and be incorporated in the DNA of actively proliferating cells with little or no toxicity, and its unique and exquisite sensitivity to UV-A radiation, an otherwise harmless frequency range, have stimulated research on its clinical employment as a new concept photosensitizer.

Results in solution, on cells and tumour biopsies have all consistently confirmed this compound's potential as a safe and effective tool to selectively target cancer cells while potentially doing away with the side effects (pain and inflammation) normally associated with classical singlet oxygen based photodynamic therapy. To summarize, Table 1 (below) lists the pros and cons of S^4dT/UV-A vs classical PDT outlining the possible advantages and challenges that this new technique presents.

Table 1. Comparisons between S^4dT/UV-A and Classical PDT

Feature	S^4dT/UV-A based PDT	Classical PDT
Intrinsic safety to patient	Yes	Yes
Localization in tumours	Complete	Partial
Need for oxygenation	No	Yes
Cell death modality	Apoptosis	Necrosis/apoptosis
Pain	None anticipated	Yes
Local Inflammation	None anticipated	Yes
Mutagenicity	None anticipated	No
Light radiation wavelength	UV-A	Red
Light penetration(approx) *	100 μm (at 340 nm)	10 mm

* Meinhardt, Krebs et al. 2008 and Stolik, Delgado et al. 2000.

The final proof of this approach will have to wait for the human clinical trials which should take place in the near future. The flexibility at position 5 of the pyrimidine ring allowed other, more effective derivatives to be synthesized and possibly more still are to come in the future. Their successful clinical employment may extend the so far limited scope of application of the exciting concept of photodynamic therapy.

REFERENCES

Allison, R. R., G. H. Downie, et al. (2004). "Photosensitizers in clinical PDT." *Photodiagnosis Photodyn Ther* 1(1): 27-42.

Attard, N. R. and P. Karran (2012). "UVA photosensitization of thiopurines and skin cancer in organ transplant recipients." *Photochem Photobiol* Sci 11(1): 62-8.

Aufderklamm, S., T. Todenhofer, et al. (2011). "Thymidine kinase and cancer monitoring." *Cancer Lett* 316(1): 6-10.

Basset-Seguin, N. (2013). "[PDT panoramic view. Principle, photosensitizers, light sources and validated indications in dermatology]." *Ann Dermatol Venereol* 140 Suppl 2: 223-8.

Batsanov, S. S. (2001). "Van der Waals Radii of Elements." *Inorganic Materials* 37(9): 871-885.

Brem, R. and P. Karran (2012). "Multiple forms of DNA damage caused by UVA photoactivation of DNA 6-thioguanine." *Photochem Photobiol* 88(1): 5-13.

Chehrehasa, F., A. C. Meedeniya, et al. (2009). "EdU, a new thymidine analogue for labelling proliferating cells in the nervous system." *J Neurosci Methods* 177(1): 122-30.

Connolly, B. A. and P. C. Newman (1989). "Synthesis and properties of oligonucleotides containing 4-thiothymidine, 5-methyl-2-pyrimidinone-1-beta-D(2'-deoxyriboside) and 2-thiothymidine." *Nucleic Acids Res* 17(13): 4957-74.

Domi, A., M. Siromachkova, et al. (1995). "Photoinactivation (365 nm) of vaccinia and herpes simplex viruses induced by a new built-in DNA photosensitizer: 4-thiothymidine." *Photochem Photobiol* 61(5): 463-70.

Edmonds, C. G., P. F. Crain, et al. (1991). "Posttranscriptional modification of tRNA in thermophilic archaea (Archaebacteria)." *J Bacteriol* 173(10): 3138-48.

Fotoohi, A. K., S. A. Coulthard, et al. (2010). "Thiopurines: factors influencing toxicity and response." *Biochem Pharmacol* 79(9): 1211-20.

Friedberg, E. C. (2003). "DNA damage and repair." *Nature* 421(6921): 436-40.

Fuente, M. J., M. Sabat, et al. (2003). "A prospective study of the incidence of skin cancer and its risk factors in a Spanish Mediterranean population of kidney transplant recipients." *Br J Dermatol* 149(6): 1221-6.

Gemenetzidis, E., O. Shavorskaya, et al. (2013). "Topical 4-thiothymidine is a viable photosensitiser for the photodynamic therapy of skin malignancies." *J Dermatolog Treat* 24(3): 209-14.

Gratzner, H. G., R. C. Leif, et al. (1975). "The use of antibody specific for bromodeoxyuridine for the immunofluorescent determination of DNA replication in single cells and chromosomes." *Exp Cell Res* 95(1): 88-94.

Hofer, B. and H. Koster (1981). "Enzymatic synthesis, ligation, and restriction of DNA containing deoxy-4-thiothymidine." *Nucleic Acids Res* 9(4): 753-67.

Iyer, S. S., W. P. Pulskens, et al. (2009). "Necrotic cells trigger a sterile inflammatory response through the Nlrp3 inflammasome." *Proc Natl Acad Sci U S A* 106(48): 20388-93.

Jack J. Fox, D. V. P., Iris Wempen, Iris L. Doerr, Loretta Cheong, Joseph E. Knoll, Maxwell L. Eidinoff, Aaron Bendich, George Bosworth Brown (1959). "Thiation of Nucleosides. II. Synthesis of 5-Methyl-2'-deoxycytidine and Related Pyrimidine Nucleosides." *J. Am. Chem. Soc.* 81(1): 178–187.

Latosinska, J. N., J. Seliger, et al. (2012). "A comparative study of the hydrogen-bonding patterns and prototropism in solid 2-thiocytosine (potential antileukemic agent) and cytosine, as studied by 1H-14N NQDR and QTAIM/ DFT." *J Mol Model* 18(1): 11-26.

Lehmann, P. (2007). "[Side effects of topical photodynamic therapy]." *Hautarzt* 58(7): 597-603.

Lozzio, C. B. and P. W. Wigler (1971). "Cytotoxic effects of thiopyrimidines." *J Cell Physiol* 78(1): 25-32.

Massey, A., Y. Z. Xu, et al. (2001). "Photoactivation of DNA thiobases as a potential novel therapeutic option." *Curr Biol* 11(14): 1142-6.

Massey, A., Y. Z. Xu, et al. (2002). "Ambiguous coding is required for the lethal interaction between methylated DNA bases and DNA mismatch repair." *DNA Repair (Amst)* 1(4): 275-86.

McKeown, S. R. (2014). "Defining normoxia, physoxia and hypoxia in tumours-implications for treatment response." *Br J Radiol* 87(1035): 20130676.

Meinhardt, M., R. Krebs, et al. (2008). "Wavelength-dependent penetration depths of ultraviolet radiation in human skin." *J Biomed Opt* 13(4): 044030.

Moloney, F. J., H. Comber, et al. (2006). "A population-based study of skin cancer incidence and prevalence in renal transplant recipients." *Br J Dermatol* 154(3): 498-504.

Munshi, P. N., M. Lubin, et al. (2014). "6-thioguanine: a drug with unrealized potential for cancer therapy." *Oncologist* 19(7): 760-5.

Nikiforov, T. T. and B. A. Connolly (1992). "Oligodeoxynucleotides containing 4-thiothymidine and 6-thiodeoxyguanosine as affinity labels for the Eco RV restriction endonuclease and modification methylase." *Nucleic Acids Res* 20(6): 1209-14.

Pridgeon, S. W., R. Heer, et al. (2011). "Thiothymidine combined with UVA as a potential novel therapy for bladder cancer." *Br J Cancer* 104(12): 1869-76.

Raab, O. (1904). "Uber die Wirkung Fluorescierenden Stoffe auf Infusorien." *Zeitschrift für Biologie* 39: 524-546.

Ramabhadran, T. V., T. Fossum, et al. (1976). "Escherichia coli mutant lacking 4-thiouridine in its transfer ribonucleic acid." *J Bacteriol* 128(2): 671-2.

Reelfs, O., P. Macpherson, et al. (2011). "Identification of potentially cytotoxic lesions induced by UVA photoactivation of DNA 4-thiothymidine in human cells." *Nucleic Acids Res* 39(22): 9620-32.

Scheit, K. G. (1968). "[The synthesis of 4-thiouridine-5'-diphosphate, 4-thiouridine-5'-triphosphate and desoxy-4-thiothymidine-5'-triphosphate]." *Chem Ber* 101(4): 1141-7.

Setlow, R. B. (1966). "Cyclobutane-type pyrimidine dimers in polynucleotides." *Science* 153(3734): 379-86.

Shigeta, S., S. Mori, et al. (1999). "Anti-herpesvirus activities and cytotoxicities of 2-thiopyrimidine nucleoside analogues in vitro." *Antivir Chem Chemother* 10(4): 195-209.

Sintim, H. O. and E. T. Kool (2006). "Enhanced base pairing and replication efficiency of thiothymidines, expanded-size variants of thymidine." *J Am Chem Soc* 128(2): 396-7.

Stolik, S., J. A. Delgado, et al. (2000). "Measurement of the penetration depths of red and near infrared light in human "ex vivo" tissues." *J Photochem Photobiol* B 57(2-3): 90-3.

Swann, P. F., T. R. Waters, et al. (1996). "Role of postreplicative DNA mismatch repair in the cytotoxic action of thioguanine." *Science* 273(5278): 1109-11.

Tappeiner, H. v. A. J. (1904). "Uber die Wirkung der photodynamischen (fluorescierenden) Stoffe auf Protozoen und Enzyme." *Deutsches Archiv für klinische Medizin* 80: 427-487.

Zhang, J., H. Gu, et al. (2014). "Exploring the binding of 4-thiothymidine with human serum albumin by spectroscopy, atomic force microscopy, and molecular modeling methods." *Carbohydr Res* 384: 102-11.

Zhang, X. and Y. Z. Xu (2011). "NMR and UV Studies of 4-Thio-2′-deoxyuridine and Its Derivatives." *Molecules* 16(7): 5655-5664.

In: Photodynamic Therapy
Editor: Adrian G. Hugo

ISBN: 978-1-63463-857-9
© 2015 Nova Science Publishers, Inc.

Chapter 9

TOWARDS MULTIFUNCTIONAL HYBRID NANOSYSTEMS FOR PDT: POLYMERIC NANOSTRUCTURES CONTAINING ZINC SELENIDE NANOPARTICLES AND PHOTOSENSITIZER

T. E. Sukhanova[1], M. L. Gelfond[2], V. A. Bershtein[3], S. V. Valueva[1], M. E. Vylegzhanina[1], A. Ya. Volkov[1], A. A. Kutin[1] and G. N. Matveeva[1]

[1]Institute of Macromolecular Compounds, Russian Academy of Sciences, St.-Petersburg, Russia
[2]N.N. Petrov Research Institute of Oncology, the Health Ministry of RF, St.-Petersburg, Russia
[3]Ioffe Physical-Technical Institute, Russian Academy of Sciences, St.-Petersburg, Russia

ABSTRACT

The use of a photodynamic therapy (PDT) is hampered in some cases by the inability to create a sufficient concentration of photosensitizer (PS) in a tumor or the inability to deliver effectively laser radiation in some localization of malignant neoplasms. A number of nosological forms of the primary tumor and its metastases (in brain, peripheral parts of the lung, pancreas, liver, kidney, and bone tissue) are not available for exposure to light, which not only limits the possibilities for PDT application but also reduces in general the effectiveness of cancer care.

One promising way to improve this situation with PDT is the creation of hybrid polymer nanosystems (HPNS) containing nanostructures from the nanoparticles (NPs) and PS, which activation is carried out without the constraints and can easily penetrate to any depth in the human body using an ionizing radiation (X-ray or gamma radiation). Under the action of ionizing radiation, NPs generate light in the spectral range required for PS activation. The nanostructures can go into the tumor itself or the blood stream with a special media such as NPs-containing colloids.

The motivation for this work was synthesizing the novel HPNSs based on zinc selenide (ZnSe) nanoparticles, stabilized by biocompatible water-soluble polymers, and a new generation PS - the Photodithazine (PD) under different conditions of their preparation. The results of PD clinical trials have demonstrated a high clinical potential of the drug, exhibiting good solubility in water and physiological media and high absorption selectivity for tumor. Our research focuses on designing water-soluble, stable in the biological environment and non-toxic HPNS. Perspective applications of prepared HPNS include, for example, their use as fluorescent cellular labels, deep-tissue and tumor imaging agents, and sensitizers for PDT in cancer treatment.

The paper briefly covers the morphology, crystalline and electronic structure of novel ZnSe-and PD-containing HPNS, their spectral characteristics and bioactivity. The combination of atomic-force microscopy (AFM), high-resolution electron microscopy (HREM), X-ray diffraction (XRD), X-ray photoelectron spectroscopy (XPS), differential scanning calorimetry (DSC), infra-red spectroscopy (IR), photoluminescence (PL), and UV-vis spectroscopy methods are used.

Our research is oriented towards the development of new generation of drugs for selective PDT in oncology.

1. INTRODUCTION

In our hard "war against cancer" [1] for the past few decades, several drastically novel approaches based on nanobiotechnological platform using NPs and quantum dots (QDs), sometimes with polymers, which can attack tumors, have appeared. Many research groups have developed multifunctional nanosystems containing NPs or QDs to seek out cancer cells and deliver imaging nanostructures and drugs to them.

Recently, nanobiotechnology- based methods for the complex diagnostics and treatment of oncological diseases based on programmed drug delivery to sick organs are being developed intensively. The most promising of them is the method of photodynamic therapy (PDT) [2, 3]. This is a much more attenuated method in clinical practice than surgery or radiation therapy, which lies in the introduction of a tumorotropic photosensitizer (PS) into the human organism. It is mainly accumulated in the lipid bilayer of the tumorous cells, actively participates in the oxidation of the biological material under the action of radiation (visible light, laser, UV or IR radiation), and generates cytotoxic singlet oxygen $^1O_2$. However, the impact of present PSs on cancerous cells is low for several reasons. First, the lifetime of $^1O_2$ in a cell does not exceed 10 μs [2, 3]. Second, porphyrin derivatives are usually used as sensitizers in PDT, the drawback of which is a tendency to aggregation in an aqueous medium; this strongly reduces their efficiency [3, 4]. As a result, the PS dose is increased in practice which leads to undesirable side effects, e.g., to the phototoxic one. Other traditional PSs are unstable and, as a rule, highly toxic limiting their use in a clinical practice. These circumstances dictate the need to both search for ways of decreasing the drug doses in PDT and create fundamentally new photosensitive materials for PDT [2]. Also, the problem of insufficient contrast between the accumulation of PD in malignant and in healthy cells has yet to be solved [3, 5].

One way to improve the efficiency of PDT drugs is to bind PS molecules to those of other substances (e.g., liposomes, nanoparticles, or polymers) in order to enhance the selectivity of PS accumulation in tumors [6], and to reduce the administration of PDT drug doses. One such drug is Photolon, a molecular complex of chlorin E6 salt and the medical polymer poly-N-vinylpyrrolidone [7]. It is therefore of great interest to find new effective hybrid polymer systems for PDT by investigating the interaction between PS and polymers of different natures, such as polyampholites and polyelectrolites, and various nanoparticles. It was founded that a complex formation of some amphiphilic polymers with PS increases the efficiency of the effect of PS on tumorous cells more than tenfold [8].

In our studies, discussed here, we have investigated the morphology, crystalline and electronic structure of novel ZnSe-containing HPNSs with water-soluble bioactive polymers as stabilizer, their spectral characteristics and bioactivity, under changing the composition and molar ratio between the components. The complex formation between several polymers, possessing the hydrophobic fragments, a second-generation photosensitizer - "Photodithazine" (PD), and between the components in the ZnSe-containing HPNSs are demonstrated.

2. STUDY OF THE COMPLEX FORMATION OF WATER-SOLUBLE POLYMERS AND PHOTOSENSITIZER

2.1. Photodithazine – A Second-Generation Photosensitizer for PDT

The design of effective photosensitizers for the PDT of oncological diseases is a topical problem now. Derivatives of porphyrin, phthalocyanine, chlorins, and bacteriochlorins are commonly used as sensitizers in PDT. An important feature of these compounds is their combination of high PS activity and the ability to absorb light in the red and near IR regions of the spectrum (i.e., in the so-called "range of the tissue transparency window" at $\lambda = 650–900$ nm). The absorption of light by biological tissues in this range is minimal and the light penetrates deeper into the tissues of the body [1, 2]. One disadvantage of these compounds, as the representatives of the first PS generation, is their tendency to aggregation in aqueous media, which lowers their efficiency [2-5]. In Russia and other countries, PSs of the second generation have recently been developed and introduced into clinical practice, e.g., Temoporfin, Photofrin, Photogem, and Photosan, along with drugs based on chlorophyll derivatives, such as Photochlorin and Photodithazine; these systems exhibit high rates of excretion in addition to strong absorption in the red region of the spectrum [9, 10].

Photodithazine (PD) is N-methyl-D-glucosamine salt of E6 chlorin [11] that is easily soluble in water without forming aggregates, ensuring its high photodynamic activity. In addition, PD has the best pharmacokinetic properties among the PSs of this series [12], as it is an effective sensitizer for treating a broad range of tumors such as skin cancer, cancer of the thyroid gland, malignant brain tumors, etc. PD is nontoxic for humans and use in PDT as active oxygen generator [10, 11, 12]. PD sensitizer has the structural formula:

It should be noted that PD molecules have a typical hydrophobic porphyrin core and peripheral hydrophilic oxygen containing groups [11]. The topical problem in our study was the investigation of mechanisms of the interaction between PD and nanoparticles stabilized by bio- and synthetic polymers in view of the need for developing new efficient therapeutic and oncologic drugs [13-15].

2.2. Water-Soluble Polymers for ZnSe Nanoparticles Stabilization

A set of ionic water-soluble polymers with hydrophobic fragments in their macromolecules were employed as polymeric stabilizers (PSts) in our work [13-16]:

4. Polycation, the biocompatible poly-*N*-methacryloyloxyethyl-*N,N,N*-trimethylammoniummethyl sulfate (PMETAMS) with molecular weight $M_w = 170 \times 10^3$.
5. The weak polyacid, poly(methacrylic acid) (PMAA) with $M_w = 35 \times 10^3$.
6. The strong polyacid, poly(2-acrylamido-2-methyl–1-propanesulfonic acid) (PAMPSA) with $M_w = 2.5 \times 10^6$.
7. Nonionic synthetic polymer - poly-N-vinyl-2-pyrrolidone (PVP).
8. Natural polymer - bovine serum albumin (BSA).

In the work [13], the complexation of above-mentioned polymers was investigated in mixtures containing ~1 wt. % of PD sensitizer.

The ZnSe-containing HPNSs were prepared in two steps process as described in [14-16]. First, to perform the hydrothermal synthesis of ZnSe nanoparticles, a sodium selenite aqueous solution was mixed with a zinc acetate $(Zn(Ac)_2 \cdot 2H_2O)$ solution. After vigorous stirring, the mixture was placed into an autoclave, and hydrazine hydrate $(N_2H_4 \cdot H_2O)$ was added afterwards. The autoclave was placed into a thermostat and kept at a temperature of 180°C for 4 h. In the second step, for the preparation of ZnSe nanosystems with polymer stabilizers, a calculated weighted amount of dried ZnSe powder was introduced into the corresponding polymer stabilizer solution and stirred intensively for 2 h [14, 15].

2.3. Spectral Characterization of Complex Formation

The absorption spectra of traditional photosensitizers including those of the porphyrin series are sensitive to complex formation in the visible region; therefore, the analysis of the absorption spectra of the studied systems was used to confirm the formation of the polymer/PD and ZnSe/polymer/PD complexes. To study the process of complex formation in these double and triple systems, we measured the curves of the dependence of the absorbance D on the wavelength λ for PD and the nanosystems (Figs. 1–3).

Figure 1 shows the results of measuring the dependencies of absorbance D on wavelength in the spectral region of 500 to 720 nm for aqueous solutions of the initial PD and PSt–PD mixtures [13]. In this region of wavelengths, the absorption band at λ= 645 nm is typical of PD (Figure 1, curve 1). For PSt/PD systems (i.e., PMETAMS/PD, PAMPSA/PD, and PMAA/PD) changes are observed in the intensity and position of the absorption bands (Figure 1, curves 2–4). For the PMETAMS/ PD system, an increase in PD peak amplitude is observed along with a bathochromic shift from $\lambda = 645$ nm to $\lambda = 660$ nm (Figure 1, curve 2). Two overlapping bands are observed for the PMAA/PD system, the first being close to the position of the pure PD absorption band, and the second one to the position of the PMETAMS/PD system's peak, with the intensities of both being substantially lower than that of the initial PD (Figure 1, curve 4).

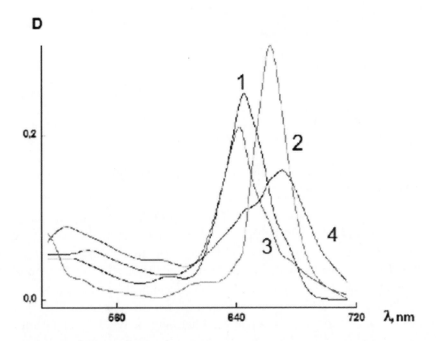

Figure 1. Spectra in the visible region for PD (1) and mixtures of polymers with PD (99 : 1) in an aqueous solution: PMETAMS/PD (2); PAMPSA/PD (3); PMAA/PD (4) [13].

As there were no absorption bands in the studied spectral region for all of neat PSts, the changes detected in the visible spectra demonstrate the ability of PMETAMS and PMAA polymers to form complexes with PD. For the PAMPSA/PD system, there is no virtually shift in the main absorption peak typical of pure PD (Figure 1, curve 3), and peak intensity is only slightly lower than that of the pure PD. This suggests that complexes do not seem to form in the PAMPSA/ PD system.

Figure 2 shows the UV-vis. spectra of aqueous solutions of binary PMAA/PD (1) and ternary ZnSe/PMAA/PD (2) nanosystems with 1 wt.% PD. PMAA/PD system manifests three absorption bands in the UV-visible range: at 280, 400 (the Soret band) and 640 nm. For the ZnSe/PMAA/PD, the peak intensity at $\lambda = 280$ nm increases, and also a considerable growth of peaks at $\lambda = 320$-460 and 600-700 nm can be seen. At last, a new low-intensity peak at $\lambda \approx 500$ nm appears in the case of the ternary system. Of a special significance, ternary nanosystem produces much stronger response in a desired for PDT spectral range of 640-670 nm ("tissue transparency window"). Such changes in the spectrum may be attributed certainly to complex formation between polymer, PD and ZnSe nanoparticles.

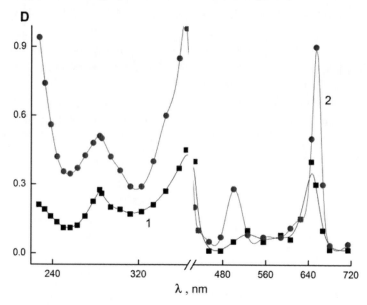

Figure 2. UV-vis. spectra of aqueous solutions of binary PMAA/PD (1) and ternary ZnSe/PMAA/PD (2) nanosystems containing 1.0 wt.% PD.

Figure 3 shows the far-IR spectra of PMAA and PMETAMS films and the mixtures of these polymers with PD [13]. Two broad absorption bands with the maxima at 188 and 356 cm^{-1} are observed in the PMAA spectrum (Figure 3a). The first maximum corresponds to the vibrational modes of double H-bonds (the cycles formed by pairs of COOH groups) although the broad absorption band is likely to include also a band of the vibrational modes of single H-bonds (~100–120 cm^{-1} [17]). The band at 356 cm^{-1} is due to mixed torsional and deformation skeletal vibrations in PMAA [18]. After introducing 1 % PD, a shift of the 356 cm^{-1} band to 390 cm^{-1} is observed along with a drop in its intensity, and the form of the band at 188 cm^{-1} changes asymmetrically toward short wavelengths. These changes may be interpreted as a consequence of PMAA–PD complex formation, in particular as some suppression of the chain dynamics. Lesser changes caused by adding PD are observed in the far-IR spectrum of PMETAMS-based nanosystem (Figure 3b). In this case, small changes are observed only in the region of skeletal vibrations of about 200 to 300 cm^{-1}.

Figure 4 shows a few mid-IR spectra for the same polymers and complexes [13]. In the spectrum of pure PMAA, a broad absorption band with a maximum at 1720 cm^{-1} and high intensity at ~1700 cm^{-1} is observed (Figure 4a, curve *1*), i.e., in the range of vibrational frequencies ν(C=O), indicating the presence of single and double H-bonds, respectively, in PMAA. An essential result is the considerable change in the IR spectrum in the presence of PD (Figure 4a, curve *2*) where the emergence of new absorption bands (not related to the pure PD) at 1550 and 1390 cm^{-1} appear. These bands correspond to the symmetrical and asymmetrical ν(C=O) vibrations in carboxylates. It clearly indicates strong interaction between certain COOH groups of PMAA and PD (most likely NH groups) with the salt formation.

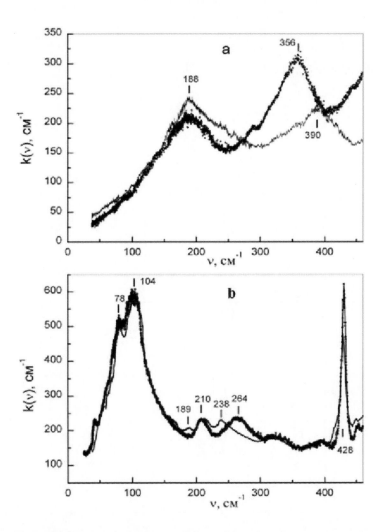

Figure 3. Far-IR spectra of films of (a) PMAA and (b) PMETAMS in their initial state (bold lines) and after adding 1 wt. % of PD (fine lines) [13].

Another spectral changes induced by PD are observed for PMETAMS (Figure 4b): a shift of the ν(C=O) band with a maximum at 1750 cm^{-1} and the =C-O-C vibration bands at 1070 and 1020 cm^{-1} by ~10 cm^{-1} to lower frequencies occurs.

2.4. Thermal Behavior of the Complexes

Figure 5 shows a few DSC curves obtained in the region of glass transition for polymers under study and their mixtures with PD [13]. In the DSC curve of pure PMAA (Figure 5, curve 1), two heat capacity ΔC_p steps (two glass transitions) are observed: the higher one at $T_{g1} = 127°C$ and the lower one at $T_{g2} = 179°C$. This could be explained in two ways: either by the presence of macromolecules with very high and very low molecular weights, or by the formation of not only double hydrogen (H) bonds between the COOH-groups (cyclic dimers) but also of partially open cycles (the formation of single H-bonds). In the PMAA/PD system (Figure 2, curve 2), both transitions (ΔC_p steps) disappear confirming the formation of the strong complexes with PD. This results in suppression of cooperative segmental dynamics within polymer glass transition. It should be indicated that two-step glass transition in the pure PMAA was also totally suppressed in ZnSe/PMAA/PD blend due to the formation of stable complexes between the components.

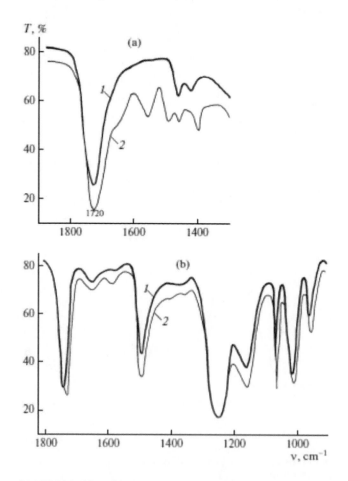

Figure 4. IR spectra of (a) PMAA (1) and PMAA+1 wt. % PD (2); (b) PMETAMS (1) and PMETAMS+1 wt.% PD (2) [13].

Other results were obtained for PMETAMS and PAMPSA systems (Figure 5, curves 3-5). For PMETAMS, adding PD resulted only in broadening glass transition toward lower temperatures due to inferior molecular packing, whereas the complicated two-step glass transition in PAMPSA remained virtually unchanged in the presence of PD. The latter confirms the absence of essential interactions and complex formation between PAMPSA and PD.

3. MORPHOLOGY OF ZNSE/POLYMER NANOSYSTEMS

Zinc selenide (ZnSe) is one of the most important wide-gap semiconductors of the group $A^{II}B^{VI}$, having high photosensitivity and transmission range of 0.5–22 μm. Its large band-gap value (2.7 eV) at room temperature and high photosensitivity make ZnSe an appropriate material for light-emitting diodes in the red, blue, and green ranges, laser displays, thin film transistors, photoelectrochemical cells, and ultrafast optoelectronic devices [14]. Zinc selenide is used as a material for the production of optical elements: windows, lenses, mirrors, prisms, beam splitters, which work in the IR range. For the preparation of ZnSe-based nanosystems, sonochemical methods, the method of reverse micelles, soft template synthesis, solvothermal or hydrothermal syntheses [refs. in 14] are used. It is shown that depending on the synthesis method, a polymer matrix is used as a stabilizer, and ZnSe/polymer nanostructures of various morphologies may be obtained, including tubes, rods, needles, plates, tors, hollow spheres.

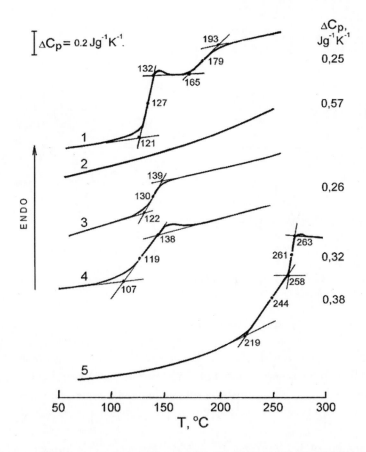

Figure 5. DSC curves of PMMA (1), PMMA/1 wt.% PD (2), PMETAMS (3), PMETAMS/1 wt. % PD (4), and PAMPSA (5). DSC curve of PAMPSA/1 wt.% PD virtually coincided with curve 5 [13].

The ZnSe-containing nanosystems were prepared in two steps [14, 15]. First, the hydrothermal synthesis of ZnSe nanoparticles is performed. In the second step, for the preparation of ZnSe nanosystems with polymer stabilizers, a certain amount of dried ZnSe powder is introduced into the polymer stabilizer solution.

Peculiar morphological character is demonstrated by nanosystems based on nanoparticles of ZnSe with PMAA. It is seen from AFM images that the nanosystem at the molar ratio ZnSe : polymer $\nu = 0.025$ has a self-assembled fibrillar network morphology with irregularly shaped nanostructures of sizes of $R = 50$–100 nm (Figs. 6, a-d), which are arranged on the surface of fibrils, "adorning" them (Figure 6, c). It is interesting that at $\nu = 0.1$, the fibrillar network becomes denser while the nanostructures become smaller; they have a mean radius of $R = 20$–40 nm. The value of estimated arithmetic average surface roughness of the ZnSe/PMAA film is $R_a = 2.1$ nm.

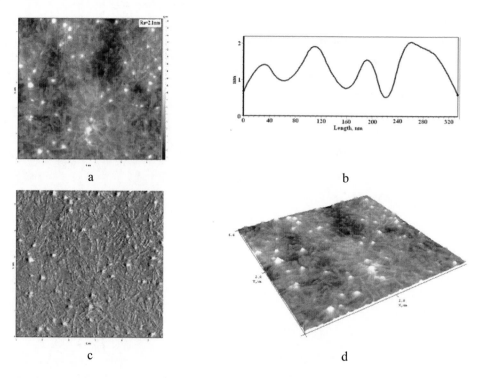

a   b

c   d

Figure 6. AFM images of ZnSe/PMAA film obtained in a tapping mode: a - topography, b - profile, c - amplitude image, d - 3D image.

Changes in morphology depending on a molar ratio and complex formation with PD in systems under study have been observed [14-16, 19]. AFM data (Figure 7) revealed that complexes of ZnSe-polymer with Photodithazine greatly differ from binary ZnSe/polymer compositions. The system generates large elliptic form nanostructures with sizes of 100-300 nm in transversal direction and 300-600 nm in the longitudinal direction. The value of estimated arithmetic average surface roughness of the ternary ZnSe/PMAA/PD composition film is $R_a = 22.3$ nm.

The introduction of the polymer BSA stabilizer leads to significant changes in the morphology of the nanosystem. It is seen in the AFM image of the topography of the film surface obtained from the ZnSe/BSA/PD solution (Figure 8) that film, consisting mainly of hybrid nanostructures with sizes of 20–50 nm and a smaller quantity (by 1–2 orders of magnitude less) of large nanostructures with a spherical shape of 70–280 nm, is formed. The 3D image (Figure 8d) clearly shows that the film covers the whole surface of the mica substrate. The triple system ZnSe/ BSA/PD system forms a very thin and flat film on the substrate surface: the value of estimated arithmetic average surface roughness of the ZnSe/BCA/PD film is R_a= 1.0 nm (Figure 8a).

The morphology of the formed films of nanosystems changes significantly upon a substantial reduction in the polymer stabilizer concentration in the system [15, 16, 19]. Also, our results show in the AFM images of the topography of the film surface obtained upon deposition of the solution of ZnSe nanoparticles stabilized first by PD and then by BSA, that the ultrathin (1–2 nm thick) and more homogeneous film evenly covering the substrate surface was formedne. It is probable that the macrocyclic PD ligand forms a stable solvate shell around ZnSe nanoparticles passivating the entire surface of zinc selenide nanoparticles preventing the BSA macromolecules approaching them and forming a complex [15].

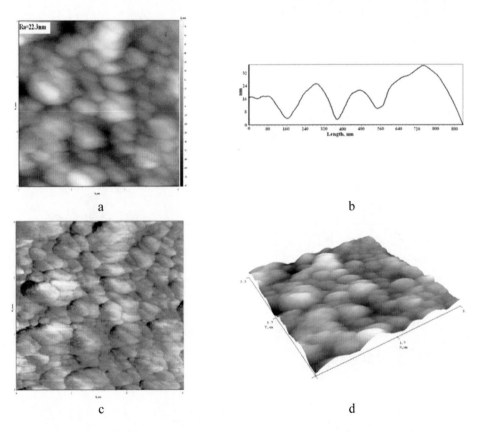

Figure 7. AFM images of ZnSe/PMAA/PD system obtained in contact mode: a-topography, b-profile, c-contrast of lateral forces (torsion), d - 3D image.

4. CRYSTAL AND ELECTRONIC STRUCTURES OF THE ZNSE/POLYMER NANOSYSTEMS

In order to determine the chemical state of Zn and Se in the ZnSe/polymer nanosystems, the XPS spectra of the $Zn2p$ and $Se2p$ inner levels were recorded [14]. As an example, the XPS spectra of ZnSe/PVP and ZnSe/PMAA nanosystems are displayed in Figure 9. The chemical shifts for both systems were estimated as $\Delta Zn2p = + 0.7$ eV and $\Delta Se3p = -0.7$ eV. It means that more electronegative Se atoms withdraw electrons of zinc atoms, i.e., Zn and Se atoms form the nanoparticles of chemical compound ZnSe in the process of synthesis, indeed, and the presence of polymer stabilizer does not influence on their state.

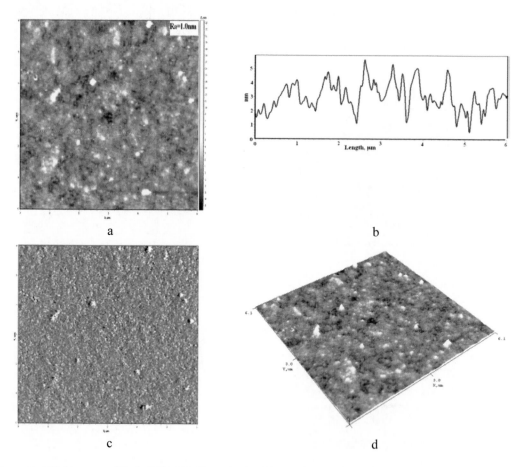

Figure 8. AFM images of ZnSe/BSA/PD film, obtained in tapping mode: a-topography, b-profile, c-amplitude image, d-3D image.

The crystal structure of nanostructures in films obtained from solutions of nanosystems was studied by the method of X-ray powder diffraction. In the diffraction pattern for the ZnSe/PVP nanosystem with $v = 0.1$ three peaks at the scattering angles $2\theta = 27.23°$, $45.21°$, and $53.59°$ are present (Figure 10). These peaks correspond to the (111), (220), (311) planes of cubic blende phase of ZnSe, respectively. Moreover, the XRD pattern exhibits broad diffraction peaks, which reveal that ZnSe might be assembled from nanoparticles with the smaller size about 2 - 4 nm. The size of the ZnSe nanocrystallites was calculated using the Scherrer's equation from the half-widths of these three peaks being equal to 6.5 ± 0.5 nm.

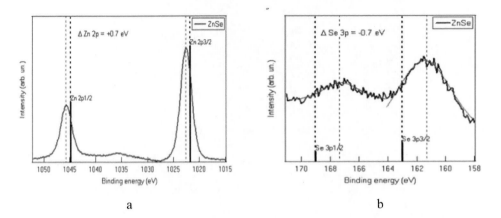

a   b

Figure 9. XPS spectra of Zn2p (a) and Se3p (b) inner levels in ZnSe nanoparticles stabilized with PVP or PMAA [14].

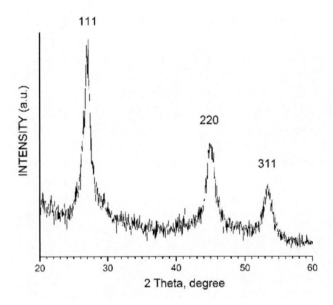

Figure 10. X-ray diffraction pattern of the ZnSe/PVP nanosystem at v = 0.1.

The presence of a cubic crystal cell of synthesized ZnSe nanoparticles is also confirmed by TEM and HREM investigations [14]. TEM images show that the populations of nanoparticles of the ZnSe/PVP nanosystem with the sizes of 5-100 nm are formed. A HREM image of one particle and the Fourier transform from the region indicated by a square on the micrograph are presented in Figure 11. The Fourier transform corresponds to the crystallographic area with the axis of a cubic crystal lattice of ZnSe with the cell parameters $a = b = c = 5.62$ Å, and $\alpha = \beta = \gamma = 90.00°$.

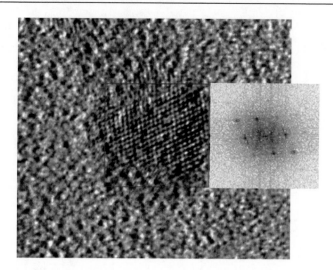

Figure 11. High resolution image of ZnSe/PVP nanosystem and Fourier transform (the right inset) of a nanocrystal ZnSe embedded into the polymer matrix of PVP [14].

5. PHOTOLUMINESCENCE PROPERTIES OF ZnSe/POLYMER/PD NANOSYSTEMS

The excitation at 415 nm and photoluminescence spectra were measured for aqueous solutions of PD and its system with ZnSe and BSA (Figure 12). The analysis of spectra presented in Figure 12 shows that the maximum in the excitation band of PD is observed at λ = 410–415 nm for neat PD and for the triple ZnSe/BSA/PD system. However, a short-wavelength shift by 23 nm from 653 to 630 nm is observed in the photoluminescence emission spectra upon the transition from PD to the triple system that may be due to the formation of stable complexes between components [15].

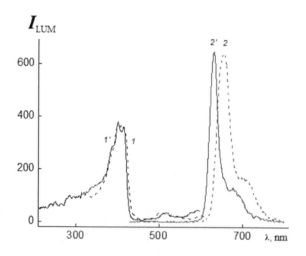

Figure 12. Excitation (*1*, *1'*) and luminescence (*2*, *2'*) spectra of PD (*1*, *2*) and the ZnSe/BSA/PD nanosystem in an aqueous solution ($c_{PD} = 8.3 \times 10^{-6}$ M) (*1'*, *2'*) [15].

An important point is that the intensity of the maximum of the photoluminescence spectrum is practically the same for the triple system and PD, though the content of PD in the triple nanosystem is three times less. This fact makes possible to reduce the dose of the PD being used during PDT without decreasing its efficiency. Moreover, ZnSe/BSA nanostructures do not quench the photoluminescence of PD in the triple system, i.e., do not affect its ability to generate active forms of oxygen.

6. BIOACTIVITY OF ZNSE/POLYMER/PD NANOSYSTEMS. PROSPECTS FOR THE DEVELOPMENT AND IMPROVEMENT OF THE PDT METHOD

The practice of using PDT in some cases is associated with the inability to create a sufficient concentration of photosensitizer in the tumor or the inability to deliver effectively laser radiation in some localization of malignant neoplasms. A number of nosological forms of the primary tumor and its metastases (in brain, peripheral parts of the lung, pancreas, liver, kidney, and bone tissue) are not available for exposure to light, which not only limits the possibilities of application of PDT but also reduces the effectiveness of cancer care in general.

In experiments on animals, we investigated the possibility in principle of management of transport and the concentration of nanoparticles, involved in the nanosystems containing PD with external X-ray irradiation. To improve the biocompatibility and solubilization of the complex PD/ZnSe nanoparticles, poly-N-vinyl-2-pyrrolidone (PVP) solution was used. PVP is widely used in pharmaceuticals because it facilitates the penetration of drugs through biological barriers, increasing the concentration of drug in tumor cells, and increases in some cases the photocatalytic activity of PD by 5-10 times [8].

Trials on NMRI mice, weighing 20-25 g were performed using an X-ray diagnostic apparatus "Electron-OKO" in doses up to 50 mZv. Ehrlich tumor cells inoculated into the plantar pad of the left and right foots by introducing 0.25 ml 20% suspension of tumor cells. Prepared drug - colloid solution containing a complex of ZnSe nanoparticles, stabilised by PVP or BSA with PD, were injected intraperitoneal. In an hour after the introduction of drug, the X-ray irradiation of the right foot only was carried out.

In the case of complex ZnSe/polymer/PD concentration of drug in the tumor increased continuously with time. The work shows the formation of complexes PD and polymer with ZnSe particles, determined the structure of the complexes. The resulting complexes are stable for a long time at 20-40°C, which is important for applications in medicine.

In experimental animals, the size of the tumors was measured diameter of the plantar footpads in mice, and the difference between the diameters of the tumor and normal plantar footpads was measured. Comparison of growth dynamics inhibition of Ehrlich tumour in control and skilled groups of animals within 25 days has shown that the sizes of a tumour in control group essentially exceed tumour volume in a group of animals for which the complex ZnSe/polymer/PD was injected and irradiated. The difference was on average 3 mm. Figure 13 shows the result of PDT application with the ZnSe/polymer/PD nanosystem.

Trials on laboratory animals, using the targeted delivery of drug to the tumor by means of

X-ray irradiation, have shown that the phototoxic properties of PD, combined with ZnSe-containing HPNS, were preserved, and the efficiency of the photosensitizer increased compared with the officinal drug; the presence of PVP increased its effectiveness. In some cases, tumor lysis resulted in spontaneous amputation of necrotic paws animal. Thus, the synthesized complexes can be used as sensitizers in PDT.

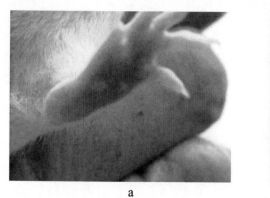 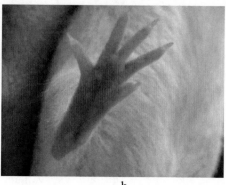

a   b

Figure 13. The right pad of skilled mouse with intertwined Ehrlich tumour for 5 days: a - the control (only X-ray irradiation), b - after injection of a drug and X-ray irradiation.

The assessment of acute and chronic toxicity of synthesized ternary nanosystems ZnSe/polymer/PD, on cells cultures of melanoma and cancer of a mammary gland has shown that cytotoxic action on tumor cells was not displayed. Efficiency determination of ternary ZnSe-containing nanosystems on oncological cellular cultures is of a fundamental value and will be a subject of detailed research at the following stage of our work [20, 21].

CONCLUSION

Hybrid nanosystems, based on ZnSe nanoparticles, various polymer stabilizers and new Photodithazine (PD) photosensitizer, were synthesized and investigated. Their morphological characteristics, i.e., the mean size and shape of the forming nanostructures, were determined. Depending on the composition and technological factors, the nanostructures with the sizes of 5 to 200 nm were formed. The effects of the polymer stabilizer nature on the structure, morphology and properties of these nanosystems were studied. The formation of stable complexes in some of these nanosystems was established experimentally. Along with different structures and morphologies, the complexes had different spectral and thermal-physical characteristics due to the different equilibrium between electrostatic and hydrophobic interactions in the systems. The preliminary estimations of the efficiency of prepared HPNSs regarding oncological cell cultures were performed and gave a positive result. Therefore, the developed nanosystems can be considered as the perspective components in designing new effective highly soluble photosensitive drugs for photodynamic therapy, the combined treatment of malignant new growths in oncology.

ACKNOWLEDGMENTS

The work is partially performed within the framework of the Scientific and Educational Center "Nanostructures and Self-Organization in Functional Macromolecular Systems and Their Diagnostics". The authors are grateful to Dr. Ute Kolb (Institute of Physical Chemistry, Johannes Gutenberg University of Mainz, Germany) for the opportunity to use the TECNAI F30 (FEI) microscope.

The authors are grateful to the Russian Foundation for Basic Researches for a financial support (project No. 10-03-01075) and OOO "VETA-GRAND" for supplying the Photodithazinee samples.

CONFLICT OF INTEREST

The authors have declared that no conflict of interest exists.

REFERENCES

[1] The War on Cancer: An Anatomy of Failure, a Blueprint for the Future (book review). *JAMA* 295 (24): 2891–2892 (2006).

[2] C. A. Robertson, E. D. Hawkins, and H. Abrahamse, *J. Photochem. Photobiol.* B: Biol. 96, 1 (2009).

[3] M. L. Gel'fond, *Prakt. Onkol.* 8 (4), 204 (2007) (in Russian).

[4] M. Kepczynski, K. Nawalany, B. Jachimska, et al., *Colloids Surf., B: Biointerf.* 49, 22 (2006).

[5] Yu. V. Kul'velis, V. A. Trunov, V. T. Lebedev, et al., *Phys. Solid State* 52, 1040 (2010).

[6] A. S. Derycke and P. A. de Witte, *Int. J. Oncol.* 20, 181 (2002).

[7] P. Petrov, T. Trukhacheva, G. Isakov, et al., *Acta Bioopt. Inform. Med.,* 10, 6 (2004).

[8] A. B. Solov'eva, N. A. Aksenova, N. N. Glagolev, et al. *Rus J Phys Chem* B, 6, 3, 433-440 (2012).

[9] E. F. Stranadko and M. V. Ryabov, *Al'manakh Klinich. Med.,* 12, 36 (2006) (in Russian).

[10] M. L. Gel'fond, *Fiz. Med. Klinich. Issled.* 15 (2), 33 (2005) (in Russian).

[11] G. V. Ponomarev, L. D. Tavrovskii, A. M. Zaretskii, V. V. Ashmarov, and R. F. Baum, R. F. Patent No. 2276976 (2006).

[12] V. A. Evtushenko, M. F. Vusik, and V. A. Chizhikov, *Ros. Bioterap. Zh.* 5 (1), 35 (2007) (in Russian).

[13] T.E. Sukhanova, V.A. Bershtein, S.V. Valueva, et al. *Rus J Phys Chem* A, 88, 3, 544-550 (2014).

[14] T. E. Sukhanova, M. E. Vylegzhanina, S. V. Valueva, et al., J. Surf. Invest.: X-Ray, Synchrotron, *Neutron Tech.* 8, 3, 484 (2014).

[15] T. E. Sukhanova, M. E. Vylegzhanina, S. V. Valueva, et al., J. Surf. Invest.: X-Ray, Synchrotron, *Neutron Tech.* 7, 4, 671 (2013).

[16] T. Sukhanova, V. Bershtein, S. Valueva, et al., in *Proceedings of the 14th IUPAC International Symposium on MacroMolecular Complexes MMC-14* (Helsinki, Finland, 2011), p. 64.

[17] V. A. Bershtein and V. A. Ryzhov, *Adv. Polym. Sci.* 114, 43 (1994).

[18] E. S. Rufino and E. E. S. Monteiro, *Polymer.* 44, 7189 (2003).

[19] T. E. Sukhanova, M. E. Vylegzhanina, S. V. Valueva, et al., in *Proceedings of the 9th International Conference on Methodological Aspects of Scanning Probe Microscopy* (Minsk, Belarus', 2010), p.35.

[20] T. E. Sukhanova, S. V. Valueva, A. Ya. Volkov, et al., in *Proceedings of the 1st International Scientific Practical Conference on Higher Technologies. Principles and Applied Researches in Physiology and Medicine* (St.-Petersburg, Russia, 2010), 4, p.174.

[21] M. L. Gel'fond, A.I. Arsenjev, E.V. Lechenko, et al., *J. Laser Medicine.* 16, 2, 25-30 (2012) (in Russian).

In: Photodynamic Therapy
Editor: Adrian G. Hugo

ISBN: 978-1-63463-857-9
© 2015 Nova Science Publishers, Inc.

Chapter 10

OCULAR PHOTODYNAMIC THERAPY

Assaf Dotan[1],[*] and Rita Ehrlich[1]
[1]Department of Ophthalmology, Rabin Medical Center,
PetachTikva, Israel

ABSTRACT

Verteporfin is a light-activated photosensitizing drug administered in a liposomal properties formulation. It is preferentially taken up by neovascular endothelium cells that have increased expression of low-density lipoprotein receptors. It is activated by non-thermal laser light to obtain endothelial damage and closure of neovascular structures.

Ocular photodynamic therapy (PDT) was approved and introduced as a novel treatment for choroidal neovascularization related to age-related macular degeneration, pathologic myopia and ocular histoplasmosis syndrome.

Other ocular pathologies had also used PDT with some remarkable results. These extended applications include choroidal neovascularization (CNV) secondary to choroiditis and retinochoroiditis, angioid streaks, central serous chorioretinopathy, retinal angiomatous proliferation, parafoveal telangiectasia or CNV associated with macular dystrophy and idiopathic CNV, as well as diseases unrelated to CNV, such as choroidal hemangioma, retinal hamartoma, choroidal melanoma and angiomatous lesions secondary to systemic diseases.

To date, with the introduction of various anti-Vascular endothelial growth factor (VEGF) and VEGF trap therapy, the role of PDT has certainly changed. It still has an important role in some diseases, such as chronic central serous chorioretinopathy and polypoidal choroidal vasculopathy. It might also maintain a role in combination therapy due to its unique properties of selective vascular targeting.

INTRODUCTION

Ocular photodynamic therapy is a treatment modality designed to selectively occlude ocular choroidal neovascular tissue.

---

[*] E-mail: docdotan@gmail.com.

Using verteporfin PDT selectively targets vascular endothelial cells. By damaging the intraluminal portion of the exposed vessels, the treatment achieves selective vascular occlusion without affecting the adjacent neural structures.

Ocular photodynamic therapy has been introduced as a treatment for choroidal neovascularization due to age-related macular degeneration (AMD), choroidal neovascularization (CNV) secondary to pathologic myopia and ocular histoplasmosis syndrome [1–5].

Studies indicate that PDT may also be used to treat CNV secondary to various vascular retinochoroidal diseases, such as choroiditis, retinochoroiditis, angioid_streaks, parafoveal telangiectasia or CNV associated with macular dystrophy, idiopathic CNV, as well as in diseases without any CNV, such as choroidal and retinal hemangioma, retinal hamartoma, choroidal melanoma, chronic CSCR, angiomatous lesions secondary to systemic diseases [6–10].

Ocular photodynamic therapy causes reduced leakage and vessel occlusion by two possible mechanisms. The specificity and uptake of verteporfin by target cells with a high expression of low-density lipoprotein receptors, such as tumor and neovascular endothelial cells, are enhanced by the use of a liposomal formulation and its rapid uptake by plasma low-density lipoprotein [11, 12].

Whereas normal vessels are usually spared from the phototoxic effect due to their intact blood retina barrier, preventing any extravasation of the photosensitization within the nonfenestrated vascular wall, pathologic leakage in choroidal and retinal hemangiomas and CNV might contribute to the vascular occlusion [13].

The main advantage of PDT over laser treatment remains the selective thrombosis of new vessels while preserving adjacent neuroretinal structures [14].

Verteporfin (Visudyne)

Photosensitizers selectively bind to abnormal neovascularization through its expression of increased numbers of lipoprotein receptors, thus achieving the desirable feature of selectivity with preservation of normal blood vessels. Most agents possess strong absorption properties in the far-red spectral region (660–780nm), where light has the greatest penetration through blood and tissue.

Most photosensitizing molecules, including verteporfin, as well as a number of agents under clinical evaluation, are structurally related to porphyrins [15].

The benzoporphyrin derivative monoacid verteporfin (Visudyne) consists of two isomers that differ in the location of the carboxylic acid and methyl ester on the lower pyrole rings of the chlorine macrocycle. Because verteporfin is hydrophobic, it requires formulation within liposomes. In addition to improving penetration into cells and delivery by an intravenous route, this may actually further enhance its selectivity. Verteporfin is activated with a monochromatic laser light in the range of approximately 689–691nm. The molecule is well tolerated following intravenous administration, and cutaneous light sensitivity is kept to a minimum compared with other molecules, which either have longer periods of photosensitization, or less favorable therapeutic indices [15].

Verteporfin photodynamic therapy (PDT) was the first photosensitizer approved for the treatment of exudative AMD in 2000. The technique involves infusion of 6 mg/m^2

verteporfin over a 10-minute period followed by laser irradiation, using a 689 nm diode laser (light dose: 50 J/cm ^{2}; power density: 600 mW/cm ^{2}; duration: 83 seconds) 15 minutes after the start of the infusion. Verteporfin demonstrated safety and efficacy in localizing choroidal neovascular membranes in preclinical trials in nonhuman primates [15].

The mechanism in which PDT induces tissue destruction is not exactly understood and appears to involve endothelial cell membrane damage by free radicals activated by the thermal laser light inducing platelet activation and blood clot formation. Activated platelets release mediators such as histamine, thromboxane and TNF-α and these mediators trigger a sequence of events, including vasoconstriction, thrombosis, increased vascular permeability, blood stasis and hypoxia [16-18].

PDT for Standard Indications

PDT for Subfoveal Choroidal Neovascularization (CNV) Secondary to Age-Related Macular Degeneration (AMD)

The hallmark of the neovascular form of AMD is the presence of CNV. Non-neovascular changes such as the presence of drusen, a thickening of the inner aspect, can predispose a break in Bruch's membrane, allowing buds of neovascular tissue from the choriocapillaris to perforate the outer aspect of Bruch's membrane. These new vessels are accompanied by fibroblasts, resulting in a fibrovascular complex that proliferates within the inner aspect of Bruch's membrane. This fibrovascular complex can disrupt and destroy the normal architecture of the choriocapillaris, Bruch's membrane, and the RPE and result in damage to the retina.

Patients with subfoveal, predominantly classic CNV (> 50% of the lesion with classic component) and those with small occult CNV (< 4 disc diameters) due to AMD may benefit from PDT.

Classic CNV is characterized by well-demarcated areas of intense hyperfluorescence appearing early and showing progressive leakage on fluorescein angiography. The appearance of occult CNV varies widely and can be difficult to identify. It can appear as irregular elevation of stained retinal pigment epithelium (RPE) with "stipples" of hyperfluorescence or poorly demarcated areas of leakage at the level of the RPE in the late phases of the angiogram.

Four large, randomized, double-masked, placebo-controlled multicenter trials[1–4] and a similarly designed but smaller single–center studies have assessed the efficacy of verteporfin in adults with subfoveal CNV secondary to AMD.

These multicenter studies are: the TAP Investigation [1], which consisted of two studies of identical design conducted in Europe and the United States of America with pooled results reported together (n=609); the VIP trial (n = 339);[2, 3] and the VIM study (n = 117) [4].

In the TAP Study [1] patients were included if they had a subfoveal CNV secondary to AMD with some classic component on fluorescein angiography (FA), lesion dimension of < 5,400 μm and best-corrected visual acuity (BCVA) between 20/40 and 20/200 Snellen equivalents. Patients were treated either with verteporfin or placebo and followed up at three-months intervals over two years. Retreatment was performed if the investigator determined persistent or recurrent leakage from CNV on FA.

The primary endpoint was the percentage of eyes for which losses of less than 15 ETDRS letters from baseline were observed at 12 and 24 months. PDT was significantly more effective than the placebo, both at 12 months (61% versus 46%) and 24 months (53% versus 38%). In a subgroup analyses for predominantly classic lesions at baseline, 59% of verteporfin-treated patients compared with 31% of placebo-treated patients lost ≤ 15 letters at the 24 months examination. Patients were treated an average of 3.5 times in the first year and a total of 5 times by the end of the second year.

The VIP Study [2, 3] a multicenter, double-masked, placebo-controlled, randomized trial, evaluated the efficacy and safety of photodynamic therapy in AMD patients with occult lesions (VIP 2) and in pathologic myopia (VIP 1). In the second arm, the VIP AMD [2] Study, visual stabilization was greater in verteporfin-treated eyes (45%) compared to the placebo-treated patients (32%). Although there was no significant difference between the treated group and the placebo group at the 12-month follow-up, a minimal but significant difference in the mean VA could be pointed out at the 24-month control. A subgroup analysis revealed a beneficial effect for occult CNV lesions < 4 disc areas or VA < 20/50 at the 12- and 24-month follow-ups. When the preoperative lesion size was > 4 disc areas and VA > 20/50, the mean postoperative VA at the 12- and 24-month follow-ups was less in the treatment group compared to the placebo group.

The VIM Study [4] objective was to determine the efficacy of photodynamic therapy in minimally classic membranes (where the classic component represents less than 50% of the neovascular lesion) sized below 6 disc area. The study results suggested that smaller minimally classic lesions <4 disc areas appeared to benefit from PDT treatment. Thus, patients with smaller minimally classic lesions may benefit to a limited degree from verteporfin PDT.

The major safety issue with PDT is choroidal hypoperfusion, documented in fluorescein and ICG angiography in the first days after treatment and, more rarely, in the following months (Figure 1). Controversy exists regarding the cumulative effect of treatment in permanent occlusion of the normal choriocapillaris and the association between this hypoperfusion and eventual functional consequences [19].

PDT for Subfoveal Choroidal Neovascularization (CNV) Secondary to Pathologic Myopia (PM)

CNV due to pathological myopia may develop in 5%–10% of eyes with an axial length of more than 26.5 mm, often in conjunction with widespread chorioretinal degeneration and lacquer cracks in the posterior pole (Figure 2).

The VIP study is the largest study to have investigated the efficacy and safety of PDT with verteporfin in the treatment of subfoveal CNV caused by pathological myopia [3]. One hundred and twenty patients were randomized into the verteporfin-treated and placebo-treated groups.

In the group of pathologic myopia (VIP PM), after a follow-up of 24 months, 36% of patients lost ≥8 letters of visual acuity in the treated group compared to 51% in the placebo group.

The change in VA between baseline and the 24-month examination was in favor of cases assigned to verteporfin. After 24 months of follow-up 40% of treated eyes gained at least 5 letters compared to 13% in the placebo group. Improvement of at least 15 letters was found in 12% of treated eyes compared to 0% in the placebo group.

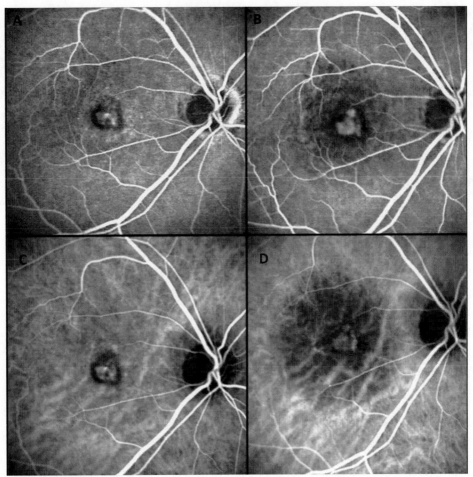

(Courtesy of Prof. R. Axer-Siegel).

Figure 1. Fluorescin angiogram shows an area of classic CNV in an AMD patient (A). Fluorescin angiogram taken two weeks after PDT treatment shows a hypofluorescent ring around the CNV (B). Indocyanine green angiography (ICGA) shows an area of hyperfluorescence corresponding to the CNV seen on the FA (C). Indocyanine green angiography (ICGA) taken two weeks after PDT treatment shows hypofluorescent area corresponding to the treatment spot and may represent area of choroidal hypoperfusion following treatment (D).

In a retrospective study on patients with pathological myopia, visual prognosis after PDT was found to be influenced by age at treatment.

Patients older than 60 years of age had a less favorable response to treatment in terms of visual acuity outcome [20].

Development of subretinal fibrosis after PDT further correlates with the size of the CNV and the refractive error [21].

PDT for Subfoveal Choroidal Neovascularization (CNV) Secondary to Ocular Histoplasmosis Syndrome (OHS)

Presumed ocular histoplasmosis involves the classic triad of discrete atrophic choroidal scars in the macula or midperiphery known as histo spots, peripapillary atrophy, and choroidal neovascularization, which leads to severe loss of central vision.

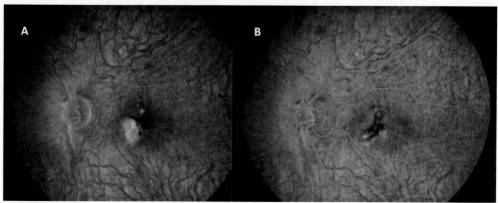

(Courtesy of Prof. R. Axer-Siegel).

Figure 2. A 25 years old high myopic patient. Fluorescin angiogram shows leakage from a predominantly classic CNV (A). Fluorescin angiogram taken one month after PDT treatment shows scarring of the CNV (B).

Photodynamic therapy for choroidal neovascularization secondary to ocular histoplasmosis was approved by the US Food and Drug Administration in August 2001 following the publication of the one-year results of the Verteporfin in Ocular Histoplasmosis study [5]. This uncontrolled, prospective study enrolled 26 patients with subfoveal CNV, of which most cases (73%) were predominantly classic. The two-year results of the study showed improvement in visual acuity as well as absence of serious adverse events following treatment [22].

The median change in visual acuity score increased by 6 letters from baseline, and the median contrast sensitivity score increased by 3.5 letters. In addition, circumstantial and temporal evidence obtained in the study points towards the existence of a causal relation between photodynamic treatment and absence of leakage and resolution of hemorrhage. No case of severe vision decrease, infusion-related back pain, or photosensitivity reaction were reported, although this comparison was limited by the small number of OHS patients studied. A mean of only 3.9 verteporfin treatments was necessary over the two years of the study to achieve an absence of fluorescein angiographic leakage in the POHS group.

PDT for Non-Standard Indications

PDT for Central Serous Chorioretinopathy (CSCR)

Central serous chorioretinopathy (CSCR) is characterized by choroidal hyperperfusion and neurosensory retinal detachment secondary to RPE lesions, and occurs most frequently in middle-aged men [23]. It usually resolves without treatment and has a good prognosis, with normal vision often returning within a few months [23].

However, visual loss or permanent symptoms may occur in cases with persistent focal leakage or chronic diffuse leakage [24]. Treatment should be considered after three months without resolution of fluids [23]. Some patients develop CNV secondary to CSCR, which is a potentially sight-threatening complication that has a tendency to develop in eyes where the RPE–Bruch's membrane complex is disrupted [25].

Several prospective [24, 26–28] and retrospective case series [29, 30] have reported PDT in CNV secondary to CSCR. The standard regimen of verteporfin PDT was evaluated in two prospective case series [24, 28].

Ergun E. et al. reported their experience with 26 eyes of 24 patients with CNV due to CSCR that were treated with verteporfin PDT and followed up for a mean of 22 months. Additional treatments were given with two- to three-month intervals if required, based on FA [28]. In these patients, VA improved by 1.6 lines at year 1 and 2.2 lines at year 2.

Encouraging results were also shown with the use of PDT in CSCR with acute or chronic leakage. Improvements in VA have been reported with the standard verteporfin PDT regimen in a retrospective case series of nine patients with acute focal RPE leaks secondary to CSCR (from 20/80 at baseline to 20/40 at month 6) [29].

In two retrospective studies in chronic CSCR, five of seven patients showed an improvement of two lines or more [31] and best-corrected visual acuity (BCVA) improved by a mean of 1.7 lines in seven of 11 eyes [32].

In a retrospective pulled data from the macula society[33], on 265 eyes of 237 patients with CSCR, the number of PDT treatments was 1 in 89%, 2 in 7%, and 3 in 3% of eyes. Post-PDT follow-up ranged from one month to more than one year.

Following PDT, VA improved $\geq$3 lines in <1%, 29%, and 48% of eyes with baseline VA $\geq$20/32, 20/40 to 20/80, and $\leq$20/100, respectively. Subretinal fluid had been resolved in 81% eyes by the last visit. They concluded that photodynamic therapy was associated with improved VA and resolution of subretinal fluid.

Severe choroidal ischemia was reported in chronic CSCR patients treated with standard verteporfin PDT [34]. This led physicians to explore reduced fluence PDT as an alternative to the standard protocol.

Two prospective studies evaluated the use of a reduced dose (3 mg/m^2, half the standard dose) of verteporfin, guided by indocyanine green angiography (ICGA), in eyes with symptomatic chronic CSCR [26, 27].

In one study, 48 eyes had a mean improvement of 1.6 lines of VA, and 45 eyes (96%) had stable or improved vision at 12 months [27]. In the other study, 20 eyes from 18 patients had an improvement in mean VA from 20/40 at baseline to 20/30 at one month [26]. There were also significant reductions in central retinal thickness (from 276 to 158 μm), and 17 eyes (85%) had complete resolution of their serous RPE detachment and/or pigment epithelial detachment. Dose optimization has also been investigated in patients with acute CSCR. In a prospective double-masked placebo-controlled trial at 12 months, 37 of 39 patients (94.9%) treated with half-dose verteporfin had no subretinal fluid at the macula, and the group's mean BCVA improved by 1.8 lines, with all verteporfin-treated patients having stable or improved VA [35].

Overall, verteporfin PDT is associated with promising outcomes in patients with CSCR (Figure 3).

PDT for Polypoidal Choroidal Vasculopathy (PCV)

Polypoidal choroidal vasculopathy is characterized by multiple and recurrent serosanguinous RPE detachments that often resemble and can be considered a subtype of AMD.

The areas of serosanguinous detachment are often peripapillary, multifocal, orange and nodular.

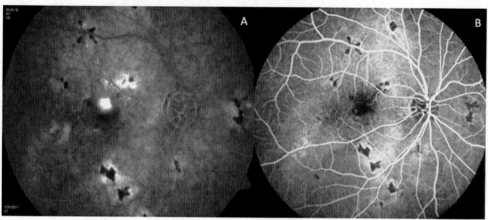

(Courtesy of Dr. K. Mimouni).

Figure 3. A 58 years old patient withchronic central serous chorioretinopathy (CSCR). Fluorescin angiogram with multiple RPE changes as well as a hot spot and early leakage (A). Fluorescin angiogram taken one month after PDT treatment shows no hot spot or fluorescein leakage (B).

The natural history and visual acuity outcome of polypoidal vasculopathy may be better than that of CNV associated with AMD. Indocyanine green angiography (ICGA) can provide accurate diagnosis of PCV, as PCV can be misdiagnosed as occult CNV when fluorescein angiography (FA) is used alone. The involvement of choroidal vessel abnormalities in PCV indicates that verteporfin PDT may have a key role in treating this disorder by occluding the vascular network and causing regression of the polyps.

Lee et al. [36] reported PDT in nine eyes with PCV. Obliterating polypoid elements was achieved in seven of the nine eyes. During the follow-up period of 3–18 months VA stabilized or improved in eight of the nine eyes and no reactivation of PCV was observed. An additional PDT was required in four eyes to decrease persisting vascular leakage.

Hussain et al. [38] retrospectively reviewed the records of nine patients after PDT in PCV. Follow-up ranged from 12 to 16 months. Visual acuity improved in four of the nine eyes (44.4%) by 1 line and remained unchanged in five (55.6%).

In a prospective, two-centered case series Chan et al. [37] found stable or improved vision in 21 (95%) of the 22 eyes at the one-year follow-up. The mean BCVA improved by 1.3 lines.

In summary, PDT offers an effective way to treat PCV by obliteration of polypoid elements and by stabilization or improvement of VA.

PDT for Choroidal Hemangioma

Isolated choroidal hemangiomas appear as reddish-orange, well-circumscribed tumors of varying thickness. They may be discovered during routine examination or due to visual symptoms related to induced hyperopia or from serous detachment. Circumscribed hemangiomas transilluminate readily and have distinctive echographic and angiographic characteristics. Large choroidal vessels are visible early during ICG angiography, and the tumors show a characteristic washed-out pattern in later phases of the angiogram.

Visual loss may be progressive and irreversible because of chronic foveal detachment, leading to loss of photoreceptor function. Verteporfin PDT was introduced as a treatment option because it occludes aberrant choroidal vasculature while sparing the overlying retina and retinal vasculature [39].

Verteporfin PDT can induce complete and irreversible occlusion of the microvasculature in choroidal tumors, although this may require more than one treatment [40]. In addition, several reports have demonstrated encouraging visual and anatomical outcomes in 150 patients with circumscribed choroidal hemangioma treated with various verteporfin PDT regimens. Verteporfin PDT safely induced persistent regression of choroidal hemangioma, and led to sustained improvement or stabilization of VA and resolution of retinal fluid in almost all cases, often after a single treatment [41–45].

Verteporfin PDT is an effective and well-tolerated option for circumscribed choroidal hemangioma, and considered the treatment of choice, especially for subfoveal tumors.

Verteporfin PDT may also be useful in diffuse choroidal hemangioma in patients with Sturge–Weber syndrome. Case reports involving two patients showed that a single verteporfin PDT treatment improved VA, resolved exudative retinal detachment associated with choroidal hemangioma, and reduced the thickness of the choroidal hemangioma [45, 46].

Combination Therapies

Combined approaches for treating exudative AMD have been investigated as a means of improving treatment efficacy and reducing treatment frequency.

Ocular photodynamic therapy produces an acute antiangiogenic effect through thrombosis, resulting in vessel closure, but it may need to be sustained chronically with antiangiogenic agents for long-term efficacy [47]. Furthermore, the hypoxia induced following PDT might increase the angiogenic factors.

Additionally, there is evidence that inflammation plays an important role in angiogenesis of CNV [48]. VEGF expression in CNV specimens from patients with AMD seems to correlate with the degree of local inflammation. Experimental studies in tissues other than ocular tissues have demonstrated that PDT itself induces an inflammatory response, characterized by leukocyte infiltration and up-regulation of cytokines, such as intracellular adhesion molecule 1 and interleukin 6 [49]. Inflammation can cause up-regulation of VEGF and significant secondary scarring. Combination treatment modalities targeting both the angiogenic and inflammatory axes of AMD could potentiate PDT's therapeutic effect and prevent recurrences.

Clinical trials have evaluated the effect of verteporfin-PDT followed by triamcinolone acetonide (TA) at various time points. In a prospective case series of 184 eyes with all types of subfoveal AMD-associated CNV, 25 mg of triamcinolone were injected intravitreally 16 hours after the verteporfin-PDT treatment [50]. VA improved in the majority of patients, with a mean increase of approximately one Snellen line with a median follow-up time of 39 weeks. The number of retreatments was less than expected but about a quarter of patients developed increased intraocular pressure. Subsequent studies have found similar results for both subfoveal and juxtafoveal CNV [51, 52].

The ANCHOR study [53] a multicenter, randomized trial compared ranibizumab to verteporfin photodynamic therapy for neovascular age-related macular degeneration. Patients were randomized to verteporfin PDT plus monthly sham intraocular injection, or sham verteporfin PDT plus monthly intravitreal ranibizumab (0.3 mg or 0.5 mg) injection.

Following 24 months, the VA benefit from ranibizumab was statistically significantly superior to PDT: 89.9% to 90.0% of ranibizumab-treated patients had lost <15 letters from baseline (vs. 65.7% of PDT patients); 34% to 41.0% had gained ≥15 letters (vs. 6.3% of PDT group); and, on average, VA was improved from baseline by 8.1 to 10.7 letters (vs. a mean decline of 9.8 letters in PDT group).

The RADICAL study was a prospective, multicenter, randomized phase 2 clinical trial that investigated whether combination therapy reduces retreatment rates compared with ranibizumab monotherapy while maintaining similar visual acuity outcomes and an acceptable safety profile. The trial included 162 patients randomized to one of four treatment arms: photodynamic therapy (PDT) with reduced-fluence verteporfin followed by ranibizumab (n=43); reduced-fluence PDT followed by ranibizumab-dexamethasone triple therapy (n=39); very low-fluence PDT followed by ranibizumab-dexamethasone triple therapy (n=39); or ranibizumab monotherapy (n=41).

Of the four treatment groups, the triple therapy half-fluence group had the fewest retreatment visits compared with ranibizumab monotherapy. Through 24 months, patients in the triple therapy half-fluence group had a mean of 4.2 retreatment visits compared with 8.9 for patients who received ranibizumab monotherapy. In the second year, the average number of retreatment visits in the triple therapy half-fluence group (1.2) was approximately one third that of the ranibizumab monotherapy group (3). At month 24, mean visual acuity in the triple therapy half-fluence group improved 1.8 letters fewer (95% confidence interval, 11.1 letters fewer to 7.6 letters better) compared with the ranibizumab monotherapy group.

The FOCUS study [54] evaluated ranibizumab in combination treatment with PDT in predominantly classic subfoveal CNV lesions in 162 patients. Patients received monthly intravitreal injections of ranibizumab 0.5 mg (n =106) or sham injections (n = 56). All patients received PDT on day zero followed by quarterly injections as needed.

At month 24, 88% of ranibizumab + PDT patients had lost <15 letters of vision (vs 75% for PDT alone), 25% had gained >15 letters (vs 7% for PDT alone). On average, ranibizumab + PDT patients exhibited less lesion growth and greater reduction of CNV leakage and subretinal fluid accumulation, and required fewer PDT retreatments, than PDT-alone patients (mean = 0.4 vs 3.0 PDT retreatments). The study concluded that ranibizumab +PDT was more effective than PDT alone and had a low rate of associated adverse events.

Kaiser et al. [55] published a retrospective study that assessed outcomes of patients with choroidal neovascularization (CNV) due to age-related macular degeneration (AMD) treated with verteporfin photodynamic therapy (PDT) and bevacizumab. At 12 months, 82% of patients (578/701) had stable or improved vision (loss of <3 lines or a gain in VA), 36% (255/701) improved by ≥3 lines, and 17% (121/701) improved by ≥6 lines. After one year, patients gained approximately 1.2 lines (6 letters) of VA. Patients who were treatment naïve gained significantly more VA (+8.4 letters) compared with those who had been previously treated (+2.4 letters). The study concluded that combination therapy with PDT and bevacizumab led to vision benefit for most patients, particularly those who were treatment naïve at baseline.

Two large multicenter studies, the DENALI [56] and the MONT BLANC [57], did not find combination therapy with anti-VEGF and PDT to show great advantage over anti-VEGF therapy alone.

In the DENALI study [56], ranibizumab was administered monthly in the monotherapy group. In both combination therapy groups (standard/reduced fluence PDT and ranibizumab)

ranibizumab was initiated with three consecutive monthly injections, followed by retreatment as needed. Verteporfin PDT was administered on day 1 and at three-month intervals as needed. All patients were evaluated monthly for 12 months.

At month 12, patients in the standard fluence combination group gained on average 5.3 letters from baseline, and patients in the reduced fluence combination group gained on average 4.4 letters. Patients in the ranibizumab monthly monotherapy group gained on average 8.1 letters. On average, patients in the combination groups required 2.2 (standard fluence) or 2.8 (reduced fluence) additional ranibizumab injections after the mandatory three loading doses as compared to an average of 7.6 additional injections in the ranibizumab monthly monotherapy cohort.

Ranibizumab monotherapy or combined with verteporfin PDT improved VA at month 12, but did not demonstrate noninferiority in terms of visual acuity gain for verteporfin PDT ranibizumab combination therapy compared with ranibizumab monthly monotherapy. Reduced fluence did not provide a clinical benefit over standard fluence in verteporfin PDT combination arms.

Similarly, in the MONT BLANC study [57], patients were randomized 1:1 to as-needed (PRN) combination (standard-fluence verteporfin PDT and ranibizumab 0.5 mg) or PRN ranibizumab monotherapy (sham infusion PDT with ranibizumab 0.5 mg) following a loading dose of three injections.

At month 12, visual improvement was +2.5 letters in the combination therapy group and +4.4 letters in the ranibizumab monotherapy group. The noninferiority limit of 7 letters was met; however, other endpoints, including the proportion of patients with a treatment-free interval of >3 months (96% vs 92%) and the number of ranibizumab retreatments (1.9 vs 2.2) were similar, suggesting that adding verteporfin PDT does not reduce the number of ranibizumab injections required.

The EVEREST study [58] assessed the effects of verteporfin photodynamic therapy (PDT) combined with ranibizumab or alone versus ranibizumab monotherapy in patients with symptomatic macular polypoidal choroidal vasculopathy. At month 6, verteporfin combined with ranibizumab or alone was superior to ranibizumab monotherapy in achieving complete polyp regression (77.8% and 71.4% vs. 28.6%). The mean change in visual acuity was 10.9 letters in the combined treatment, 7.5 letters with PDT and 9.2 letters with ranibizumab monotherapy.

CONCLUSION

In response to recent advances in therapeutic options for CNV, such as anti-VEGF and VEGF trap agents, studies have been conducted examining combination treatments and comparing different therapy agents to photodynamic therapy.

Adding an anti-VEGF agent to PDT has theoretical merit. Combining anti-VEGF therapy and photodynamic therapy (with or without steroids) is thought to reduce the number of treatments needed to stabilize the CNV, although this benefit has not been observed in all studies. Studies such as RADICAL and FOCUS [54] compared combination treatment of PDT with anti-VEGF/ anti-VEGF-dexamethasone triple therapy to PDT treatment alone, and found the combination treatment to be superior.

The RADICAL study showed, at month 24 of follow-up, an improvement in mean visual acuity in the triple therapy half-fluence group of 1.8 letters compared with the ranibizumab monotherapy group. Similarly, the FOCUS study [54] concluded that ranibizumab and PDT was more effective than PDT alone.

Anti-VEGF monotherapy with ranibizumab showed superiority over PDT monotherapy and began a new era in the management of CNV. Off-label monotherapy with intravitreal bevacizumab has also gained widespread acceptance, and positive visual and anatomic results have been reported in the CATT and IVAN studies [59, 60] with similar results to ranibizumab treatment. Unfortunately, anti-VEGF monotherapy necessitates multiple, sometimes monthly injections.

Unfortunately both the DENALI [56] and MONT BLANC [57] showed in their 12-month results that the combination of anti-VEGF therapy and PDT have no greater advantage over anti-VEGF therapy alone.

PDT can be considered in cases in which anti-VEGF treatment is contraindicated and might be considered as an adjuvant treatment in patients unresponsive to anti-VEGF treatment, or uncompliant patients.

Clinical studies have been published on the effect of PDT in various choroidal vascular disorders rather than CNV, with promising results.

Studies on chronic CSCR indicate that verteporfin standard or half-fluence PDT is associated with promising outcomes. Photodynamic therapy treatment in PCV patients causes an obliteration of the polypoidal elements. In choroidal hemangioma it was shown to improve vision, resolve exudative retinal detachment and reduce the thickness of the choroidal hemangioma after a single verteporfin PDT treatment.

To date, with the introduction of various anti-VEGF and VEGF trap therapy, the role of PDT has certainly changed. PDT still has an important role in some diseases, such as chronic central serous chorioretinopathy and polypoidal choroidal vasculopathy. It might also maintain a role in combination therapy due to its unique properties of selective vascular targeting.

REFERENCES

[1]   Treatment of Age-Related Macular Degeneration with Photodynamic Therapy (TAP) Study Group: Photodynamic therapy of subfoveal choroidal neovascularization in age-related macular degeneration with verteporfin: one-year result of 2 randomized clinical trials – TAP report. *Arch. Ophthalmol.*, 1999; 117: 1329–1345.

[2]   Verteporfin in Photodynamic Therapy Study Group: Verteporfin therapy of subfoveal choroidal neovascularization in age-related macular degeneration: two-year result of a randomized clinical trial including lesions with occult with no classic choroidal neovascularization – verteporfin in photodynamic therapy report 2. *Am. J. Ophthalmol.*, 2001; 131: 541–560.

[3]   Blinder K. J., Blumenkranz M. S., et al. Verteporfin therapy of subfoveal choroidal neovascularization in pathologic myopia: 2-year results of a randomized clinical trial – VIP report No 3. *Ophthalmology*, 2003; 110: 667–673.

[4] Visudyne in Minimally Classic Choroidal Neovascularization Study Group. Verteporfin therapy of subfoveal minimally classic choroidal neovascularization in age-related macular photodydegeneration: 2-year results of a randomized clinical trial. *Arch. Ophthalmol.*, 2005 Apr.; 123(4): 448–57.

[5] Saperstein D. A., Rosenfeld P. J., et al. Photodynamic therapy of subfoveal choroidal neovascularization with verteporfin in the ocular histoplasmosis syndrome. *Ophthalmology*, 2002 Aug.; 109(8): 1499–1505.

[6] Lim J. I., Glassman A. R., et al. Collaborative retrospective Macula Society Study of photodynamic therapy for chronic central serous chorioretinopathy. *Ophthalmology*, 2014 May; 121(5): 1073–1078.

[7] Chan W. M., Lim T. H., et al. Verteporfin PDT for non-standard indications—a review of current literature. *Graefe's Arch. Clin. Exp. Ophthalmol.*, 2010 Jul.; 248(7): 943–956.

[8] Porrini G., Giovannini A., et al. Photodynamic therapy of circumscribed choroidal hemangioma. *Ophthalmology*, 2003; 110: 674–680.

[9] Muller-Velten R., Michels S., et al. Photodynamic therapy: extended indication. *Ophthalmologe*, 2003; 100: 384–390.

[10] Mennel S., Schmidt J. C., et al. Therapeutic strategies in choroidal neovascularizations secondary to angioid streaks. *Am. J. Ophthalmol.*, 2003; 136: 580–582.

[11] Schmidt-Erfurth U., Hasan T., et al. Vascular targeting in photodynamic occlusion of subretinal vessels. *Ophthalmology*, 1994; 101: 1953–1961.

[12] Noske U. M., Schmidt-Erfurth U., et al. Lipid metabolism in retinal pigment epithelium: possible significance of lipoprotein receptors. *Ophthalmologe*, 1998; 95: 814–819.

[13] Schmidt-Erfurth U., Hasan T., et al. In vivo uptake of liposomal benzoporphyrin derivative and photothrombosis in experimental corneal neovascularization. *Lasers Surg. Med.*, 1995; 17: 178–188.

[14] Kramer M., Miller J. W., et al. Liposomal benzoporphyrin derivate verteporfin photodynamic therapy: selective treatment of choroidal neovascularization in monkeys. *Ophthalmology*, 1996; 103: 427–438.

[15] Ryan S. J. RETINA. 5th edition. Elsevier: 2013.

[16] Miller J. W., Walsh A. W., et al. Photodynamic therapy of experimental choroidal neovascularization using lipoprotein-delivered benzoporphyrin. *Arch. Ophthalmol.*, 1995; 113(6): 810–8.

[17] Kramer M., Miller J. W., et al. Liposomal benzoporphyrin derivative verteporfin photodynamic therapy. Selective treatment of choroidal neovascularization in monkeys. *Ophthalmology*, 1996; 103(3): 427–38.

[18] Henderson B. W., Dougherty T. J. How does photodynamic therapy work? *Photochem. Photobiol.*, 1992; 55(1): 145–57.

[19] Ahmadieh H., Taei R., et al. Single-session photodynamic therapy combined with intravitreal bevacizumab and triamcinolone for neovascular age-related macular degeneration. *BMC Ophthalmol.*, 2007; 7:10.

[20] Axer-Siegel R., Ehrlich R., et al. Photodynamic therapy *Am. J. Ophthalmol.*, 2004 Oct.;138(4): 602–7.

[21] Ruiz-Moreno J. M., Montero J. A. Subretinal fibrosis after photodynamic therapy in subfoveal choroidal neovascularisation in highly myopic eyes. *Br. J. Ophthalmol.*, 2003; 87: 856–9.

[22] Rosenfeld P. J., Saperstein D. A., et al. Photodynamic therapy with verteporfin in ocular histoplasmosis: uncontrolled, open-label 2-year study. *Ophthalmology*, 2004; 111:1725–1733.

[23] Wang M., Munch I. C., et al. Central serous chorioretinopathy. *Acta. Ophthalmol.*, 2008; 86:126–145.

[24] Chan W. M., Lam D. S., et al. Choroidal vascular remodelling in central serous chorioretinopathy after indocyanine green guided photodynamic therapy with verteporfin: a novel treatment at the primary disease level. *Br. J. Ophthalmol.*, 2003; 87:1453–1458.

[25] Chan W. M., Lam D. S., et al. Treatment of choroidal neovascularization in central serous chorioretinopathy by photodynamic therapy with verteporfin. *Am. J. Ophthalmol.*, 2003; 136: 836–845.

[26] Lai T. Y., Chan W. M., et al. Safety-enhanced photodynamic therapy with half-dose verteporfin for chronic central serous chorioretinopathy: a short-term pilot study. *Br. J. Ophthalmol.*, 2006; 90: 869–874.

[27] Chan W. M., Lai T. Y., et al. Safety-enhanced photodynamic therapy for chronic central serous chorioretinopathy: one-year results of a prospective study. *Retina*, 2008; 28: 85–93.

[28] Ergun E., Tittl M., et al. Photodynamic therapy with verteporfin in subfoveal choroidal neovascularization secondary to central serous chorioretinopathy. *Arch. Ophthalmol.*, 2004; 122: 37–41.

[29] Ober M. D., Yannuzzi L. A., et al. Photodynamic therapy for focal retinal pigment epithelial leaks secondary to central serous chorioretinopathy. *Ophthalmology*, 2005; 112: 2088–2094.

[30] Moon J. W., Yu H. G., et al. Prognostic factors related to photodynamic therapy for central serous chorioretinopathy. *Graefe's Arch. Clin. Exp. Ophthalmol.*, 2009; 247: 1315–1323.

[31] Ozmert E., Batioglu F. Fundus autofluorescence before and after photodynamic therapy for chronic central serous chorioretinopathy. *Ophthalmologica*, 2009; 223: 263–268.

[32] Tarantola R. M., Law J. C., et al. Photodynamic therapy as treatment of chronic idiopathic central serous chorioretinopathy. *Lasers Surg. Med.*, 2008; 40: 671–675.

[33] Lim J. I., Glassman A. R., et al. Collaborative retrospective Macula Society Study of photodynamic therapy for chronic central serous chorioretinopathy. *Ophthalmology*, 2014; 121: 1073–1078.

[34] Lee P. Y., Kim K. S., et al. Severe choroidal ischemia following photodynamic therapy for pigment epithelial detachment and chronic central serous chorioretinopathy. *Jpn. J. Ophthalmol.*, 2009; 53: 52–56.

[35] Chan W. M., Lai T. Y., et al. Half-dose verteporfin photodynamic therapy for acute central serous chorioretinopathy: one-year results of a randomized controlled trial. *Ophthalmology*, 2008; 115: 1756–1765.

[36] Lee S. C., Seong Y. S., et al. Photodynamic therapy with verteporfin for polypoidal choroidal vasculopathy of the macula. *Ophthalmologica*, 2004; 218: 193–201.

[37] Chan W. M., Lam D. S., et al. Photodynamic therapy with verteporfin for symptomatic polypoidal choroidal vasculopathy: one-year results of a prospective case series. *Ophthalmology,* 2004; 111: 1576–1584.

[38] Hussain N., Hussain A., et al. Role of photodynamic therapy in polypoidal choroidal vasculopathy. *Indian J. Ophthalmol.,* 2005; 53: 101–104.

[39] Schmidt-Erfurth U., Hasan T. Mechanisms of action of photodynamic therapy with verteporfin for the treatment of age-related macular degeneration. *Surv. Ophthalmol.,* 2000; 45: 195–214.

[40] Schmidt-Erfurth U., Bauman W., et al. Photodynamic therapy of experimental choroidal melanoma using lipoprotein-delivered benzoporphyrin. *Ophthalmology,* 1994; 101: 89–99.

[41] Guagnini A. P., De Potter P., et al. Photodynamic therapy of circumscribed choroidal hemangiomas. *J. Fr. Ophtalmol.,* 2006; 29: 1013–1017.

[42] Michels S., Michels R., et al. Verteporfin therapy for choroidal hemangioma: a long-term follow-up. *Retina,* 2005; 25: 697–703.

[43] Verbraak F. D., Schlingemann R. O., et al. Longstanding symptomatic choroidal hemangioma managed with limited PDT as initial or salvage therapy. *Graefe's Arch. Clin. Exp. Ophthalmol.,* 2003; 241: 891–898.

[44] Jurklies B., Anastassiou G., et al. Photodynamic therapy using verteporfin in circumscribed choroidal hemangioma. *Br. J. Ophthalmol.,* 2003; 87: 84–89.

[45] Huiskamp E. A., Muskens R. P., et al. Diffuse choroidal hemangioma in Sturge–Weber syndrome treated with photodynamic therapy under general anaesthesia. *Graefe's Arch. Clin. Exp. Ophthalmol.,* 2005; 243: 727–730.

[46] Anand R. Photodynamic therapy for diffuse choroidal hemangioma associated with Sturge–Weber syndrome. *Am. J. Ophthalmol.,* 2003; 136: 758–760.

[47] Woodburn K. W., Engelman C. J., et al. Photodynamic therapy for choroidal neovascularization. *Retina,* 2002; 22: 391–405.

[48] Oh H., Takagi H., Tagaki C., et al. The potential angiogenic role of macrophages in the formation of choroidal neovascular membranes. *Invest. Ophthalmol. Vis. Sci.,* 1999; 40: 1891–1898.

[49] Gollnick S. O., Evans S. S., et al. Role of cytokines in PDT-induced local and systemic inflammation. *Br. J. Cancer,* 2003; 88: 1772–1779.

[50] Augustin A. J., Schmidt-Erfurth U. Verteporfin therapy combined with intravitreal triamcinolone in all types of choroidal neovascularization due to AMD. *Ophthalmology,* 2006; 113: 14–22.

[51] Rechtman E., Danis R. P., et al. Intravitreal triamcinolone with photodynamic therapy for subfoveal choroidal neovascularization in AMD. *Br. J. Ophthalmol.,* 2004; 88: 344–347.

[52] Spaide R. F., Sorenson J., et al. Combined photodynamic therapy and intravitreal triamcinolone acetonide for nonsubfoveal choroidal neovascularization. *Retina,* 2005; 25: 685–690.

[53] Brown D. M., Michels M., et al. Ranibizumab versus verteporfin photodynamic therapy for neovascular age-related macular degeneration: two-year results of the ANCHOR Study. *Ophthalmology,* 2009; 116: 57–

[54] Antoszyk A. N., Tuomi L., et al. Ranibizumab combined with verteporfin photodynamic therapy in neovascular age-related macular degeneration (FOCUS): year 2 results. *Am. J. Ophthalmol.*, 2008; 145: 862–874.

[55] Kaiser P. K., Registry of Visudyne AMD Therapy Writing Committee, et al. Verteporfin photodynamic therapy combined with intravitreal bevacizumab for neovascular age-related macular degeneration. *Ophthalmology*, 2009; 116: 747–755.

[56] Kaiser P. K., Boyer D. S., et al. Verteporfin plus ranibizumab for choroidal neovascularization in age-related macular degeneration: twelve-month results of the DENALI Study. *Ophthalmology*, 2012; 119: 1001–1010.

[57] Larsen M., Schmidt-Erfurth U., et al. Verteporfin plus ranibizumab for choroidal neovascularization in age-related macular degeneration: twelve-month MONT BLANC Study results. *Ophthalmology*, 2012; 119: 992–1000.

[58] Koh A., Lee W. K., et al. Efficacy and safety of verteporfin photodynamic therapy in combination with ranibizumab or alone versus ranibizumab monotherapy in patients with symptomatic macular polypoidal choroidal vasculopathy. *Retina*, 2012; 32: 1453–1464.

[59] CATT Research Group. Ranibizumab and Bevacizumab for Neovascular Age-Related Macular Degeneration. *N. Engl. J. Med.*, 2011 May 19; 364(20):1897-908.

[60] IVAN Study Investigators. Ranibizumab versus bevacizumab to treat neovascular age-related macular degeneration: one-year findings from the IVAN randomized trial. *Ophthalmology*, 2012 Jul.; 119(7):1399-411.

INDEX

D

E

F

G

H

Q

R

T

U

V

W

X

Y

Z